Pregnancy Metabolism, Diabetes and the Fetus

The Ciba Foundation for the promotion of international cooperation in medical and chemical research is a scientific and educational charity established by CIBA Limited – now CIBA-GEIGY Limited – of Basle. The Foundation operates independently in London under English trust law.

Ciba Foundation Symposia are published in collaboration with Excerpta Medica in Amsterdam

Excerpta Medica, P.O. Box 211, Amsterdam

Pregnancy Metabolism, Diabetes and the Fetus

Ciba Foundation Symposium 63 (new series)

1979

Excerpta Medica

Amsterdam · Oxford · New York

ISBN 0-444-90054-3
ISBN 90-219-4069-8

Published in April 1979 by Excerpta Medica, P.O. Box 211, Amsterdam and Elsevier/North-Holland Inc., 52 Vanderbilt Avenue, New York, N.Y. 10017.

Suggested series entry for library catalogues: Ciba Foundation Symposia.
Suggested publisher's entry for library catalogues: Excerpta Medica

Ciba Foundation Symposium 63 (new series)

334 pages, 55 figures, 50 tables

Library of Congress Cataloging in Publication Data
Main entry under title:

Pregnancy metabolism, diabetes, and the fetus.

   (Ciba Foundation symposium; 63 (new ser.))
   Bibliography: p.
   Includes index.
   1. Pregnancy–Congresses. 2. Maternal–fetal exchange–Congresses. 3. Metabolism–Congresses. 4. Diabetes in pregnancy–Congresses. I. Ciba Foundation. II. Title. III. Series: Ciba Foundation. Symposium; new ser., 63.
RG558.P73   612.6'3   78-32046
ISBN 0-444-90054-3 (Elsevier/North-Holland)

Printed in The Netherland by Casparie, Heerhugowaard

Contents

Participants

Symposium on Pregnancy Metabolism, Diabetes and the Fetus held at the Ciba Foundation, London, 30 March–1 April 1978

R. W. BEARD *(Chairman)* Department of Obstetrics & Gynaecology, St Mary's Hospital Medical School, Norfolk Place, London W2 1PG, UK

F. C. BATTAGLIA Department of Pediatrics, University of Colorado Medical Center, 4200 East Ninth Avenue, Denver, Colorado 80262, USA

P. H. BENNETT Epidemiology & Field Studies Branch, National Institute of Arthritis, Metabolism and Digestive Diseases, 1440 East Indian School Road, Phoenix, Arizona 85014, USA

N. A. M. BERGSTEIN Department of Obstetrics & Gynaecology, Hospital Zevenaar, Kampsingel 72, 6901 JJ Zevenaar, The Netherlands

E. BLÁZQUEZ Centro de Investigaciones Biologicas, Instituto 'G. Marañón', Velázquez 144, Madrid 6, Spain

J. M. BRUDENELL Department of Obstetrics & Gynaecology, King's College Hospital, Denmark Hill, London SE5 9RS, UK

R. A. CHEZ Department of Obstetrics–Gynecology, The Milton S. Hershey Medical Center, Hershey, Pa. 17033, USA

Æ. M. DEUCHAR Department of Biological Sciences, University of Exeter, Hatherly Laboratories, Prince of Wales Road, Exeter EX4 4PS, UK

N. FREINKEL Center for Endocrinology, Metabolism & Nutrition, Northwestern University Medical School, 303 East Chicago Avenue, Chicago, Illinois 60611, USA

J. W. GARROW Division of Clinical Investigation, MRC Clinical Research Centre, Northwick Park Hospital, Watford Road, Harrow, Middlesex HA1 3UJ, UK

M. D. G. GILLMER Department of Obstetrics & Gynaecology, St Mary's Hospital Medical School, Norfolk Place, London W2 1PG, UK

J. R. GIRARD   Laboratory of Developmental Physiology, Collège de France, 11 Place Marcelin-Berthelot, 75231 Paris, Cedex 05, France

J. J. HOET   Laboratoire de Recherches de la Clinique Médicale, Catholic University of Louvain 54.29, Avenue Hippocrate 54, Louvain en Woluwe, 1200 Brussels, Belgium

D. HULL   Department of Child Health, University of Nottingham, Clifton Boulevard, Nottingham NG7 2UH, UK

R. K. KALKHOFF   Endocrine-Metabolic Section, Department of Medicine, The Medical College of Wisconsin, Milwaukee County General Hospital, 8700 West Wisconsin Avenue, Milwaukee, Wisconsin 53226, USA

R. D. G. MILNER   Department of Paediatrics, University of Sheffield, Children's Hospital, Sheffield S10 2TH, UK

R. L. NAEYE   Department of Pathology, The Milton S. Hershey Medical Center, The Pennsylvania State University, Hershey, Pa. 17033, USA

D. J. NAISMITH   Department of Nutrition, Queen Elizabeth College, Atkins Building, Campden Hill, London W8 7AH, UK

J. B. O'SULLIVAN   Diabetes & Arthritis Unit, Boston University Medical Center, 408 Atlantic Avenue (Room 815), Boston, Mass. 02210, USA

*J. PEDERSEN   Medical Department T, Bispebjerg Hospital, Bispebjerg Bakke 23, 2400 Copenhagen NV, Denmark

B. PERSSON   Department of Pediatrics, Karolinska Institute, St Göran's Children's Hospital, Box 12500, S-112 81 Stockholm, Sweden

N. RÄIHÄ   Department of Obstetrics & Gynecology and Pediatrics, University Central Hospital, 00290 Helsinki 29, Finland

E. SHAFRIR   Department of Clinical Biochemistry, The Hebrew University-Hadassah Medical School, PO Box 1172, Jerusalem, Israel

J. M. STOWERS   Diabetic Clinic, Aberdeen Royal Infirmary, Woolmanhill, Aberdeen AB9 1GS, Scotland, UK

D. H. WILLIAMSON   Metabolic Research Laboratory, Nuffield Department of Clinical Medicine, Radcliffe Infirmary, Oxford OX2 6HE, UK

M. YOUNG   Department of Gynaecology, St Thomas's Hospital Medical School, Lambeth Palace Road, London SE1 7EH, UK

Editors: KATHERINE ELLIOTT *(Organizer)* and MAEVE O'CONNOR

---

* Died 21 November 1978

Introduction

R.W. BEARD and J.J. HOET*

St Mary's Hospital Medical School, London and *Université Catholique de Louvain, Brussels

The Ciba Foundation has always had a scientific tradition of bringing to the forefront essential issues for mankind.   In recent years several Ciba Foundation symposia have been devoted to elucidating the fundamental causes of, and ways of reducing, perinatal wastage and morbidity – in 1960 *Congenital Malformations,* 1965 *Preimplantation Stages of Pregnancy,* 1969 *Foetal Autonomy,* 1973 *Intrauterine Infections,* 1974 *Size at Birth,* 1977 *The Fetus and Birth,* 1978 *Major Mental Handicap,* and now this symposium on *Pregnancy Metabolism, Diabetes and the Fetus.*

The past 20 years have seen a steady fall in perinatal mortality throughout the western world.   The precise reasons for this are still being debated but it seems likely to be due to better health, following a rise in standards of living, combined with improved medical care.   Technological advances have provided the obstetrician and paediatrician with much greater insight into the development and day-to-day health of the fetus, and early detection of conditions such as hypoxia has increased the possibility of reducing morbidity as well as mortality at the time of delivery.   The unchanging incidence of congenital malformations in our society, however, still constitutes a major moral and social problem.   Early detection of abnormalities, with subsequent termination of pregnancy, is no solution to this problem.   More often than not, malformations are unsuspected during pregnancy and many malformed babies survive into later life with varying degrees of serious handicap; in addition, many parents regard legal abortion as unacceptable.   It is therefore essential for the origins of malformations to be better defined. The cause may well be multifactorial, and the actual conditions leading to a particular malformation are known in only a small percentage of cases.

Diabetes is a well-defined metabolic disorder, complicating pregnancy, in which the incidence of malformations is up to three times higher than the

1

normal rate. Thus it is reasonable to suggest that it is the abnormal metabolism of the mother at the time of implantation and organogenesis that may, in some way, be responsible for many of these anomalies. The fetus is to a certain extent autonomous, but its selective metabolic requirements may not be met by the abnormal metabolism of a diabetic mother. Diabetes may therefore serve as a useful, naturally occurring model which can be used to study the evolution of congenital abnormalities. If it can be demonstrated that the metabolic milieu may be responsible for the development of fetal anomalies, then the wider possibility must exist that other forms of metabolic disturbance, for example nutritional deprivation, may increase the possibility of fetal abnormality.

Little is known of the influence of the mother's metabolism on her fetus, and the main aim of this symposium is to lay the foundation for investigations of a possible link between metabolic disturbance in the mother and fetal anomaly. A first step towards achieving this objective is to characterize metabolic interrelationships within the mother, and between the mother and the fetus, in normal pregnancy, particularly in the early, possibly critical, months. From this information it should then be possible to determine the selective metabolic needs of the embryo and fetus. The implications of possessing such knowledge are considerable. Not only may it give us insight into aberrations of fetal development but it could also provide a basis for determining the nutritional requirements of pregnancy that may be of extreme importance to women in the Third World.

References

CIBA FOUNDATION (1960) *Congenital Malformations (Ciba Found. Symp.)*, Churchill, London
CIBA FOUNDATION (1965) *Preimplantation Stages of Pregnancy (Ciba Found. Symp.)*, Churchill, London
CIBA FOUNDATION (1969) *Foetal Autonomy (Ciba Found. Symp.)*, Churchill, London
CIBA FOUNDATION (1973) *Intrauterine Infection (Ciba Found. Symp. 10)*, Elsevier/Excerpta Medica/North-Holland, Amsterdam
CIBA FOUNDATION (1974) *Size at Birth (Ciba Found. Symp. 27)*, Elsevier/Excerpta Medica/North-Holland, Amsterdam
CIBA FOUNDATION (1977) *The Fetus and Birth (Ciba Found. Symp. 47)*, Elsevier/Excerpta Medica/North-Holland, Amsterdam
CIBA FOUNDATION (1978) *Major Mental Handicap: methods and costs of prevention (Ciba Found. Symp. 59)*, Elsevier/Excerpta Medica/North-Holland, Amsterdam

Pregnancy as a tissue culture experience: the critical implications of maternal metabolism for fetal development

NORBERT FREINKEL and BOYD E. METZGER

Center for Endocrinology, Metabolism and Nutrition and Departments of Medicine and Biochemistry, Northwestern University Medical School, Chicago, Illinois

Late pregnancy is attended by significant changes in maternal intermediary metabolism. We have summarized these *in extenso* elsewhere (Freinkel *et al.* 1979). They include an enhanced maternal transfer to the metabolism of fat whenever food is withheld ('accelerated starvation' [Freinkel 1965]) and mechanisms for conserving ingested nutrients for delivery to the conceptus when the mother eats again ('facilitated anabolism' [Freinkel *et al.* 1974]). By sampling circulating fuels in normal gravid and non-gravid volunteers during regular alimentation (with three liquid formula feedings per day), we have been able to demonstrate that the disposition of every major class of nutrient is altered in late gestation (Freinkel *et al.* 1979). We have emphasized that each of these major fuels is responsive to the action of insulin and that late pregnancy poses significant challenges to maternal insulinogenic reserve.

However, none of these alterations in the mother's metabolism would be nearly as interesting if it were not for the role that maternal fuels play in a unique tissue culture experience. During pregnancy, the conceptus develops from a fertilized egg into a multicellular structure with complex functions. The building blocks are derived entirely from the mother and ultimately determined by what she eats, how she handles these nutrients, and how they are stored and recalled. In essence, then, in the tissue culture system that constitutes pregnancy, the composition of the incubation medium for all newly developing cells is determined in large measure by the vagaries of maternal metabolism.

Four rate-limiting factors can be identified in establishing the conditions for tissue culture. Firstly, the absolute concentration of individual metabolites in the maternal circulation determines the quantitative availability of individual substrates. Secondly, access of these substrates to the conceptus depends upon placental blood flow. As yet, the precise factors which regulate

3

placental perfusion have not been well delineated; the possibility that ambient fuels and their intraplacental disposition may modulate placental haemo-dynamics remains an area for potentially fruitful inquiry.   Thirdly, the fate of individual fuels can be modified by the concurrent availability of other fuels ('substrate interactions' [Freinkel 1978]).   For example, increases in ambient free fatty acids (FFA) can promote steatosis in the placenta (Freinkel 1965; Herrera & Freinkel 1975) and enhance intraplacental formation of lactic acid from glucose (Freinkel 1965).   Similarly, ketones, when present, can sup-plant glucose or lactic acid as placental oxidative fuels (Shambaugh *et al.* 1977*a,b*).   Thus, structure and function in the conceptus may be altered by the qualitative as well as quantitative characteristics of the prevailing substrate mixture.   Finally, transplacental transfer mechanisms (Cornblath & Schwartz 1976; Pedersen 1977*a*) are the ultimate arbiters of what is available to the fetus.   The relationships are summarized in Fig. 1.   Maternal glucose crosses the placenta freely by facilitated diffusion and is abstracted conti-nuously in direct proportion to maternal blood sugar levels. Amino acids cross the placenta by active transport systems and differential concentration gra-dients within the fetal circulation may be influenced by transport competitions as well as substrate interactions.   Data concerning FFA are controversial and vary in different species; some transplacental flux appears to be operative in all.   Ketones traverse the placenta freely so that the fetus is presented with abundant ketones once an adequate ketonaemia has been established in the mother (Scow *et al.* 1958; Girard *et al.* 1973, 1977; Shambaugh *et al.*

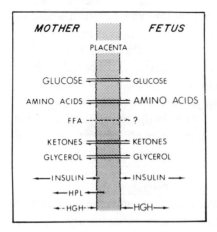

FIG. 1. Placental permeability and the relationships between maternal and fetal fuels and hormones.

1977*a*). Some fuels such as lactic acid may originate directly within the placenta (Freinkel 1965; Burd *et al.* 1975) and thus do not depend upon concentrations in the maternal circulation. Moreover, it is becoming increasingly apparent that the fetus is not wholly passive in these exchanges and that the fetus may autoregulate its metabolic mixture by influencing transplacental transfer, or by forming some new fuels from stored fetal precursors (Goodner & Thompson 1967; Jost & Picon 1970; Girard *et al.* 1977; Battaglia & Meschia 1978).

However, despite the many limitations of existing knowledge, it may not be inappropriate to view circulating metabolites in the mother as an index of the substrates that are available to the developing fetus. In this special relationship, certain additional features should also be underscored. For example, the conceptus *per se* can modify the maternal environment through its endocrine functions. The placenta elaborates hormones (e.g. placental lactogen [HPL], and sex steroids) into the maternal circulation in ever-increasing amounts which parallel placental growth and development (as reviewed elsewhere [Freinkel *et al.* 1979]). These hormones do not cross the placenta (Fig. 1); they do, however, exert lipolytic and contrainsulin actions in the mother and thereby provide a permissive setting for such special maternal metabolic adaptations of late pregnancy as 'accelerated starvation' (Freinkel *et al.* 1979).

The placenta also constitutes an impermeable barrier to insulin. The early observations that maternal insulin does not cross the placenta although it may be sequestered (i.e. bound) within the placenta (Goodner & Freinkel 1961) and actively degraded there (Freinkel & Goodner 1960) have now been confirmed in many laboratories (Cornblath & Schwartz 1976; Pedersen 1977*a*). Since the disposition of most maternal fuels is intimately linked to the adequacy of insulin secretion in the mother (Freinkel *et al.* 1979), this means that maternal insulinization may be the prepotent arbiter of the incubation medium in which the conceptus develops. Excursions in maternal fuels should exhibit the greatest swings when maternal insulin is most deficient – and the presentation of substrates to the conceptus should display the greatest lability under such circumstances (Freinkel *et al.* 1979). In this context, diabetes in pregnancy constitutes a fascinating experiment in cell biology, with ramifications extending far beyond that disease entity *per se*. It may well provide the best insights into the factors that regulate the tissue culture aspects of gestation.

GESTATIONAL DIABETES

To assess whether even the most minor limitations of maternal insulinization can unmask the dependencies of the conceptus upon maternal fuels, we have been conducting studies in women with gestational diabetes; that is, asymptomatic gravida discovered to have mild glucose intolerance by routine screening during pregnancy, i.e. White Class A (White 1949).

We feel that definitions must be extremely rigorous for such clinical subgroups. We diagnose gestational diabetes according to the glucose tolerance criteria of O'Sullivan & Mahan (1964). However, we further subdivide gestational diabetics on the basis of the manifest severity of their disturbance in carbohydrate metabolism. Those with fasting plasma glucose below 105 mg/dl (5.8 mmol/l) are designated Class A_1; those with fasting plasma glucose slightly above normal, that is, between 105 and 130 mg/dl (5.8 and 7.2 mmol/l), are classified as A_2 and those whose fasting plasma glucose exceeds 130 mg/dl (7.2 mmol/l) we categorize as Class B. Since postprandial blood sugar, that is, blood sugar after alimentary challenge, is conditioned by the disposition (i.e. 'utilization') of exogenous fuels, whereas fasting blood sugar reflects the regulation of endogenous fuel traffic (i.e. restraints to 'production' of glucose from endogenous precursors), the distinctions provide pathophysiological as well as clinical insights. We would suggest that 'underutilization' constitutes the principal metabolic disturbance in Class A_1, whereas Classes A_2 and B are experiencing varying degrees of 'overproduction' in addition to 'underutilization'.

What is the basic defect in Class A_1 subjects? By plasma fractionation techniques, we have been able to demonstrate that they do not elaborate abnormal secretory products: the relationships between circulating insulin and proinsulin in Class A_1 gestational diabetics are the same as in pregnant women with normal carbohydrate metabolism (Phelps et al. 1975). Gestational diabetics also do not display abnormal feedback relationships between insulin and glucagon; their values for basal plasma glucagon are not disturbed and we have shown that suppressibility of circulating glucagon by oral glucose is well preserved (Daniel et al. 1974; Nitzan et al. 1975). All these characterizations have been corroborated in other laboratories (Luyckx et al. 1975; Kühl 1976; Kühl & Holst 1976). Our ongoing studies suggest that faulty insulin secretory kinetics may be implicated in most Class A_1 gestational diabetics (Metzger et al. 1975). We have been finding sluggish responsiveness to secretory stimulation in most of them as judged by subnormal increases in plasma immunoreactive insulin (i.e. above normal fasting levels) during the first 15 min after oral glucose – a time when their increments in plasma glucose are not significantly different from those in pregnant women with normal carbohydrate metabolism (Metzger et al. 1975).

In collaboration with Dr Richard L. Phelps we have initiated 'around the clock' studies in Class A_1 gestational diabetics to assess whether their minor disturbances in oral glucose tolerance are also attended by detectable disturbances in general fuel traffic during meal-eating. It should be recalled that such gestational diabetics have much smaller disturbances in glucoregulation than the pregnant chemical diabetics in whom diurnal observations have been reported previously (Persson 1974; Gillmer *et al.* 1975*a,b;* Persson & Lunell 1975; Lewis *et al.* 1976). For our studies we confine subjects to a Metabolism Ward, as described elsewhere (Freinkel *et al.* 1979), and administer 2110 kcal (8860 kJ) per day (containing 275 g carbohydrate and 76 g protein) in three equal feedings at 8:00 a.m., 1:00 p.m. and 6:00 p.m. Subjects remain recumbent for a 24-hour period while blood is sampled from indwelling venous catheters at hourly intervals between 8:00 a.m. and midnight and at 2:00 a.m., 4:00 a.m. and 6:00 a.m.

To date, six women with normal oral glucose tolerance and seven Class A_1 gestational diabetics have been studied in this fashion in week 32–39 of pregnancy. In the A_1 gestational diabetics, the rises in plasma glucose are greater within one hour after every meal than in the control subjects, and persist longer; the concurrent increases in plasma insulin appear to be less at one hour, but later values for insulin tend to exceed control values in association with the prolongation of the postprandial hyperglycaemia. Other fuels also show distinct, albeit more subtle, abnormalities in the A_1 gestational diabetics. Thus, values for FFA after overnight fast tend to be higher and decrements in response to meal-eating smaller; absolute values for triglycerides tend to be higher at most times although meal-eating does not appear to elicit appreciably greater acute increments. Certain of the individual amino acids also show distinct changes. For example, plasma values for the gluconeogenic amino acid, serine, tend to stabilize at slightly higher levels during overnight fasting, whereas postprandial increments in the plasma values for the branched chain amino acid, isoleucine, seem to persist longer after every meal.

These preliminary data suggest that even those minimal derangements of maternal insulin that characterize Class A_1 gestational diabetes *are already attended by some demonstrable disturbances in the metabolism of every class of foodstuff.* Thus, any analysis of maternal insulinization that is confined to carbohydrate metabolism alone is simplistic and inconsistent with the broader dimensions of reality.

What about the consequences? Can one demonstrate any changes in the progeny of mothers who displayed such minimal changes in fuel metabolism during pregnancy? The published criteria for gestational diabetes have varied so widely that critical analysis has been difficult and, at times, controversial. Accordingly, for the purposes of this conference, we have reviewed our own recent experiences with Class A_1 gestational diabetics. None of these patients have been treated with insulin and we question whether any conventional form of insulin delivery can rectify the faulty acute insulin secretory response of the Class A_1 subjects. For our analysis, we have not included patients with added 'risk factors', i.e. patients under the age of 20, over the age of 40, and those in whom obesity was sufficient for antepartum weights to have exceeded 150% of ideal body weight. Within these rigid criteria, the birth weights of infants from our Class A_1 gestational diabetics, when corrected for age at delivery (Lubchenco et al. 1966), have been minimally but significantly ($P < 0.05$; Table 1) greater than those of offspring from age-matched gravida with normal carbohydrate metabolism whom we have followed at the same time.

The syndrome of 'large babies' (Pedersen 1977b) thus already may be present even in the most mild forms of gestational diabetes (see above). Macrosomia has been long recognized as one of the hallmarks of diabetes in pregnancy and explained by the classical 'Hyperglycaemia–Hyperinsulinism' hypothesis of Pedersen (1977b) (Fig. 2): herein diminished insulin secretion in the mother leads to maternal hyperglycaemia. The glucose freely crosses the placenta, causing hyperglycaemia in the fetus, stimulation of fetal insulin secretion, increased deposition of fat and glycogen (which carcass analyses have corroborated), and the formation of large babies (Fig. 2).

To what extent does birth weight in the offspring of our Class A_1 gestational diabetics conform to the Pedersen theory? We have been examining the relationships between weights of the newborn and antepartum circulating maternal fuels as judged by blood samples secured after 14-hour overnight fast

TABLE 1

The effect of mild diabetes on birth weight

Population: age: 20–40
          Prepregnancy weight: less than 150% of ideal body weight

	Infant weight	Observed (g)	Corrected[a] (ratio)
Normal carbohydrate metabolism	($n = 77$)	3221 ± 59	1.051 ± 0.19
Gestational diabetes class A_1	($n = 38$)	3480 ± 98	$1.122 \pm .028$
	P	N.S.	< 0.05

[a] Weights have been adjusted according to the Colorado Scale (Lubchenco et al. 1966) by the ratio: Weight at birth/Expected weight for gestational age

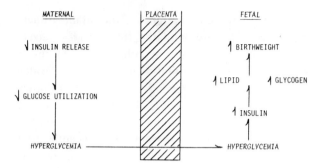

FIG. 2. Fetal development in pregnant diabetics. The classical 'hyperglyaemia–hyperinsulinism' hypothesis of Pedersen.

during weeks 32 to 36 of gestation and during tests of oral glucose tolerance. Our preliminary analyses have disclosed that the birth weights (corrected for gestational age [Lubchenco *et al.* 1966]) of infants of Class A_1 gestational diabetics appear to correlate with fasting maternal plasma glucose ($P < 0.05$), plasma triglyceride ($P < 0.05$), and plasma alanine ($P < 0.05$), serine ($P < 0.05$), valine ($P < 0.10$), isoleucine ($P < 0.05$), and glycine ($P < 0.05$)

It is not completely understood how all these fuels could contribute to macrosomia. The role of glucose is readily encompassed by the Pedersen hypothesis. Similarly, concentration-dependent increased transfer of amino acids across the placenta (Young & McFadyen 1973) could provide the fetus with more building blocks for protein anabolism, gluconeogenesis, or even direct insulinogenic stimulus (especially in the case of the branched-chain amino acid [Fajans & Floyd 1972]). The possible relationships between birth weight and triglycerides are somewhat more tenuous since direct transplacental transfer of triglycerides has been questioned (Dawes 1968). However, we have found that fasting levels for FFA (Freinkel & Metzger 1975) as well as triglycerides (B.E. Metzger & N. Freinkel, unpublished observations, 1978) correlate directly with the total integrated increase in plasma glucose during oral glucose tolerance in weeks 32 to 36 of pregnancy. Therefore, if FFA and/or triglycerides served as alternative oxidative fuels in the mother, they could retard the disposition of ingested glucose and prolong its availability for transplacental delivery to the fetus. On the other hand, slow hydrolysis of esterified lipids in the maternal circulation or within the placenta could effect a sustaining infusion of fatty acids and glycerol for direct utilization in the fetus (Koren & Shafrir 1964).

In any event, our demonstration that even the mildest of gestational diabetes can disturb the traffic in every insulin-dependent fuel in the mother, and our statistical correlations between the birth weights of the infants of such mothers and the antepartum levels of many circulating fuels besides glucose, prompt the following expansion of the Pedersen hypothesis (Fig. 3): inadequate acute insulin release in response to alimentation may cause 'underutilization' of many ingested nutrients so that postprandial increments for lipids, and selected amino acids as well as glucose, can be greater and more prolonged in the maternal circulation. The fetus thereby would be provided with potential access to more abundant mixed nutrients. Conceivably, placental structure and/or function might also be modified via the increased availability of certain maternal fuels (Freinkel 1965).

The expanded theory could find fuller expression in more severe chemical diabetes (Fig. 4). In such mothers, the limitations in basal insulin output as well as in their acute secretory response to meal-eating would result in maternal 'overproduction' as well as 'underutilization'. Thus, circulating glucose, lipids, and selected amino acids would be raised (and more available to the conceptus) in the fasted state as well as after eating.

Moreover, heightened ketonaemia could be another expression of the 'overproduction' so that the conceptus might be presented with marked qualitative as well as quantitative changes in the substrate mixture (Fig. 4). Allusion has already been made to the potential implications of altered substrate mixtures for the placenta (Freinkel et al. 1979); as will be discussed later, similar considerations may obtain for the fetus.

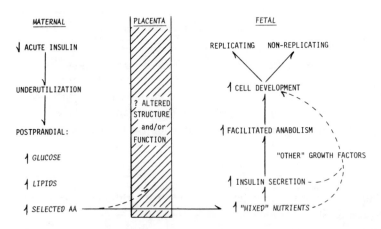

FIG. 3. Fetal development in mild gestational diabetes (maternal 'underutilization' only). The Pedersen hypothesis expanded as described in text.

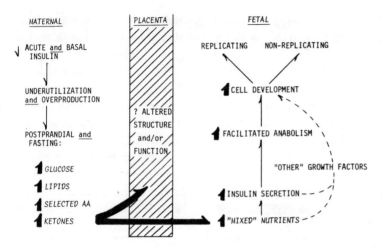

FIG. 4. Fetal development in more severe diabetes in pregnancy (maternal 'underutilization and overproduction'). The Pedersen hypothesis expanded as described in text.

THE ROLE OF FETAL INSULIN

In each of the above formulations for macrosomia (Figs. 2–4), more fetal growth should be possible, even without hormonal facilitation, as a simple consequence of the increased provision of substrate(s)*. However, as shown in Figs. 2–4, all the formulations presuppose that fetal anabolism is enhanced further by fetal insulin. The premise of insulin participation is supported by the finding that visceromegaly of all the insulin-sensitive structures contributes to the macrosomia (Fee & Weil 1963; Naeye 1965). Nonetheless, the precise manner in which more fetal insulin becomes available has not been clarified fully. Although fetal islets appear to be capable of adequate insulin synthesis in response to secretory stimulation (Asplund 1973; Heinze *et al.* 1975), their capacity to release insulin acutely may be developed less fully. Despite conflicting data (Kervran & Girard 1976), most evidence

---

* Intrinsic to all the 'increased substrate' theories of macrosomia is the assumption that the higher concentrations of nutrients in the maternal circulation can gain access to the conceptus. This need not always be the case. Clinicians have long appreciated that the offspring of long-standing diabetics may be 'small for gestational age' (SGA). The SGA offspring are particularly common in diabetics with calcific changes in pelvic vasculature. Clearly, substrates can only exert meaningful impact when delivery is not compromised by anatomical or functional restraints to placental blood flow and/or permeability.

suggests that nutrient secretagogues elicit limited acute increases in insulin release from fetal islets even during the period of greatest fetal growth, that is late in gestation (see Milner *et al*. 1975 for detailed review). This implied lack of maturation of stimulus–secretion coupling in fetal islets has been documented by a number of other metabolic parameters besides insulin release. For example, we found that the poorly responsive islets of the 21.5-day-old rat fetus also display a diminished capacity to accumulate and retain orthophosphate and an attenuated phosphate efflux and nucleotide turnover during acute stimulation with glucose (Asplund & Freinkel 1978)

For humans, much of our knowledge concerning intrauterine islet secretory performance has been based on inferences derived from experiences with neonates. Thus, using analysis for plasma C-peptide, we have been able to confirm (Phelps *et al*. 1978) the earlier observations based on assays for immunoreactive insulin (Isles *et al*. 1968; Falorni *et al*. 1972; Mølsted–Pedersen & Jørgensen 1972) that the newborn of mothers with normal carbohydrate metabolism secrete insulin sluggishly when challenged with intravenous glucose during the first few hours of life (Fig. 5). However, some increment

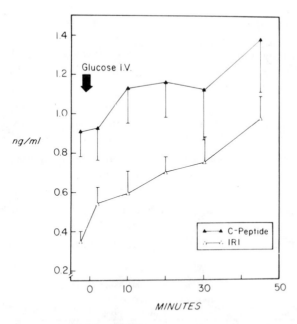

FIG. 5. Beta cell response to intravenous glucose in normal neonates. The heavy arrow denotes the 2–min interval during which glucose was infused into normal infants 2–4 h after birth. Mean ± S.E.M. values for IRI and C-peptide are presented. Each point is based on observations secured in nine infants. (Reprinted from Phelps *et al*. 1978.) IRI: immunoreactive insulin.

does occur (Isles *et al.* 1968; Falorni *et al.* 1972; Mølsted–Pedersen & Jørgensen 1972; Phelps *et al.* 1978) so that, presumably, the levels of circulating insulin in the fetus before delivery should also be increased coincident with the augmented delivery of nutrient secretagogues from the mother.   Much evidence suggests that additional mechanisms become operative in the fetus when maternal insulinization is deficient.   The islets of infants from diabetic mothers display clear-cut histological evidence of hyperplasia (Dubreuil & Anderodias 1920; Cardell 1953; Driscoll *et al.* 1960; Naeye 1965).   We have found that basal plasma levels of C-peptide at two to three hours after birth in the offspring of diabetic mothers are generally not outside the range of values seen in infants of mothers with normal carbohydrate metabolism (Phelps *et al.* 1978) (Fig. 6).   However, the concomitant basal values for plasma glucose are lower (Fig. 6) so that prevailing 'steady-state' ratios for plasma C-peptide/glucose are increased (Phelps *et al.* 1978).   We feel that these seemingly altered feedback relationships between basal insulin secretion and ambient glucose in the offspring of diabetic mothers may, perhaps, reflect an increase in the absolute number of islets – and, hence, an increased matrix of secretory tissue already available during intrauterine life.   The ratios need not connote full secretory maturation of the individual islets.   The latter can only be evaluated by acute secretory challenge.   As shown in Fig. 7, we have encountered an adult-type of acute insulin release, that is, a maximal outpour-

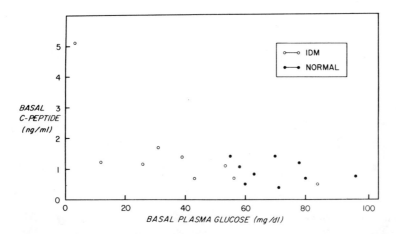

FIG. 6.   Relationships between basal plasma glucose and basal plasma C-peptide.   Blood samples were secured at 2–4 h of age in nine newborn infants of diabetic mothers (IDM) and nine infants from mothers with normal carbohydrate metabolism and similar socioeconomic backgrounds.   (Adapted from Phelps *et al.* 198.)

ing of insulin already evinced in the earliest sample of blood during intravenous tests of glucose tolerance two hours after birth in only about half of
the infants of diabetic mothers (Phelps *et al.* 1978). These have also been
the infants in whom subsequent rates of disposition of intravenous glucose (K_t)
were most rapid (Fig. 7).

From all the foregoing, it follows that fetal insulin deserves inclusion in any
analysis of fetal contributions to the tissue culture aspects of gestation. However, it may be helpful to differentiate between several possible levels of
impact. Firstly, a sluggish release of insulin from a normal complement of
fetal islets could abet macrosomia without any mechanisms beyond heightened substrate delivery having to be invoked. (Although data are sparse, an
adequate number of insulin receptors appear to be present in the peripheral
tissues of the human fetus in late gestation [Thorsson & Hintz 1977] so that
responsiveness of fetal tissues to insulin action need not be restricted by lack of
receptors.) Secondly, in most infants of diabetic mothers, the absolute complement of islets appears to be increased so that the total elaboration of insulin
at any level of substrate may be augmented disproportionately. Finally, in a
finite proportion of the infants, an adult-type pattern of acute insulin release

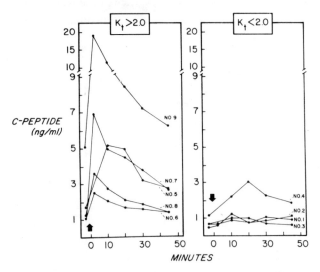

FIG. 7. Pattern of β cell secretory response in infants of diabetic mothers. Subjects have been
subdivided on the basis of fractional rates of glucose disposition which exceed values in normal
neonates $(K_t > 2.0)$ or fall within the normal range $(K_t < 2.0)$. Mothers of all infants except
infant 6 had received insulin treatment during pregnancy. Plasma C-peptide measurements
were secured after removing potentially cross-reacting, antibody-bound proinsulin. (Reprinted
from Phelps *et al.* 1978.)

can be elicited.   Presumably, this type of secretory responsiveness *in utero* could enable the normal adult 'fed state' (Freinkel 1978) to be replicated in the fetus.   In other words, such infants should be able to respond to an acute influx of nutrients from the mother with an acute outpouring of insulin and thereby effect maximal fetal anabolism.   In so far as somatomedin-type growth factors are responsive to nutrient and insulin interactions (Phillips *et al.* 1978), one may even hypothesize that such relationships could favour the formation of additional 'growth factors' in the fetus (Figs. 3 and 4).   Soma-tomedin bioactivity has already been demonstrated in cord serum and found to correlate with birth weight and gestational age in normal human pregnancy (Gluckman & Brinsmead 1976).

It remains to be established which of the components of the fetal fuel mixture (e.g. glucose; selected amino acids; other nutrients) acting alone, additively or synergistically are responsible for the induction of extra islets and the secretory maturation of some of them when delivery of substrate is heightened.   Ongoing studies with tissue culture of fetal islets (Hellerstrom *et al.* 1978) should provide clarification.

IMPLICATIONS FOR CELL BIOLOGY

Our formulation has implications far beyond the 'large baby' syndro-me.   In essence, we have postulated that the formation (and perhaps matura-tion) of certain cells during fetal life can be influenced by altered nutrient flux.   Certain ramifications of this postulate must be recognized: although all cells are formed *in utero,* not all cells have the same life cycle or replicative potential (Fig. 8).   Some are 'terminal' cells which persist through most of the life of the host and can be established only during finite periods in human development.   For example, it has been suggested that much of the total complement of adipocytes is laid down during late intrauterine and early neonatal life, and during a brief interval in adolescence (Knittle & Hirsch 1968; Hirsch & Knittle 1970).   Similarly, although some regenerative capa-city may be operative (Hay 1971), it is felt that differentiation and replication of muscle cells may occur chiefly during intrauterine life, late childhood and adolescence (Cheek 1968).   In contrast, the cells of tissues such as the gas-trointestinal tract, liver, kidney, skin or blood, etc. retain replicative potential throughout life and may be renewed continuously (Fig. 8).

Within this framework, what have we achieved with the 'large babies'?   In accordance with current concepts of cell biology, supranormal endowment may have been effected for certain 'terminal' cells during their intrauterine

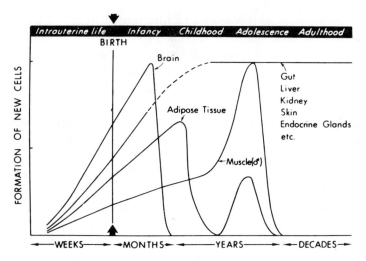

FIG. 8. Cycles of cell development.

phase of differentiation and formation.   Adipocytes must be included in this category.   Although data on the number of fat cells in large babies from diabetic mothers are sparse, carcass analyses would indicate that adipose tissue is indeed increased (Fee & Weil 1963).   We do not know whether this relative plethora persists or whether compensating cut-backs during the other periods of cell formation eventually result in a normal complement of adipocytes.   However, *pro tem.*, one may ask whether recipients of intrauterine surfeit are more vulnerable to obesity in adult life?   In other words, has nurture conspired with nature to make these offspring more susceptible to maturity-onset diabetes in later life by influencing the number of adipocytes that are formed *in utero?*   Prospective data are limited and inconclusive.   However, some suggestive evidence has accrued with regard to the opposite side of the coin: significantly less obesity has been found in 19-year-old men subjected to food shortage during the last trimester of intrauterine life and the first few neonatal months in the Dutch famine of 1944–45 (Ravelli *et al.* 1976).   (In the same series, significantly higher rates of obesity were encountered when famine had occurred during the first half of pregnancy [Ravelli *et al.* 1976].   It has been postulated that this may have coincided with a critical period in intrauterine life during which hypothalamic centres regulating food intake are differentiating.)

What does this mean with regard to the development of pancreatic islets?   Studies increasingly suggest that β cells may also constitute 'terminal' or 'near-terminal' cells with finite and limited replicative capacity (Logotheto-poulos 1972).   If so, increased formation of β cells, premature maturation of some of them, and attendant reduction in the secretory potential of other islet components, such as the α cells, could have meaningful consequences.   It could result in a form of premature β cell ageing and contribute to diminished insulinogenic reserve in later life.   Data concerning the incidence of maturity-onset diabetes in the offspring of diabetic mothers *vis-à-vis* diabetic fathers would be particularly interesting with regard to this example of nurture influencing nature during a critical period of cell differentiation and replication.

The possible implications are perhaps most intriguing for brain.   Although not considered to be responsive to insulin action, brain cells represent classical 'terminal', non-replicative structures.   As reviewed recently (Nowak & Munro 1977; Winnick & Morgan 1979), brain development is completed during the perinatal period in most laboratory animals and structural as well as functional changes have been elicited by manipulating maternal nutrition during this interval.   Even neurohumoral components within the brain may be affected: for example, long-range deficits in hypothalamic thyrotropin-releasing hormone have been reported after neonatal caloric deprivation in rats (Shambaugh & Wilber 1974).   It is commonly believed that the full complement of brain cells in humans is formed during intrauterine life and the first few neonatal months (Fig. 8).   Whether ambient fuels can influence the development of the human brain remains controversial.   Some suggestive data warrant citation.   Brain weights below the average figure for more normal infants of similar body weights have been found in infants of diabetic mothers (Cardell 1953), even when corrected for dry weight (Fee & Weil 1963).   Although macrosomia affecting all viscera except the brain could account for some of these differences (Naeye 1965), Gruenwald has reported that brains from infants of diabetic mothers are smaller on an absolute as well as a relative basis (Gruenwald 1966).   Moreover, survey data from largely urban populations in the United States (Churchill & Berendes 1969; Churchill *et al.* 1969) and a recent confirmatory report dealing with American rural subjects (Stehbens *et al.* 1977) have indicated that ketonuria in the mother (and the implied increased delivery of ketones to the developing fetus) may be followed by documentable reductions in I.Q. when offspring are tested during early childhood.   By contrast, the offspring of mothers deprived of food during the Dutch famine of 1944–1945 have not demonstrated significant reductions in I.Q. when tested at the time of induction into the military (Stein *et al.* 1972).

The qualitative aspects of the fetal fuel mixture may be particularly relevant to brain cells. Many laboratories (as reviewed in Shambaugh *et al.* 1977*a*) have shown that fetal brain can oxidize ketones. We are currently trying to assess the implications of this for the disposition of other fuels (Shambaugh *et al.* 1977*b*). As summarized in Fig. 9, Shambaugh has established that added ketones can depress oxidation of fuels such as glucose, lactic acid and amino acids (not shown) when surviving fetal brain slices are incubated with substrate mixtures that simulate the relationships that obtain *in vivo* (Shambaugh *et al.* 1977*b*). Ongoing efforts are directed at trying to determine whether ketones also modify the disposition of such fuels along other biosynthetic pathways. The question assumes particular importance during fetal life. Whereas the oxidative potential of ketones can effectively *sustain* function in adult brain (Owen *et al.* 1967), the metabolic desiderata may be quite different when new non-replicating brain cells are being formed.

The concept of 'terminal' cells, responsive to the composition and disposition of ambient nutrients during their period of induction, is one that has not received sufficient attention in the past. We have conjectured about a few possibilities above; the list could be expanded to include many other, perhaps transcendent, possibilities.

Each possibility can only be evaluated by carefully designed *prospective* studies in which correlations are sought between appropriate antepartum and perinatal events, and the subsequent performance of 'terminal' cells in the progeny. Such longitudinal efforts are currently under way in our laboratory.

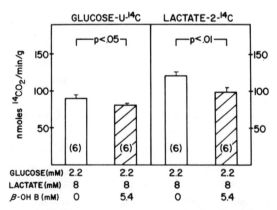

FIG. 9. Effect of β-hydroxybutyrate (β-OH B) on glucose and lactate oxidation by fetal brain. Fetal rat brains were derived from fed mothers on day 20 of gestation. Brain slices were incubated with glucose, lactate and 0 (open bars) or 5.4 mM (cross-hatched bars) D,L-β-hydroxybutyrate, as shown above. Heights of the bars denote the evolution of $^{14}CO_2$ from [U-^{14}C]glucose or [2-^{14}C] lactate. (Adapted from Shambaugh *et al.* 1977*b*.)

SUMMARY AND CONCLUSIONS

Maternal insulin may be the prepotent arbiter of fuel metabolism during late pregnancy. Diurnal observations have disclosed that even the most minor disturbances in maternal insulinization are attended by demonstrable changes in the disposition of every major class of nutrients. However, the implications extend far beyond the fuel economy of the mother. Pregnancy represents a type of tissue culture in which the conceptus develops *de novo* and the composition of the tissue culture medium is determined by the maternal fuels which gain access to the conceptus. As in all tissue culture exercises, the developing cells may be greatly influenced by the nature of the incubation medium. For many of the developing fetal cells, this carries few long-range implications since they will be undergoing continuous renewal throughout the lifetime of the offspring. Other cells, however, are more 'terminal' structures. They have limited replicative capacity and some of the total endowment and function of these cells in the offspring may be influenced by intrauterine and perinatal events. These include brain cells, fat cells, muscle cells and perhaps the β cells of the pancreatic islets. Thus, pregnancy constitutes a unique opportunity for nutritional and biochemical engineering. It is the arena *par excellence* in which nurture, as exemplified by the character of maternal fuels, may influence nature, as represented by the intrinsic genetic endowment of the fetus. No single period in human development provides a greater potential for long-range 'pay-off' via a relatively short-range period of enlightened metabolic manipulation.

ACKNOWLEDGEMENTS

Our studies of intermediary metabolism in pregnancy have spanned almost two decades. We would be remiss if we failed to express our gratitude to the numerous colleagues with whom we have enjoyed so many stimulating collaborations during this interval. We should also like to acknowledge Research Grants AM 10699 and MRP HD11021 and Training Grants AM 05071 and AM 07169 from the National Institutes of Health; Research Grant 6–136 from The National Foundation–March of Dimes, and a Research Grant from the Kroc Foundation for partial support for the present efforts.

References

ASPLUND, K. (1973) Effects of glucose on insulin biosynthesis in fetal and newborn rats. *Horm. Metab. Res. 5*, 410–415

ASPLUND, K. & FREINKEL. N. (1978) Phosphate metabolism and glucose-initiated efflux of phosphate ions in islets of fetal pancreas. *Diabetes 27*, 611–619

BATTAGLIA, F. C. & MESCHIA, G. (1978) Principal substrates of fetal metabolism. *Physiol. Rev.* *58*, 499–527

BURD, L. I., JONES, M.D. JR., SIMMONS, M. A., MAKOWSKI, E. L., MESCHIA, G. & BATTAGLIA, F. C. (1975) Placental production and foetal utilisation of lactate and pyruvate. *Nature (Lond.)* *254*, 710–711

CARDELL, B. S. (1953) The infants of diabetic mothers: a morphological study. *J. Obstet. Gynaecol. Br. Commonw. 60*, 834–853

CHEEK, D. B. (1968) Muscle cell growth in normal children, in *Human Growth, Body Composition, Cell Growth, Energy, and Intelligence* (Cheek, D. B., ed.), pp. 337–351, Lea & Febiger, Philadelphia

CHURCHILL, J. A. & BERENDES, H. W. (1969) Intelligence of children whose mothers had acetonuria during pregnancy, in *Perinatal Factors Affecting Human Development (Sci. Pub. 185)*, p. 30, Pan American Health Organization, Washington, D. C.

CHURCHILL, J. A., BERENDES, H. W. & NEMORE, J. (1969) Neuropsychological deficits in children of diabetic mothers: a report from the collaborative study of cerebral palsy. *Am. J. Obstet. Gynaecol. 105*, 257–268

CORNBLATH, M. & SCHWARTZ, R. (1976) *Disorders of Carbohydrate Metabolism in Infancy*, 2nd edn., pp. 29–71, Saunders, Philadelphia

DANIEL, R. R., METZGER, B. E., FREINKEL, N., FALOONA, G., UNGER, R. H. & NITZAN, M. (1974) Carbohydrate metabolism in pregnancy. XI. Response of plasma glucagon to overnight fast and oral glucose during normal pregnancy and in gestational diabetes. *Diabetes 23*, 771–776

DAWES, G. S. (1968) *Foetal and Neonatal Physiology*, pp. 210–222, Year Book Medical Publishers, Chicago

DRISCOLL, S. G., BENERSCHKE, K. & CURTIS, G.W. (1960) Neonatal deaths among infants of diabetic mothers. *Am. J. Dis. Child. 100*, 818–835

DUBREUIL, G. & ANDERODIAS, J. (1920) Islets de Langerhans glands chez un nouveau-né issu de mère glycosurique. *C. R. Soc. Biol. 83*, 1490–1493

FAJANS, S. S. & FLOYD, J. C. JR. (1972) Stimulation of islet cell secretion by nutrients and by gastrointestinal hormones released during digestion, in *Handb. Physiol. Sect. 7: Endocrinology,* vol. 1: *Endocrine Pancreas* (Steiner, D. & Freinkel, N., eds.) pp. 473–493, Williams & Wilkins, Baltimore

FALORNI, A., FRACASSINI, F., MASSI-BENEDETTI, F. & AMICI, A. (1972) Glucose metabolism, plasma insulin and growth hormone secretion in newborn infants with erythroblastosis fetalis compared with normal newborns and those born to diabetic mothers. *Pediatrics 49*, 682–693

FEE, B. A. & WEIL, W. B. JR. (1963) Body composition of infants of diabetic mothers by direct analysis. *Ann. N. Y. Acad. Sci. 110*, 869–897

FREINKEL, N. (1965) Effects of the conceptus on maternal metabolism during pregnancy, in *On the Nature and Treatment of Diabetes* (Leibel, B. S. & Wrenshall, G. A., eds.) *(Int. Congr. Ser. 84)*, pp. 679–691, Excerpta Medica, Amsterdam

FREINKEL, N. (1978) The role of nutrition in medicine: recent developments in fuel metabolism. *J. Am. Med. Assoc. 239*, 1868–1872

FREINKEL, N. & GOODNER, C.J. (1960) Carbohydrate metabolism in pregnancy. I. The metabolism of insulin by human placental tissue. *J. Clin. Invest. 39*, 116–131

FREINKEL, N. & METZGER, B. E. (1975) Some considerations of fuel economy in the fed state during late human pregnancy, in *Early Diabetes in Early Life* (Camerini–Davalos, R. A. & Cole, H.S., eds.), pp. 289–301, Academic Press, New York

FREINKEL, N., METZGER, B.E., NITZAN, M., DANIEL, R., SURMACZYNSKA, B. & NAGEL, T. (1974) Facilitated anabolism in late pregnancy: some novel maternal compensations for accelerated starvation, in *Proc. 8th Congr. Diabetes Fed.* (Malaise, W.J. & Pirart, J., eds.) *(Int. Congr. Ser. 312)*, pp. 474–488, Excerpta Medica, Amsterdam

FREINKEL, N., PHELPS, R. L. & METZGER, B.E. (1979) Intermediary metabolism during normal pregnancy, in *Carbohydrate Metabolism in Pregnancy and the Newborn* (Sutherland, H. W. & Stowers, J. M., eds.) *(2nd Aberdeen Int. Colloq.)*, Springer, Berlin

GILLMER, M.D.G., BEARD, R. W., BROOKE, F.M. & OAKLEY, N. W. (1975a) Carbohydrate metabolism in pregnancy. Part I. Diurnal plasma glucose profile in normal and diabetic women. *Br. Med. J. 3*, 399–402

GILLMER, M. D. G., OAKLEY, N. W., BROOKE, F. M. & BEARD, R. W. (1975b) Metabolic profiles in pregnancy. *Isr. J. Med. Sci. 11*, 601–608

GIRARD, J. R., CUENDET, G. S., MARLISS, E. B., KERVRAN, A., RIEUTORT, M. & ASSAN, R. (1973) Fuels, hormones, and liver metabolism at term and during the early postnatal period in the rat. *J. Clin. Invest. 52*, 3190–3200

GIRARD, J. R., FERRE, P., GILBERT, M., KERVRAN, A., ASSAN, R. & MARLISS, E. B. (1977) Fetal metabolic response to maternal fasting in the rat. *Am. J. Physiol. 232*, E456–E463

GLUCKMAN, P. D. & BRINSMEAD, M. W. (1976) Somatomedin in cord blood: relationship to gestational age and birth size. *J. Clin. Endocrinol. Metab. 43*, 1378–1381

GOODNER, C. J. & FREINKEL, N. (1961) Carbohydrate metabolism in pregnancy. IV. Studies on the permeability of the rat placenta to I^{131} insulin. *Diabetes 10*, 383–392

GOODNER, C. J. & THOMPSON, D. J. (1967) Glucose metabolism in the fetus in utero: the effect of maternal fasting and glucose loading in the rat. *Pediatr. Res. 1*, 443–451

GRUENWALD, P. (1966) Growth of the human fetus. II. Abnormal growth in twins and infants of mothers with diabetes, hypertension, or isoimmunization. *Am. J. Obstet. Gynecol. 94*, 1120–1132

HAY, E. D. (1971) Skeletal-muscle regeneration. *N. Engl. J. Med. 284*, 1033–1034

HEINZE, E., SCHATZ, H., NICOLE, C. & PFEIFFER, E. F. (1975) Insulin biosynthesis in isolated pancreatic islets of fetal and newborn rats. *Diabetes 24*, 373–377

HELLERSTROM, C., LEWIS, N. J., JOHNSON, R. & FREINKEL, N. (1978) Maturation of insulin release and phosphate metabolism in fetal rat islets maintained in tissue culture. *Diabetes 27 (Suppl. 2)*, 456 (abstr.)

HERRERA, E. & FREINKEL, N. (1975) Metabolites in the liver, brain and placenta of fed or fasted mothers and fetal rats. *Horm. Metab. Res. 7*, 247–249

HIRSCH, J. & KNITTLE, J. L. (1970) Cellularity of obese and nonobese human adipose tissue. *Fed. Proc. 29*, 1516–1521

ISLES, T. E., DICKSON, M. & FARQUHAR, J. W. (1968) Glucose tolerance and plasma insulin in newborn infants of normal and diabetic mothers. *Pediatr. Res. 2*, 198–208

JOST, A. & PICON, L. (1970) Hormonal control of fetal development and metabolism, in *Advances in Metabolic Disorders*, vol. 4 (Levine, R. & Luft, R., eds.), pp. 123–184, Academic Press, New York

KERVRAN, A. & GIRARD, J.R. (1976) Time course of a glucose-induced increase in plasma insulin in the rat foetus *in utero*. *J. Endocrinol. 70*, 519–520

KNITTLE, J. L. & HIRSCH, J. (1968) Effect of early nutrition on the development of rat epididymal fat pads. Cellularity and metabolism. *J. Clin. Invest. 47*, 2091–2098

KOREN, Z. & SHAFRIR, E. (1964) Placental transfer of free fatty acids in the pregnant rat. *Proc. Soc. Exp. Biol. Med. 117*, 411–414

KÜHL, C. (1976) Serum proinsulin in normal and gestational diabetic pregnancy. *Diabetologia 12*, 295–300

KÜHL, C. & HOLST, J.J. (1976) Plasma glucagon and the insulin: glucagon ratio in gestational diabetes. *Diabetes 25*, 16–23

LEWIS, S.B., WALLIN, J.D., KUZUYA, H., MURRAY, W.K., COUSTAN, D.R., DAANE, T.A. & RUBENSTEIN, A.H. (1976) Circadian variation of serum glucose, C-peptide immunoreactivity and free insulin in normal and insulin-treated diabetic pregnant subjects. *Diabetologia 12*, 343–350

LOGOTHETOPOULOS, J. (1972) Islet cell regeneration and neogenesis, in *Handb. Physiol.* Sect. 7: *Endocrinology*, vol. 1: *Endocrine Pancreas* (Steiner, D. & Freinkel, N., eds.), pp. 67–76, Williams & Wilkins, Baltimore

LUBCHENCO, L. O., HANSMAN, C. & BOYD, E. (1966) Intrauterine growth in length and head circumference as estimated from live births at gestational ages from 26 to 42 weeks. *Pediatrics 37*, 403–408

LUYCKX, A.S., GERARD, J., GASPARD, U. & LEFEBVRE, P. J. (1975) Plasma glucagon levels in normal women during pregnancy. *Diabetologia 11,* 549–554

METZGER, B. E., NITZAN, M., PHELPS, R.L. & FREINKEL, N. (1975) The beta cell in gestational diabetes: victim or culprit? *Clin. Res. 23,* 445A

MILNER, R. D. G., LEACH, F. N. & JACK, P.M.B. (1975) Reactivity of the fetal islet, in *Carbohydrate Metabolism in Pregnancy and the Newborn* (Sutherland, H.W. & Stowers, J.M., eds.), pp. 83–104, Churchill Livingstone, Edinburgh

MØLSTED–PEDERSEN, L. & JØRGENSEN, K. R. (1972) Aspects of carbohydrate metabolism in newborn infants of diabetic mothers. III. Plasma insulin during intravenous glucose tolerance test. *Acta Endocrinol. 71,* 115–125

NAEYE, R. L. (1965) Infants of diabetic mothers: a quantitative morphologic study. *Pediatrics 35,* 980–988

NITZAN, M., FREINKEL, N., METZGER, B. E., UNGER, R. H., FALOONA, G. R. & DANIEL, R. R. (1975) The interrelations of glucose, insulin and glucagon after overnight fast and in response to oral glucose during late pregnancy. *Isr. J. Med. Sci. 11,* 617–622

NOWAK, T. S. JR. & MUNRO, H. N. (1977) Effects of protein–calorie malnutrition on biochemical aspects of brain development, in *Nutrition and the Brain,* vol. 2 (Wurtman, R.J. & Wurtman, J. J., eds.), pp. 193–260, Raven Press, New York

O'SULLIVAN, J. B. & MAHAN, C.M. (1964) Criteria for the oral glucose tolerance test in pregnancy. *Diabetes 13,* 278–285

OWEN, O.E., MORGAN, A. P., KEMP, H.G., SULLIVAN, J. M., HERRERA, M.G. & CAHILL, G. F. JR. (1967) Brain metabolism during fasting. *J. Clin. Invest. 46,* 1589–1595

PEDERSEN, J. (1977a) *The Pregnant Diabetic and Her Newborn,* 2nd edn., pp. 106–122, Williams & Wilkins, Baltimore

PEDERSEN, J. (1977b) *The Pregnant Diabetic and Her Newborn,* 2nd edn., pp. 211–220, Williams & Wilkins, Baltimore

PERSSON, B. (1974) Assessment of metabolic control in diabetic pregnancy, in *Size at Birth (Ciba Found. Symp. 27),* pp. 247–273, Elsevier/Excerpta Medica/North–Holland, Amsterdam

PERSSON, B. & LUNELL, N.O. (1975) Metabolic control in diabetic pregnancy: variations in plasma concentrations of glucose, free fatty acids, glycerol, ketone bodies, insulin, and human chorionic somatomammotropin during the last trimester. *Am. J. Obstet. Gynaecol. 122,* 737–745

PHELPS, R. L., BERGENSTAL, R., FREINKEL, N., RUBENSTEIN, A.H., METZGER, B. E. & MAKO, M. (1975) Carbohydrate metabolism in pregnancy. XIII. Relationships between plasma insulin and proinsulin during late pregnancy in normal and diabetic subjects. *J. Clin. Endocrinol. Metab. 41,* 1085–1091

PHELPS, R. L., FREINKEL, N., RUBENSTEIN, A. H., KUSUYA, H., METZGER, B. E., BOEHM, J. J. & MØLSTED–PEDERSEN, L. (1978) Carbohydrate metabolism in pregnancy. XV. Plasma C-peptide during intravenous glucose tolerance in neonates from normal and insulin-treated diabetic mothers. *J. Clin. Endocrinol. Metab. 46,* 61–68

PHILLIPS, L. S., ORAWSKI, A. T. & BELOSKY, D. C. (1978) Somatomedin and nutrition. IV. Regulation of somatomedin activity and growth cartilage activity by quantity and composition of diet in rats. *Endocrinology 103,* 121–127

RAVELLI, G–P., STEIN, Z. A. & SUSSER, M. W. (1976) Obesity in young men after famine exposure in utero and early infancy. *N. Engl. J. Med. 295,* 349–353

SCOW, R. O., CHERNICK, S. S. & SMITH, B. B. (1958) Ketosis in the rat fetus. *Proc. Soc. Exp. Biol. Med. 98,* 833–835

SHAMBAUGH, G. E. III & WILBER, J. F. (1974) The effect of caloric deprivation upon thyroid function in the neonatal rat. *Endocrinology 94,* 1145–1149

SHAMBAUGH, G. E. III, MROZAK, S. C. & FREINKEL, N. (1977a) Fetal fuels. I. Utilization of ketones by isolated tissues at various stages of maturation and maternal nutrition during late gestation. *Metabolism 26,* 623–636

SHAMBAUGH, G. E. III, KOEHLER, R. A. & FREINKEL, N. (1977b) Fetal fuels. II. Contributions of selected carbon fuels to oxidative metabolism in the rat conceptus. *Am. J. Physiol. 233,* E457–E461

STEHBENS, J. A., BAKER, G. L. & KITCHELL, M. (1977) Outcome at ages 1, 3, and 5 years of children born to diabetic women. *Am. J. Obstet. Gynecol. 127,* 408–413

STEIN, Z., SUSSER, M., SAENGER, G. & MAROLLA, F. (1972) Nutrition and mental performance: prenatal exposure to the Dutch famine of 1944–1945 seems not related to mental performance at age 19. *Science (Wash. D.C.) 178,* 708–713

THORSSON, A.V. & HINTZ, R. L. (1977) Insulin receptors in the newborn: increase in receptor affinity and number. *N. Engl. J. Med. 297,* 908–912

WHITE, P. (1949) Pregnancy complicating diabetes. *Am. J. Med. 7,* 609–616

WINNICK, M. & MORGAN, B. L. G. (1979) Nutrition and cellular growth of the brain, in *The Year in Metabolism 1978* (Freinkel, N., ed.), Plenum Press, New York

YOUNG, M. & MCFADYEN, I.R. (1973) Placental transfer and fetal uptake of amino acids in the pregnant ewe. *J. Perinat. Med. 1,* 174–182

Discussion

Williamson: I have a philosophical question about the accelerated starvation theory. There is a tremendous metabolic drain on the mother when the fetus is there. In starvation lactating rats cease milk production and prevent the loss of glucose carbon (Williamson & Robinson 1977). By analogy, if the human mother is starved is there any mechanism by which the mother can decide to jettison the fetus and save herself?

Freinkel: Resorption of fetuses has been described in some studies with starved animals. However, there may be some less severe mechanisms for conserving maternal reserves during more conventional dietary deprivation. The hypoglycaemia of fasting in pregnancy (Scow *et al.* 1964; Herrera *et al.* 1969a; Felig & Lynch 1970) is one such possibility (Freinkel *et al.* 1972; Metzger & Freinkel 1975). Hypoglycaemia supervenes whenever food is withheld from pregnant subjects (see Freinkel *et al.* 1979 for review). It occurs more rapidly and to a far greater degree than the fall in blood sugar that is seen when non-gravid females are starved for 36 hours or longer (Merimee & Fineberg 1973; Fajans & Floyd 1976; Tyson *et al.* 1976). As judged from animal models, the hypoglycaemia of fasting in pregnancy appears to threaten homeostasis because heightened catecholamine secretion is seen as soon as it becomes manifest (Herrera *et al.* 1969b). Some time ago we showed that the hypoglycaemia seems to be due to a disparate decline in the circulating level of gluconeogenic amino acids (Metzger *et al.* 1971). Thus, despite the fact that the maternal liver is revved up for heightened gluconeogenesis (Herrera *et al.* 1969a; Metzger *et al.* 1973), intrahepatic potential seems to be thwarted by limitations in the generation of gluconeogenic precursors. Similar conclu-

sions have been reached by Felig and co-workers (1972).   We have designated the fasting hypoglycaemia of pregnancy a 'substrate deficiency syndrome'
(Freinkel 1975).   It is as if at some point the mother says, 'I will stop tearing
myself apart to support the demands of the conceptus'.   We are still trying to
delineate the mediating factors.   Direct effects of circulating ketones and
catechols on maternal muscle, and braking of maternal muscle catabolism via
the persistent insulin, all appear to be contributory.   However, in the broader
sense, the hypoglycaemia of fasting in pregnancy must be recognized as a
mechanism by which some conservation is effected.   Since the gradients for
facilitated diffusion of glucose are concentration-dependent and usually pro-
portional to blood sugar level in the mother, the hypoglycaemia restricts the
rate of removal of maternal glucose.   The fall in circulating amino acids can
also effectively diminish access of maternal amino acids to the fetus (Freinkel
et al. 1972).

Williamson: I normally think of ketone bodies as being an important
fuel.   In the fetus they might also be a signal for glucose utilization to fall and
in this way also prevent the drain of glucose from the mother.

Freinkel: We agree completely that the ketones serve as a signal for a decline
in glucose utilization.   However, this poses unique, and as yet unanswered,
questions when it occurs in a setting of newly developing cells.   Here one may
ask whether other biosynthetic or anabolic processes are also modified coincident with substituting ketones for other oxidative fuels.

Battaglia: It is clear that if the mother undergoes some sort of cardiovascular
stress, all the defence mechanisms are in the direction of quickly sacrificing the
fetus and preserving maternal viability.   Starvation is different in this regard
because even with prolonged starvation, the potential for fetal survival continues for a long time and the metabolic demands on the mother imposed by
pregnancy are still increasing.   I believe there are at least two aspects related
to the question of fetal survival during maternal starvation.   One is that the
fetus alters its caloric requirements, which benefits the mother.   That aspect
hasn't yet been discussed.   The second aspect is that you have been discussing
concentration changes in the mother's blood but what we are really after is an
assessment of the umbilical uptake of solutes, i.e. quantities of amino acid or
glucose delivered to the fetus.   This takes us into considerations of the impact
of uterine blood flow changes upon solute flow.   The mechanisms that would
quickly and markedly reduce uterine blood flow would quickly sacrifice the
fetus, probably through hypoxia rather than a reduction in amino acids, keto
acids or other substrate transfer to the fetus.

You mentioned that if the keto acid concentrations are increased, glucose is
being spared in the fetus, but you presented no data on umbilical uptake of

solutes such as glucose.   One needs some fixed reference point against which to judge whether transfer of solutes such as keto acids is of any quantitative significance, a reference point such as total CO_2 production in the fetus or total caloric requirements of the fetus – some rigid yardstick against which we can judge how quantitatively important a switch in metabolism is.   Certainly I do not believe one can make the assumption that changes in solute concentration in the maternal circulation can be interpreted as reflecting similar changes in placental transport of the same solutes to the fetus.   Furthermore, it is already clear that the placental transport of some solutes will not be affected appreciably by changes in uterine blood flow.

Freinkel: With regard to your last point, the preliminary data which Shambaugh has been securing with the oxygen electrode (G.E. Shambaugh III, unpublished observations, 1977) would suggest that diversion to ketones does not alter total oxygen consumption in isolated preparations of fetal tissues appreciably.   However, this still does not provide us with all of the necessary information.   We really must learn how much of the integrated caloric expenditure is being deployed for a given anabolic event or for modifying biosynthetic pathways in specific components of individual structures.   What I am really asking is whether anabolic events in newly developing cells can be altered when caloric expenditure remains relatively constant but substrate mixtures change.   I agree fully that blood flow must be recognized as a rate-limiting variable.   However, here again it will be important to establish whether weak organic acids (such as ketones, lactic acid, etc.) can influence structure *in vivo* as *in vitro*.   I view these questions as challenges that are relatively unique for perinatal metabolism (Freinkel 1978).

Beard: So in general terms, would you agree that the first sacrifice the fetus makes is that it stops growing – it goes into hibernation before eventually death supervenes?

Freinkel: Yes indeed, especially in late gestation during the period of the most active fetal growth.   And yet, it is quite surprising how relatively little compromise of weight actually occurs.   For example, complete fast effects no change in total fetal weight when the pregnant rat is fasted from day 16 to 18 of gestation and only 14% reduction during fasting from day 18 to 20 of gestation (Shambaugh *et al.* 1977).

Williamson: Fain & Scow (1966) showed that in rats two days' starvation did not affect fetal weight.   As far as I know nobody has starved them for longer than that.

Räihä: There is some evidence that changes in the amino acid environment in the fetus and amino acid imbalance in the newborn infant might affect intellectual development.   Have you any information about the amino acid concentrations in the fetus of a diabetic mother versus the normal fetus?

Freinkel: We do not have any data on human fetuses. However, we have been exploring these parameters in the offspring of rats who were rendered mildly diabetic with streptozotocin before mating (L. Airoldi *et al.,* unpublished observations, 1977–1978). We have been particularly interested in tyrosine, tryptophan, noradrenaline (norepinephrine) and serotonin in the fetal brains to assess to what extent alterations in circulating amino acids can compromise the development of neurotransmitters in fetal brain. Observations to date would indicate that serotonin and norepinephrine in fetal brain are influenced very little by substantial excursions in the ambient precursor amino acids. Thus, our preliminary findings suggest that development of these neurotransmitters in the rat fetus appears to be delimited by maturation of biosynthetic enzymes rather than the availability of appropriate building blocks.

Girard: We found (Girard *et al.* 1977) that starvation of pregnant rats during the last four days of gestation (day 17.5 to 21.5) produced a decrease in fetal weight. This was associated with an increase in the activity of liver gluconeogenic enzymes in the fetus. Maternal glucose might be saved from depletion if the fetus produced its own glucose, and so decreased the maternal glucose gradient.

Freinkel: You will recall that Goodner also secured evidence for activation of fetal gluconeogenesis during starvation in the pregnant rat, using equilibrium infusion techniques about a decade ago (Goodner & Thompson 1967). Ogata has been obtaining similar findings in our laboratories with infusions of labelled glucose into conscious fed and fasted pregnant rats (Ogata *et al.* 1978). I fully agree that fetal gluconeogenesis could be a mechanism for conserving maternal fuels. However, it has to be viewed as a very finite defence at best since the fetus is still using building blocks originally derived from the mother.

Girard: The metabolic adaptations occurring in the fetus during maternal starvation are probably very important in saving maternal glucose. If the fetus synthesizes glucose through gluconeogenesis, there is a decrease in the maternal – fetal gradient of glucose, so glucose production by the mother can be decreased and maternal amino acids spared.

Shafrir: Adult brain has been shown to utilize ketone bodies very effectively as a fuel. The reduction in lactate utilization and glucose production that you find in the fetus may be just a switch-over from glucose to ketone body metabolism without any detrimental effect on brain development.

Freinkel: I tried to emphasize some of the distinctions between the fetal and the adult brain. The adult brain has one major objective for its energy consumption, that is, to maintain function. The fetal brain, on the other hand, has additional jobs. It has to form new cells of various types, to myelinate some of them, to provide supporting structures for others, etc. In other words, whereas adult brain is concerned with preserving the *status quo,* the fetal brain is also undergoing proliferation. The proliferative aspects are particularly important to cells that I have designated as 'non-replicating'. These cells have only a finite period for proliferation and it is conceivable that long-range consequences may supervene when substrate mixtures are compromised during this interval.

References

FAIN, J. N. & SCOW, R. O. (1966) Fatty acid synthesis in vivo in maternal and fetal tissues in the rat. *Am. J. Physiol. 210,* 19–25

FAJANS, S.S. & FLOYD, J. C. JR. (1976) Fasting hypoglycemia in adults. *N. Engl. J. Med. 294,* 766–772

FELIG, P. & LYNCH, V. (1970) Starvation in human pregnancy: hypoglycaemia, hypoinsulinemia, and hyperketonemia. *Science (Wash. D. C.) 170,* 990–992

FELIG, P., JIN KIM, Y., LYNCH, V. & HENDLER, R. (1972) Amino acid metabolism during starvation in human pregnancy. *J. Clin. Invest. 51,* 1195–1201

FREINKEL, N. (1975) Hypoglycemic disorders, in *Textbook of Medicine* (Beeson, P.B. & McDermott, W., eds.), pp. 1619–1624, Saunders, Philadelphia

FREINKEL, N. (1978) The role of nutrition in medicine: recent developments in fuel metabolism. *J. Am. Med. Assoc. 239,* 1868–1872

FREINKEL, N., METZGER, B. E., NITZAN, M., HARE, J. W., SHAMBAUGH, G. E. III, MARSHALL, R. T., SURMACZYNSKA, B. Z. & NAGEL, T. C. (1972) 'Accelerated starvation' and mechanisms for the conservation of maternal nitrogen during pregnancy. *Isr. J. Med. Sci. 8,* 426–439

FREINKEL, N., PHELPS, R. L. & METZGER, B. E. (1979) Intermediary metabolism during normal pregnancy, in *Carbohydrate Metabolism in Pregnancy and the Newborn* (Sutherland, H. W. & Stowers, J. M., eds.) *(2nd Aberdeen Int. Colloq.),* Springer, Berlin

GIRARD, J. R., FERRÉ, P., GILBERT, M., KERVRAN, A., ASSAN, R. & MARLISS, E. B. (1977) Fetal metabolic response to maternal fasting in the rat. *Am. J. Physiol. 232,* E456–E463

GOODNER, C. J. & THOMPSON, D.J. (1967) Glucose metabolism in the fetus in utero: the effect of maternal fasting and glucose loading in the rat. *Pediatr. Res. 1,* 443–451

HERRERA, E., KNOPP, R. H. & FREINKEL, N. (1969a) Carbohydrate metabolism in pregnancy. VI. Plasma fuels, insulin, liver composition, gluconeogenesis and nitrogen metabolism during late gestation in the fed and fasted rat. *J. Clin. Invest. 48,* 2260–2272

HERRERA, E., KNOPP, R. H. & FREINKEL, N. (1969b) Urinary excretion of epinephrine and norepinephrine during fasting in late pregnancy in the rat. *Endocrinology 84,* 447–450

MERIMEE, T. J. & FINEBERG, S. E. (1973) Homeostasis during fasting. II. Hormone substrate differences between men and women. *J. Clin. Endocrinol. Metab. 37,* 698–702

METZGER, B. E. & FREINKEL, N. (1975) Regulation of maternal protein metabolism and gluconeogenesis in the fasted state, in *Early Diabetes in Early Life* (Camerini–Davalos, R. A. & Cole, H. S., eds.), pp. 303–311, Academic Press, New York

METZGER, B. E., HARE, J. W. & FREINKEL, N. (1971) Carbohydrate metabolism in pregnancy. IX. Plasma levels of gluconeogenic fuels during fasting in the rat. *J. Clin. Endocrinol. 33,* 869–873

METZGER, B. E., AGNOLI, F., HARE, J. W. & FREINKEL, N. (1973) Carbohydrate metabolism in pregnancy. X. Metabolic disposition of alanine by the perfused liver of the fasting pregnant rat. *Diabetes 22,* 601–608

OGATA, E. S., SANDERS, L., METZGER, B. & FREINKEL, N. (1978) Effects of the conceptus on glucose kinetics during fasting in pregnancy. *Pediatr. Res. 12,* 54 (abstr.)

SCOW, R. O., CHERNICK, S.S. & BRINLEY, M. S. (1964) Hyperlipemia and ketosis in the pregnant rat. *Am. J. Physiol. 206,* 796–804

SHAMBAUGH, G. E. III, MROZAK, S. C. & FREINKEL, N. (1977) Fetal fuels. I. Utilization of ketones by isolated tissues at various stages of maturation and maternal nutrition during late gestation. *Metabolism 26,* 623–636

TYSON, J. E., AUSTIN, K., FARINHOLT, J. & FIEDLER, J. (1976) Endocrine–metabolic response to acute starvation in human gestation. *Am. J. Obstet. Gynecol. 125,* 1073–1084

WILLIAMSON, D. H. & ROBINSON, A.M. (1977) Control of glucose metabolism in lactating-rat mammary gland: effects of other substrates, insulin and starvation. *Biochem. Soc. Trans. 5,* 829–834

The influence of hormonal changes of pregnancy on maternal metabolism

RONALD K. KALKHOFF and HAK–JOONG KIM

Endocrine-Metabolic Section, Department of Medicine, Medical College of Wisconsin and Clinical Research Center, Milwaukee County Medical Complex, Milwaukee, Wisconsin

Abstract   Mammalian pregnancy is characterized by progressive hyperinsulinaemia, raised plasma lipids and increased vulnerability to ketosis after food deprivation.   The present investigations were performed to assess the role of two placental steroids, oestradiol and progesterone, in the development of these changes, since plasma titres of these hormones progressively increase during human gestation.

In both human subjects and adult female rats it was demonstrated that these two steroids, separately or in combination, augment plasma insulin concentration *in vivo*, cause hypertrophy of pancreatic islets and promote exaggerated secretion of insulin, but not glucagon, by pancreatic islets *in vitro*.   Hypertriglyceridaemia induced by oestrogen alone or combined with progesterone was associated with increased splanchnic production of triglyceride as well as altered tissue lipoprotein lipase (EC 3.1.1.34) and circulating apoproteins that influence activity of this enzyme.   The combined regimen also increased hepatic glycogen storage and suppressed gluconeogenesis *in vivo* in the rat while accelerating the onset of ketosis during starvation in human subjects and in the animal model.

Oestradiol and progesterone appear to effect metabolic changes in non-pregnant animals and human subjects that simulate maternal adaptations to advancing gestation, including altered endocrine pancreatic function, triglyceride metabolism and metabolic fuel storage and mobilization.

In early gestation and long before the fetus places significant demands on maternal nutrients, the placenta and, to some extent, the pituitary begin to elaborate hormones that anticipate the metabolic requirements of two individuals instead of one.   An orderly maternal–fetal adaptation and coexistence is contingent upon the establishment of maternal hyperinsulinaemia and predominance of insulin-mediated anabolism in the fed state.   In the absence of this adjustment the sequence of other necessary metabolic events becomes disturbed, diabetes supervenes, and the health of mother and fetus becomes jeopardized.   It is the purpose of this discussion to demonstrate how certain placental hormones serve maternal needs by dictating critical alterations in the

29

endocrine pancreas, lipid metabolism and fuel storage and release so that maternal–fetal wellbeing is ensured throughout gestation and parturition.

PREGNANCY AND THE PANCREATIC ISLET

Several investigators, including those in our own group, have documented the presence of basal hyperinsulinaemia and exaggerated plasma insulin responses to oral and intravenous glucose and tolbutamide in normal human pregnancy.

To explore the relationship between high plasma concentrations of progesterone in gestation and hyperinsulinaemia, we gave non–pregnant adult volunteers between 300 and 500 mg of progesterone in oil intramuscularly for six days. From day 3 through day 6 urinary pregnanediol levels were in the range of late human pregnancy (25–50 mg/24 h). Throughout the six-day period there were no significant changes in basal plasma glucose, free fatty acids, cortisol or growth hormone concentrations. However, after day 3, fasting insulin levels significantly increased. Fig. 1 depicts, on the right, the results of glucose tolerance tests (100 g orally) and plasma insulin responses in the volunteers before and during progesterone administration. For purposes of comparison, similar tests done on normal pregnant women are shown on the left. These data demonstrate that progesterone augments both basal and post-challenge insulin concentrations in a manner resembling late pregnancy. Similar changes were observed after we gave intravenous tolbutamide to the same individuals. However, unlike what occurs in pregnancy, basal glucose levels were not depressed by progesterone nor was the glucose curve significantly altered (Kalkhoff *et al.* 1970).

Pancreatic islet function was examined *in vitro* as well (Costrini & Kalkhoff 1971). Pancreatic islets were isolated by a collagenase technique from pregnant and control rats and groups of 10 islets were incubated for 90 min in a 16.7 mM-glucose medium. Fig. 2 reveals that during the three-week gestational period, insulin secretion increased significantly during the second week. We succeeded in reproducing this effect in non-pregnant adult female rats with daily parenteral doses of oestradiol (5 μg) or progesterone (5 mg) separately or in combination for 21 days as well as when we gave half the combined dose for the same period of time. Fig. 3 illustrates this effect with the dosage regimens.

The data in Figs. 2 and 3 also related to significant increases in pancreatic islet diameter and protein content and to hyperinsulinaemia *in vivo* in similar groups of rats during intravenous glucose tolerance testing. Progesterone alone was without effect on carbohydrate tolerance whereas oestradiol improved it. These latter findings are highly consistent with the classic studies of

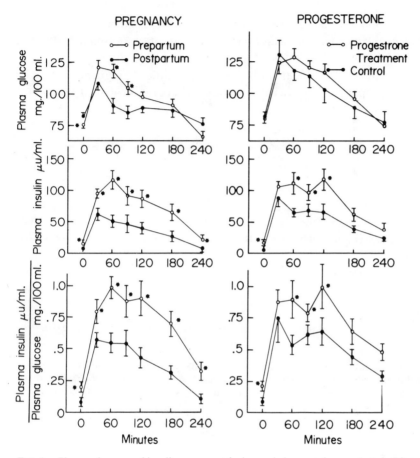

FIG. 1.   Plasma glucose and insulin responses during oral glucose tolerance tests in 10 pregnant women before and after delivery (left) and in 7 normal adults before and on day 5 of progesterone administration (right).   Values are mean ± S.E.M. *: $P < 0.05$ with respect to differences from control values.   From Kalkhoff *et al.* (1970) with permission of the publishers.

Houssay and co-workers (1954) who reported an ameliorative effect of oestrogens on diabetes in association with pancreatic islet hypertrophy in the rat.   Similar effects of natural oestrogens have been found in a variety of mammalian species including rabbits and man, as reviewed elsewhere (Kalkhoff 1972).

From these observations it is difficult to justify the classification of either oestradiol or progesterone as insulin antagonists.   It is also not possible to define whether their separate or combined actions on the pancreatic islet are direct, indirect or both.   Recently, Howell and coworkers (1977) reported that incubation of isolated rat islets with progesterone and oestradiol for 20 h resulted in enhanced insulin secretion by different substrate stimuli.   Thus, at least one laboratory has provided evidence for a direct effect.

The physiological significance of hyperinsulinaemia of pregnancy cannot be placed in a proper perspective without some consideration of α-cell glucagon, a

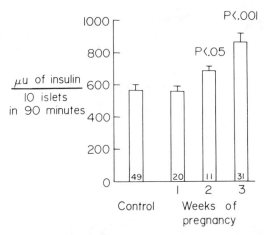

FIG. 2.   *In vitro* insulin secretion in response to 16.7 mM–glucose by isolated pancreatic islets obtained from control rats and pregnant animals at different weeks of gestation.   Values are mean ± S.E.M.   Numbers of experiments are indicated within bars.   Data from Costrini & Kalkhoff (1971).

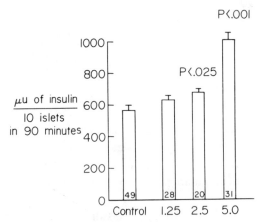

FIG. 3.   *In vitro* insulin secretion in response to 16.7 mM–glucose by isolated pancreatic islets obtained from control rats and animals injected daily with a combined regimen of oestradiol (in μg) and progesterone (in mg) for three weeks.   Values are mean ± S.E.M.   Numbers within bars denote numbers of experiments.   Data from Costrini & Kalkhoff (1971).

known insulin antagonist.   In our more recent studies the perifusion technique of Lacy and co-workers (1972) was employed to assess pancreatic islet
insulin and glucagon secretory rates in late gestation in rats (Kalkhoff & Kim
1978).   One hundred islets from control or pregnant rat pancreases were
isolated by a collagenase method and perifused in chambers side by side in a
buffered medium containing 2.8 mM-glucose for 30 min.   Subsequently,
different substrate stimuli were introduced and the stimulus was sustained for
an additional 50 min.   Effluent was collected at 1- or 5- min intervals for
measurement of insulin and glucagon.

Fig. 4 illustrates the bihormonal response to a high glucose (16.7 mM)
concentration.   Both acute (0–9 min) and second phase (10–50 min) insulin
secretion in pregnancy islets significantly exceeded control values.   Suppression of glucagon secretion tended to be slightly greater in the islets from
pregnant rats during the second phase.

When a 6 mM-challenge consisting of 20 amino acids was introduced,
insulin and glucagon secretory rates were comparable (Fig. 5).   When 16.7

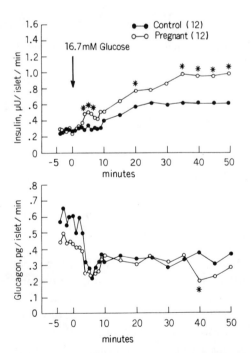

FIG. 4.   Insulin and glucagon secretion by perifused pancreatic islets from control and pregnant
rats after a 16.7 mM-glucose stimulus.   Values are mean ± S.E.M.   *: $P < 0.05$, the significance
of differences between corresponding means.   From Kalkhoff & Kim (1978) with permission of
the publishers.

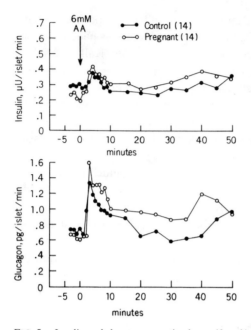

FIG. 5.   Insulin and glucagon secretion by perifused islets from control and pregnant rats after a 6 mM stimulus containing 20 amino acids.   See legend for Fig. 4 for further explanations.   From Kalkhoff & Kim (1978) with permission of the publishers.

mM-glucose and 6 mM amino acid mixtures were combined (Fig. 6), much more insulin was secreted by control and pregnancy islets than was secreted in response to either substrate challenge alone.   Moreover, acute and second phase insulin secretion was considerably higher in perifused islets from the pregnant group than from the control group, whereas no differences existed between groups with respect to the glucagon secretory profiles, i.e. acute phase glucagon release was suppressed to a comparable extent relative to peak values observed with amino acids alone.

Calculations of insulin/glucagon molar ratios at each interval for the control and pregnancy islets revealed no differences when 6 mM amino acids alone were used.   However, whenever glucose was introduced as a stimulus alone or in combination with amino acids, significantly higher ratios were observed in the pregnant group than in the controls.   These data suggest that during pregnancy insulin secretion predominates over that of glucagon whenever a glucose signal appears and that no evidence for excessive glucagon secretion exists in normal gestation in rats.   The results are relevant to reports of an increased β to α cell ratio and β cell hypertrophy in late gestation (Hellman

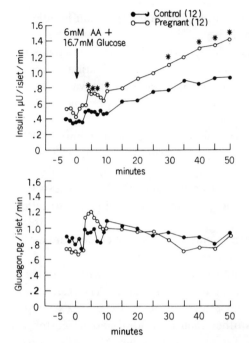

FIG. 6. Insulin and glucagon secretion by perifused islets from control and pregnant rats following a 16.7 mM-glucose + 6 mM amino acid challenge. See Fig. 4 for further explanations. From Kalkhoff & Kim (1978) with permission of the publishers.

1960; Aerts & Van Asshe 1975). They also support conclusions derived from clinical studies of pregnant women in which plasma glucagon responses to mixed meals were not excessive (Metzger & Freinkel 1975) and responses to glucose administration revealed greater than normal suppression (Daniel *et al.* 1974; Luyckx *et al.* 1975; Kuhl & Holst 1976). Since we have succeeded in reproducing these effects of pregnancy in perifused islets obtained from non-pregnant rats receiving combined oestradiol and progesterone, this also emphasizes the importance of placental steroid effects on the pancreatic islet α–β cell couple.

HEPATIC CARBOHYDRATE METABOLISM

If an increased insulin/glucagon molar secretory ratio is a physiologically meaningful response of islets to glucose-containing nutrients in pregnancy, and if it is mediated in part by placental oestrogen and progesterone, then evidence of substrate storage should exist. Insulin is the principal anabolic hormone for hepatic glycogen formation, triglyceride deposition in adipose tissue and protein synthesis in lean tissue.

In earlier work (Matute & Kalkhoff 1973) it was demonstrated that oestradiol and progesterone, especially when administered in combination, promote an increased deposition of hepatic glycogen that exceeds control values by 1.5 to over twofold. These observations are reminiscent of a previous study of oestradiol action by Walaas (1952).

In addition we reported that intravenous [U–^{14}C]alanine and [3–^{14}C] pyruvate are incorporated into liver glycogen to a significantly greater extent in the rats treated with sex steroids than in untreated rats whereas the percentage appearing in plasma glucose is significantly reduced. This suggests that glycogen synthesis and/or turnover is increased in this condition in association with impaired hepatic gluconeogenesis. Since these are insulin-like effects and the steroid regimen induces hyperinsulinaemia, we conclude that oestradiol and progesterone do facilitate glycogen storage in liver.

However, liver glycogen is not raised in pregnancy, and with short-term fasting gluconeogenic capacity appears to be augmented (Herrera et al. 1969). These discrepancies between effects of gestation and sex steroid administration suggest that factors other than oestradiol and progesterone modify these parameters in the gravid state. Nevertheless, the facilitation of glycogen anabolism by placental steroids may play an important role in offsetting catabolic events that work against nutrient fuel storage in pregnancy.

ACCELERATED STARVATION

The term accelerated starvation was coined and conceptualized by Freinkel to denote metabolic events that evolve during fasting in the pregnant state. Briefly, in a variety of mammalian species, including the rat, baboon and pregnant women, food withdrawal results in a more rapid fall in plasma glucose, insulin and glucogenic amino acids and an exaggerated rise in free fatty acids and ketone bodies, as compared with non-pregnant controls. These interrelationships have been reviewed recently by Metzger & Freinkel (1975).

Factors responsible for this increased sensitivity to a fast are not clear but must include the competition for and extraction of glucose and amino acids by the fetus, increased mobilization of free fatty acids to liver for ketogenesis and the loss of the insulin-braking effect against other catabolic events. The more rapid fall of plasma alanine could also represent a restrained release of this amino acid by skeletal muscle, since ketone bodies *per se* exert this effect in non-pregnant individuals (Sherwin et al. 1975) and simulate altered fuel homeostasis in mid-pregnancy (Felig & Lynch 1970). Thus, a true gluconeogenic substrate deficiency syndrome could exist in the pregnant fasted woman for more than one reason and contribute to maternal hypoglycaemia in this setting.

Nevertheless, and from a more simplistic point of view, there is some evidence that non-pregnant women are also more sensitive to fasting than are men from the standpoint of rates of decrease of plasma glucose and rates of increments in plasma free fatty acid (Merimee & Fineberg 1973). Since this has obvious relevance to differences in sex steroid complement, we have embarked on a study to test whether sex steroids can influence ketogenesis (Morrow *et al.* 1978).

In groups of postmenopausal women, total plasma ketones in a control state of fasting were significantly lower at 36 h than after five days of administration of a combined oral oestrogen–progestin and a repeated fast. At 36 h plasma alanine was also significantly lower during sex steroid treatment. Moreover, similar findings were observed after a 24-h starvation in rats receiving the combined oestrogen–progesterone regimen for four days as compared to control groups. A similar trend was observed in young women on combined oral contraceptives as compared to fasted women not on these agents. Thus, it appears that combinations of oestrogen and progesterone may condition a setting for accelerated ketogenesis and hypoalaninaemia independent of influences of the fetus.

MATERNAL LIPID METABOLISM

Although most plasma lipids are raised during human pregnancy, changes in triglyceride are among the most striking and may exceed non-pregnant levels by twofold or more. In recent years lipoproteins of the very low density, low density and high density (VLDL, LDL and HDL) classes have been found to be increased in gestation, with the content of triglyceride in each fraction being significantly augmented (Warth *et al.* 1975; Hillman *et al.* 1975). Since oestrogens or conventional oral contraceptive agents are known to induce increases in plasma triglyceride (Hillyard *et al.* 1956; Rössner *et al.* 1971), it was logical for research in this area to centre on the role of oestrogens in the development of hyperlipaemia of pregnancy. Moreover, the modification of oestrogen action by progesterone required elucidation.

During initial studies (Kim & Kalkhoff 1975) our animal model was used to assess the effects of oestradiol and progesterone, separately and in combination, on plasma substrate and insulin concentrations, triglyceride entry into the

TABLE 1

Plasma substrate and insulin concentrations in fed and fasted animals. (From Kim & Kalkhoff 1975 with permission of the publishers.)

	Animal group [a]			
	C	E	P	E + P
Glucose (mg/100 ml)	140 ± 8 (118 ± 4)	146 ± 6 (125 ± 6)	135 ± 6 (115 ± 3)	138 ± 5 (120 ± 6)
Free fatty acids (μequiv./l)	192 ± 7 (529 ± 30)	263 ± 26 (612 ± 55)*	162 ± 23 (580 ± 42)	245 ± 29 (598 ± 48)
Insulin (μU/ml)	26 ± 3 (11 ± 1)	37 ± 4* (30 ± 4)*	36 ± 4* (27 ± 5)*	46 ± 5* (21 ± 3)*
Triglyceride (μmol/ml)	1.94 ± 0.26 (1.16 ± 0.11)	4.49 ± 0.59* (2.32 ± 0.23)*	1.78 ± 0.21 (1.22 ± 0.13)	2.79 ± 0.27* (2.34 ± 0.27)*
Weight gain (%)	22 ± 2 (7 ± 1)	13 ± 3* (9 ± 2)	32 ± 2* (17 ± 1)*	37 ± 1* (12 ± 1)*

* Significance of the difference between means ± S.E.M. of control rats and corresponding means of rats treated with sex steroids, $P < 0.05$.

[a]There were 10 animals in each fed group and 25 animals in each fasted group. Values for fasted animals are parentheses.

C: control; E: oestrogen-treated; P. progesterone-treated; E + P: treated with oestrogen + progesterone.

plasma compartment, and alterations of tissue lipoprotein lipase (LPL) (EC 3.1.1.34).

Table 1 reveals that sex steroid treatment had little effect on plasma glucose or free fatty acids in fed or 12-hour fasted states. During the three weeks of hormonal administration both oestradiol (E) and combined regimens (E + P) significantly increased plasma triglyceride concentrations. In the fed state, the magnitude of the change was greatest with oestradiol alone; in the fasted state, E and E + P regimens produced comparable effects. These results did not correlate with the degree of induced hyperinsulinaemia or with body weight gain, since progesterone administration was without effect on this plasma lipid despite comparable increases in insulin and the greatest average gain in body weight. It is likely that the influence of oestrogens on plasma triglyceride is independent of food intake and not directly related to circulating insulin concentrations.

Endogenous triglyceride production was determined with the intravenous Triton technique (40 mg/100 g body weight) as described by Otway & Robinson (1968). LPL measurements were done on dried residues of acetone–ether extracts of parametrial fat and breast tissue. The latter method presumably provides an index of triglyceride breakdown and removal at these sites. Hepatic LPL was measured indirectly by determining protamine-resistant post-heparin lipolytic activity in plasma (Krauss et al. 1973).

Fig. 7 shows that increases in plasma triglyceride after administration of oestradiol alone or in combination with progesterone relate rather well to augmented triglyceride entry. It is also of interest that a similar relationship has been reported in the pregnant rat by Otway & Robinson (1968). These findings suggest that the hypertriglyceridaemia of gestation can be explained, in part, by an oestrogen action which is expressed via effects on splanchnic bed synthesis and release of this lipid. In the fasting state, this would represent predominantly a hepatic contribution.

Interpretation of LPL measurements, however, is more difficult. Marked suppression of the enzyme by oestradiol in adipose tissue, a major locus of plasma triglyceride catabolism, is consistent with an impairment of peripheral removal which could also effect increased circulating concentrations. However, greatly increased activities of LPL induced by progesterone alone had little influence on triglyceride levels in plasma. With the combined E+P treatment, adipose LPL was also increased. This could have a bearing on the degree of the increase in plasma triglycerides, since the latter was not as great as with oestradiol treatment alone in the presence of comparable rates of triglyceride entry.

At this point it should be mentioned that Otway & Robinson (1968) found suppressed adipose LPL in late gestation in rats. Thus, the E+P regimen, as opposed to E alone, did not reproduce this effect. This difference might be explained by extraplacental factors, including prolactin (Zinder et al. 1974) and prostaglandins (Spooner et al. 1977), that tend to suppress this lipase in pregnancy.

In the mammary glands, LPL activity was significantly increased by each of the three sex steroid regimens and was greatest with combined administration. Similar changes in breast LPL have been reported in late gestation and post partum by McBride & Korn (1963). In late pregnancy this increase in LPL activity is very probably relevant to partial amelioration of hypertriglyceridaemia with diversion of glyceride fatty acid to breast tissue in preparation for lactation. Again, prolactin and prostaglandin effects on mammary gland

LPL also very probably contribute to this phenomenon (Zinder *et al.* 1974; Spooner *et al.* 1977), in concert with the actions of oestradiol and progesterone.

Although the significance of altered hepatic LPL during treatment with these regimens is unknown, it probably contributes greatly to total post-heparin lipolytic activity (PHLA) in plasma and its inhibition by oestrogen may be one reason why PHLA decreases in this situation. Cardiac and lung LPL are unchanged in pregnancy (Otway & Robinson 1968) and after oestradiol treatment according to Hamosh & Hamosh (1975), whereas others report increased activity in heart and diaphragm with administration of oestradiol (Wilson *et al.* 1976).

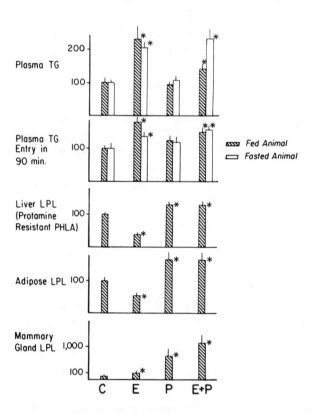

FIG. 7. Influence of the administration of oestradiol (E, 5 µg daily), progesterone (P, 5 mg daily) or the combined regimen (E + P) for 21 days on plasma triglyceride (TG), triglyceride entry and tissue lipoprotein lipases (LPL). Values are expressed as a percentage change from control (C) and asterisks denote a significant difference, $P < 0.05$. Data from Kim & Kalkhoff (1975).

We can conclude from these studies that sex steroids reproduce most, but not all, of the patterns of tissue LPL observed in pregnancy.   However, there is no significant correlation between altered plasma concentrations of triglyceride and any one of the changes in LPL measured *in vitro*.   There was a significant relationship between triglyceride entry and plasma levels of the lipid when linear regression analyses were applied.

To complicate matters further, it is known that circulating apoproteins of various types may modify tissue LPL activity.   In a subsequent investigation we explored the nature of this effect in sex-steroid-treated animals (Kim & Kalkhoff 1978).

In Fig. 8 the effects of serum obtained from the various animal groups on *in vitro* adipose LPL (normal male rat epididymal fat pad) was studied.   Differences between sera from control and from progesterone-treated rats on this parameter were not great with increasing concentrations.   However, oestradiol alone or the combined steroid regimen had significant inhibitory effects.   This is somewhat of a paradox in view of the fact that the E + P regimen augmented tissue LPLs when studied *in vitro* in the absence of this serum.

Fig. 9 reveals that when serum was fractionated into d <1.21 and d >1.21, it

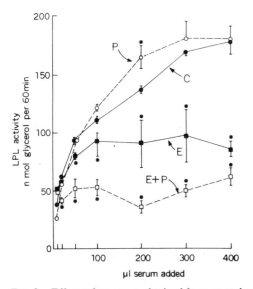

FIG. 8.   Effects of rat serum obtained from control rats (C) and animals treated with oestradiol (E) alone or combined with progesterone (E + P) on *in vitro* adipose tissue lipoprotein lipase (LPL) activity.   Each point is mean ± S.E.M. of four experiments.   *: significance of the difference between control and other group means, P < 0.05.   From Kim & Kalkhoff (1978) with permission of the publishers.

was the lower density fraction containing apoproteins such as the VLDL or HDL class that would be under suspicion.   The $d > 1.21$, containing predominantly serum proteins, was without effect on adipose LPL.   Since VLDL is the principal endogenous carrier protein for triglyceride, both it and HDL were isolated from serum by ultracentrifugation, delipidation and reconstitution in buffered 8 M-urea.   Aliquots were subjected to polyacrylamide gel electrophoresis and various apoprotein bands were identified.

In the VLDL portion (Fig. 10), there was a substantial increase in density of the arginine-rich peptide band and in those containing apo CII and apo CIIIs.   All apo C fractions were significantly increased above control values in the E and E+P treatment groups when quantitative measurements were performed with photodensitometry and appropriate standards.   Moreover, utilizing the double isotope technique of Schimke and co-workers (1968), it was also demonstrated that apo C turnover in the rats receiving the oestradiol and combined treatments significantly exceeded control values by 1.5 to over twofold.

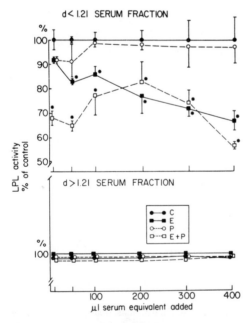

FIG. 9.   Effects of $d < 1.21$ and $d > 1.21$ serum fractions obtained from control (C) rats and animals receiving oestradiol (E) or progesterone (P), separately and in combination (E + P) on *in vitro* LPL activity in adipose tissue.   Each point is mean ± S.E.M. of four experiments and asterisks denote a significant difference between control and other group means, $P < 0.05$.

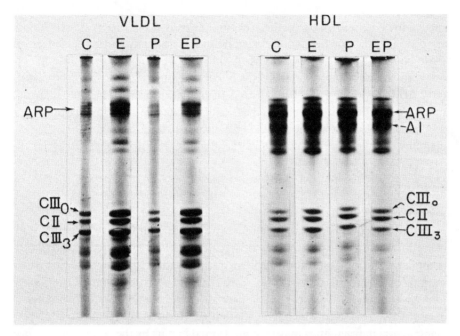

FIG. 10. Polyacrylamide gel electrophoresis of VLDL and HDL apoproteins of sex-steroid-treated rats. ARP refers to arginine-rich peptides; A1 to Apo A1; and C to apo C fractions. From Kim & Kalkhoff (1978) with permission of the publishers.

In human serum apo CII is known to be an activator of adipose LPL and apo CIIIs are inhibitors (La Rosa *et al.* 1970; Brown & Baginsky 1972). In human pregnancy Montes & Knopp (1977) have reported that apo CII/apo CIII ratios are decreased, which may favour the development of increased plasma triglyceride concentrations (Carlson & Ballantyne 1976). Although this ratio was actually increased by oestrogen treatment in our studies, this does not exclude the possibility that an overall increase of apo C may have an inhibitory effect on LPL in the rat, since the absolute effects of either CII or CIII have not been reported to date in this species.

It is also of interest that provisional evidence for suppression of LPL activity by arginine-rich peptides has been reported (Ekman & Nilsson-Ehle 1975), since this fraction in VLDL was distinctly raised in E or E+P treated rats in our investigation.

We can only speculate about the role of these steroids in maternal lipid metabolism at this time. Oestradiol and progesterone probably have direct effects on many tissue LPLs as measured by *in vitro* studies of the enzyme. In addition, the augmentation of lipoprotein delivery into the plasma by the splanchnic bed in response to these hormones provides a variety of circulating apoproteins that further modify peripheral LPL activity. The net effect of these changes in late pregnancy is to shift the lipid reservoir from adipose tissue to the circulation and selectively control sites of removal of glyceride fatty acid in preparation for parturition and lactation. The actual quantitative contribution of each process requires considerable investigation, as do the roles of other hormones and biologically active substances like prostaglandins.

CONCLUSIONS

Placental synthesis and release of oestrogens and progesterone have a profound effect on pancreatic islet function and appear to have a distinct role in the emergence of hyperinsulinaemia, pancreatic islet hypertrophy and β cell dominance during gestation. Evidence is presented that the raised concentrations of plasma insulin after sex steroid administration to rats is translated into an anabolic effect on hepatic carbohydrate metabolism. Preliminary data are also reviewed which indicate that accelerated ketogenesis and hypoalaninaemia in pregnancy may be conditioned in part by the combined actions of oestrogen and progesterone. Finally, the important role of these steroids in maternal lipid metabolism is emphasized, since there are multicentric actions on splanchnic synthesis and release of triglyceride, on peripheral tissue lipoprotein lipases and on apoproteins that modulate these lipases.

ACKNOWLEDGEMENTS

Research cited in this presentation that was performed in the authors' laboratories was supported by research grant AM 10305 and clinical research centre grant RR 00058 from the United States Public Health Service, Bethesda, Maryland, and by TOPS Club, Inc., Obesity and Metabolic Research Program, Milwaukee. Wisconsin.

References

AERTS, L. & VAN ASSHE, F. A. (1975) Ultrastructural changes of the endocrine pancreas in pregnant rats. *Diabetologia 11*, 285–289
BROWN, W. V. & BAGINSKY, M.L. (1972) Inhibition of lipoprotein lipase by an apoprotein of human very low density lipoprotein. *Biochem. Biophys. Res. Commun. 46*, 375–382
CARLSON, L. A. & BALLANTYNE, D. (1976) Changing relative proportions of apolipoproteins CII and CIII of very low density lipoproteins in hypertriglyceridemia. *Atherosclerosis 23*, 563–568

COSTRINI, N. V. & KALKHOFF, R. K. (1971) Relative effects of pregnancy, estradiol and progesterone on plasma insulin and pancreatic islet insulin secretion. *J. Clin. Invest. 50*, 992–999

DANIEL, R. R., METZGER, B. E., FREINKEL, N., FALOONA, G. R. & UNGER, R. H. (1974) Carbohydrate metabolism in pregnancy. XI. Response of plasma glucagon to overnight fast and oral glucose tolerance during normal pregnancy and in gestational diabetes. *Diabetes 23*, 771–776

EKMAN, R. & NILSSON-EHLE, P. (1975) Effects of apolipoproteins on lipoprotein lipase activity of human adipose tissue. *Clin. Chim. Acta 63*, 29-35

FELIG, P. & LYNCH, V. (1970) Starvation in human pregnancy: hypoglycemia, hypoinsulinemia, and hyperketonemia. *Science (Wash. D.C.) 170*, 990–992

HAMOSH, M. & HAMOSH, P. (1975) The effect of estrogen on the lipoprotein lipase activity of adipose tissue. *J. Clin. Invest. 55*, 1132–1135

HELLMAN, B. (1960) The islets of Langerhans in the rat during pregnancy and lactation, with special reference to the changes in the B/A cell ratio. *Acta Obstet. Gynecol. Scand. 39*, 331–349

HERRERA, E., KNOPP, R.H. & FREINKEL, N. (1969) Carbohydrate metabolism in pregnancy. VI. Plasma fuels, insulin, liver composition, gluconeogenesis, and nitrogen metabolism during late gestation in the fed and fasted rat. *J. Clin. Invest. 48*, 2260–2272

HILLMAN, L., SCHONFELD, G., MILLER, J. P. & WULFF, G. (1975) Apoproteins in human pregnancy. *Metabolism 24*, 943–952

HILLYARD, L. A., ENTENMAN, C. & CHAIKOFF, I. L. (1956). Concentration and composition of serum lipoproteins of cholesterol-fed and stilbestrol-injected birds. *J. Biol. Chem. 223*, 359–368

HOUSSAY, B. A., FOGLIA, V. G. & RODRIGUEZ, R. R. (1954) Production or prevention of some types of experimental diabetes by estrogens or corticosteroids. *Acta Endocrinol. 17*, 146–164

HOWELL, S. L., TYHURST, M. & GREEN, I. C. (1977) Direct effects of progesterone on rat islets of Langerhans in vivo and in tissue culture. *Diabetologia 13*, 579, 583

KALKHOFF, R.K. (1972) Effects of oral contraceptive agents and sex steroids on carbohydrate metabolism *Annu. Rev. Med. 23*, 429–438

KALKHOFF, R. K. & KIM, H.-J. (1978) Effects of pregnancy on insulin and glucagon secretion by perifused rat pancreatic islets. *Endocrinology 102*, 623–631

KALKHOFF, R. K., JACOBSON, M. & LEMPER, D. (1970) Progesterone, pregnancy and the augmented plasma insulin response. *J. Clin. Endocrinol. Metab. 31*, 24–28

KIM, H.-J. & KALKHOFF, R.K. (1975) Sex steroid influence on triglyceride metabolism. *J. Clin. Invest. 56*, 888–896

KIM, H.-J. & KALKHOFF, R. K. (1978) Altered apolipoproteins in sex steroid-treated rats. *Metabolism 27*, 571–587

KRAUSS, R. M., WINDMUELLER, H. G., LEVY, R. I. & FREDRICKSON, D. S. (1973) Selective measurement of two different triglyceride lipase activities in rat post-heparin plasma. *J. Lipid Res. 14*, 286–295

KUHL, C. & HOLST, J. J. (1976) Plasma glucagon and insulin: glucagon ratio in gestational diabetes. *Diabetes 25*, 16–23

LACY, P. E., WALKER, M. M. & FINK, C. J. (1972) Perifusion of isolated rat islets in vitro. Participation of the microtubular system in the biphasic release of insulin. *Diabetes 21*, 987–995

LA ROSA, J. C., LEVY, R. I., HERBERT, P., LUX, S. E. & FREDRICKSON D. S. (1970) A specific lipoprotein activator for lipoprotein lipase. *Biochem. Biophys. Res. Commun. 41*, 47–52

LUYCKX, A. S., GERARD, J., GASPARD, U. & LEFEBVRE, P.J. (1975) Plasma glucagon levels in normal women during pregnancy. *Diabetologia 11*, 549–554

MATUTE, M. L. & KALKHOFF, R. K. (1973) Sex steroid influence on hepatic gluconeogenesis and glycogen formation. *Endocrinology 92*, 762–768

MCBRIDE, O. W. & KORN, E. D. (1963) The lipoprotein lipase of mammary gland and the correlation of its activity to lactation. *J. Lipid Res. 4*, 17–20

MERIMEE, T. J. & FINEBERG, S. E. (1973) Homeostasis during fasting. II. Hormone substrate differences between men and women. *J. Clin. Endocrinol. Metab. 37,* 698–702

METZGER, B. E. & FREINKEL, N. (1975) Regulation of maternal protein metabolism and gluconeogenesis in the fasted state, in *Early Diabetes in Early Life* (Camerini-Davalos, R. A. & Cole, H. S., eds.), pp. 303–311, Academic Press, New York

MONTES, A. & KNOPP, R.H. (1977) Lipid metabolism in pregnancy. IV. C-apoprotein changes in very low and intermediate density lipoproteins. *J. Clin. Endocrinol. Metab. 45,* 1060–1063

MORROW, P. G., MARSHALL, W. P., KIM, H.-J. & KALKHOFF, R.K. (1978) Influence of sex steroids on the metabolic response to starvation. *Proc. 60th Annu. Meet. Endocr. Soc.,* Miami Beach, Florida, June 14–16, 1978, abstr. 363, p. 256

OTWAY, S. & ROBINSON, D.S. (1968) The significance of changes in tissue clearing-factor lipase activity in relation to lipemia of pregnancy. *Biochem. J. 106,* 677–682

RÖSSNER, S., LARSSON-COHN, U., CARLSON, L. A. & BOBERG, J. (1971) Effects of an oral contraceptive agent on plasma lipids, plasma lipoproteins, the intravenous fat tolerance and the postheparin lipoprotein lipase activity. *Acta Med. Scand. 190,* 301–305

SCHIMKE, R. T., GANSCHOW, R., DOYLE, D. & ARIAS, I. M. (1968) Regulation of protein turnover in mammalian tissues. *Fed. Proc. 27,* 1223–1230

SHERWIN, R. S., HENDLER, R. G. & FELIG, P. (1975) Effect of ketone infusions on amino acid and nitrogen metabolism in man. *J. Clin. Invest. 55,* 1382–1390

SPOONER, P. M., GARRISON, M. M. & SCOW, R. O. (1977) Regulation of mammary gland and adipose tissue lipoprotein lipase and blood triacylglycerol in rats during late pregnancy. Effect of prostaglandins. *J. Clin. Invest. 60,* 702–708

WALAAS, O. (1952) Effect of estrogens on the glycogen content of rat liver. *Acta Endocrinol. 10,* 193–200

WARTH, M. R., ARKY, R. A. & KNOPP, R. H. (1975) Lipid metabolism in pregnancy. III. Altered lipid composition in intermediate, very low, low, and high density lipoprotein fractions. *J. Clin. Endocrinol. Metab. 41,* 649–655

WILSON, D. E., FLOWERS, C. M., CARLILE, S. I. & UDALL, K. S. (1976) Estrogen treatment and gonadal function in the regulation of lipoprotein lipase. *Atherosclerosis 24,* 491–499

ZINDER, O., HAMOSH, M., FLECK, T. R. C. & SCOW, R.O. (1974) Effect of prolactin on lipoprotein lipase in mammary gland and adipose tissue of rats. *Am. J. Physiol. 226,* 744–748

Discussion

Williamson: We are led to believe that free fatty acids are the major precursors of ketone bodies. Your postmenopausal women had lower free fatty acid concentrations and higher ketone bodies than pregnant women. What were the triglyceride levels in those women?

Kalkhoff: Data for plasma triglyceride are not yet available to us. Specifically, six non-obese postmenopausal women were fasted for 36 h. Plasma and serum samples were obtained at 12, 24 and 36 h. After a suitable recovery period they were given oral micronized 17β-oestradiol, 2 mg, and oral medroxyprogesterone acetate, 5 mg, daily for seven days. The fast was reinstituted on days 6 and 7.

The 12-h fasting concentrations of total serum ketone bodies, plasma free fatty acids and alanine were not different before and during treatment with sex steroids. At 36 h of fasting, however, the oestrogen-progestin treatment resulted in significantly higher total serum ketone body concentrations (2157 ± 390 vs. 1645 ± 282 μmol/l, $P < 0.025$), whereas plasma free fatty acids (1212 ± 173 vs. 1530 ± 22 μmol/l, $P < 0.025$) and plasma alanine (188 ± 11 vs. 225 ± 17 μmol/l, $P < 0.05$) were significantly lower during fasting on the steroid regimen at 36 h.

We have no explanation for the lesser increment of plasma FFA concentrations in association with higher plasma ketone body responses during fasts carried out with the oestrogen–progestin regimen. Similar patterns were observed in intact female rats given short-term pharmacological doses of oestradiol and progesterone. The degree of ketonaemia that was observed in premenopausal women on oral contraceptive agents who were fasted significantly exceeded that of age and weight-matched fasted women who had never received these agents.

Williamson: When you give oestradiol are you also increasing prolactin?

Kalkhoff: I wish to emphasize two things. Administration of oestradiol or a progestin alone had no stimulatory effect on ketogenesis during fasting. In our investigations the two steroids had to be given together for this phenomenon to occur. Secondly, oestrogens may increase pituitary secretion of prolactin at lower pharmacological doses as seen in women receiving oral contraceptive agents (Tyson *et al.* 1975). Higher doses may suppress serum prolactin. Your question implies that there may be indirect effects of this regimen on ketogenesis that are mediated via other induced hormonal changes. We cannot exclude the possibility that other factors may be involved. We did not measure serum prolactin concentrations in our animal or human studies. It is of interest that others have shown a suppression of hepatic ketone body release *in vitro* in the rat after oestrogen treatment alone (Weinstein *et al.* 1977). Also, during later stages of lactation in the postpartum rat, ketogenesis also is suppressed (Whitelaw & Williamson 1977). Obviously prolactin may be implicated in these effects but its precise role requires more study.

Williamson: I am thinking mainly of your lipoprotein lipase studies. Scow's group (Spooner *et al.* 1977) have shown that the initial increase in mammary gland lipoprotein lipase after parturition may be due to the increased concentration of one of the prostaglandins.

Kalkhoff: As shown in Fig. 7 (p. 40) the combined regimen of oestradiol plus progesterone (E + P) given to female rats resulted in an increase of both adipose tissue and mammary gland LPL. We conclude that these two hormones in combination may have a role in the facilitation of triglyceride accumulation at these two sites during pregnancy.   This is consistent with the reported accretion of fat in the adipocyte and breast during the first two-thirds of human and rat gestation (Pitkin 1977; Knopp *et al.* 1973).   During late gestation, however, other events develop which may further modify tissue LPL activity.   As pointed out in our discussion, these include heightened prostaglandin and prolactin activity as well as peak action of human chorionic somatomammotropin (HCS), otherwise also known as human placental lactogen (HPL).   In late pregnancy accumulation of lipid in adipose tissue levels off (Pitkin 1977) and plasma free fatty acid concentrations are markedly increased.   This, in part, may reflect the lipolytic action of HCS on adipose tissue (Turtle & Kipnis 1967), together with the possible inhibitory effects of prostaglandins and prolactin on adipose LPL (Zinder *et al.* 1974; Spooner *et al.* 1977).   Since prolactin 'turns on' breast LPL, the net effect of these events in late gestation is expressed as diversion of free fatty acid storage away from the adipocyte and towards the breast in preparation for lactation.   In other words, the facilitated fat tissue anabolism promoted by oestrogens and progesterone in early and midpregnancy is ultimately offset in late pregnancy by catabolic actions of HCS, prolactin and prostaglandins on adipose tissue.

Milner: In the early part of your presentation you expressed all your results on hormone secretion per islet.   You also stated that islets were morphologically different in the test and control group, pregnancy being characterized by hypertrophy and hyperplasia.   Do you think that in these circumstances you might be tending to obscure significant differences between control and test groups, since you are not comparing like with like?

Kalkhoff: I don't think we are obscuring differences within the scope of this study.   As pointed out in the presentation, the increased secretion of insulin in pregnancy relates, in part, to an increased β cell mass in individual islets, since the β to α cell ratio is increased in this situation.   The purpose of the investigation was to define patterns of islet hormonal secretion *in vitro* by the perifusion technique and to seek differences between islets obtained from pregnant and control groups during exposure to various substrate stimuli.   Such an investigation will not allow us to state whether individual β cells also may be hypersecreting insulin and contribute to the hyperinsulinaemia of pregnancy over and above that due to their increased number in the pregnant state.

Freinkel: I agree completely with your presentation.   We have always emphasized that the placenta developing in parallel to the fetus provides exactly the hormonal juxtaposition that makes 'accelerated starvation' possible (Freinkel 1965; Freinkel *et al.* 1970).   Several groups (Merimee & Fineberg 1973; Fajans & Floyd 1976; Tyson *et al.* 1976), including ours, have found that blood sugar falls more during fasting in females than in males. Thus, some difference in the response to fasting seems to arise simply as a consequence of being female. However, it takes 36 hours for these differences to become manifest. We wondered whether one can show different responses to dietary deprivation more rapidly during pregnancy and whether 'accelerated starvation' can be seen in the type of conditions that are encountered during late gestation in normal clinical practice. Accordingly, we have been comparing gravid women with normal carbohydrate metabolism in week 32 to 38 of gestation and age- and weight-matched normal non-gravid females (Ravnikar *et al.* 1978). We admit them to our Clinical Research Center and withhold food after the 6 p.m. feeding after three days of equilibration on diets of 2210 kcal (9280 kJ) per day containing 250 g carbohydrate. The following day blood samples are secured from indwelling venous catheters at 6 a.m., 8 a.m., 10 a.m. and 12 noon to monitor the effects of 12, 14, 16 and 18 hours of fasting respectively. We are finding that plasma glucose is significantly lower in the pregnant subjects at 6 a.m. after 12 hours of fast but that values for FFA and β-hydroxybutyrate do not differ in the pregnant and non-pregnant populations at this time. However, significant changes occur later: FFA and β-hydroxybutyrate are increased significantly in the pregnant subjects between 8 a.m. and 10 a.m. (i.e. after 14–16 hours of fasting) and all the features of 'accelerated starvation' are very pronounced by noon (i.e. just before lunch, after 18 hours fast). Contrariwise, metabolic parameters remain quite stable during the same interval in the non-gravid subjects (Ravnikar *et al.* 1978). Clearly, therefore, 'accelerated starvation' is a very real event even under conditions of normal carbohydrate metabolism in late pregnancy, and some of the conflicting reports concerning FFA and ketones after overnight fast in normal pregnancy (as reviewed in Freinkel *et al.* 1979) must be ascribed to relatively minor variations in the temporal definitions of 'overnight fast' by different authors.

The question then is, as Ron Kalkhoff has put it so well, how much of the 'accelerated starvation' is due to the sex steroid *per se* and how much is due to the added factors introduced by the conceptus. One can't answer that with certitude in humans but we do have some relevant observations in the rat. We have performed experiments in which fetuses have been removed and placentas left intact or placentas plus fetuses removed (Freinkel *et al.* 1972; Freinkel *et al.* 1979). In the same studies, we have also removed ovaries and provided constant replacement doses of oestrogen and progesterone (since these hormones originate almost entirely in the ovary in the pregnant rat). These experiments with partial extirpation of the products of conception have documented that the presence of the fetus (and the presumed attendant removal of glucose and gluconeogenic precursors by the fetus) is necessary for the full expression of 'accelerated starvation' in late gestation. They thus confirm some of the earlier findings of others (Campbell *et al.* 1953; Bourdel & Jacquot 1956; Curry & Beaton 1958; Scow *et al.* 1964). However, they have also demonstrated that some of the hormonal changes of pregnancy, particularly the placental elaborations, establish an appropriate permissive setting and may, of themselves, effect important metabolic realignments (Freinkel *et al.* 1972; Metzger *et al.* 1975; Freinkel *et al.* 1979).

Kalkhoff: In our studies the administration of oral 17β-oestradiol and medroxyprogesterone acetate to postmenopausal women heightens the serum concentrations of ketones during fasting. The point we are making is that these two steroids may condition the liver to synthesize and release more β-hydroxybutyrate and acetoacetate during fasting and contribute to the exaggerated ketosis observed during gestation when food is withheld. This effect appears to be independent of raised plasma free fatty acids, major precursors for hepatic ketone body synthesis, since the plasma FFA response during fasting was somewhat lower in postmenopausal women on the steroid regimen than it was without this hormonal treatment.

However, the serum ketone body excursions of the treated women are not nearly as great as in the fasted, pregnant state. This difference may relate to the greater flux of plasma FFA precursors to liver in pregnancy during starvation, a phenomenon that is partly a result of enhanced adipose tissue lipolysis and turnover. Nevertheless, if our conclusion is correct, it would appear that the combined oestrogen–progestin exposure has an additional effect on ketogenesis regardless of substrate precursor availability. The phenomenon of 'accelerated starvation' observed in pregnancy, then, may not be strictly dependent on fetal extraction of nutrients as opposed to metabolic changes induced by the changing maternal hormonal milieu.

Freinkel: There is no doubt about that. I completely agree that the hormones of pregnancy *per se* have significant metabolic properties and that these actions can be elicited to an even more marked degree when more hormones are given. However, I feel that the magnitude and rapidity of the changes that we see in our normal pregnant women in late gestation when overnight fast is extended from 6 a.m. to noon can only be explained by invoking additional factors. In other words, the human observations combined with the rat data (see above) suggest to me that this rapidly induced hyperketonaemia and hypoglycaemia necessitates the additional features of removal of maternal substrates by the conceptus. There is a biological continuum with the hormones of pregnancy providing a metabolic setting of activated lipolysis, intrahepatic realignments, and insulin antagonism which, when combined with transplacental losses, give rise to what we call 'accelerated starvation' of pregnancy.

Blázquez: Dr Kalkhoff, you have found *in vitro* that pancreatic islets of pregnant rats secrete glucagon in a different manner to those from non-pregnant animals, which contrasts with the *in vivo* results obtained by other workers (Daniel *et al.* 1974). This difference may be related to the metabolic dynamics of glucagon in pregnant rats *in vivo*, in which, for example, there may be greater degradation or a different population of glucagon receptors on target organs than in non-pregnant animals. Have you any information about that?

Kalkhoff: The results of our pancreatic islet perifusion studies are consistent with many *in vivo* studies of plasma glucagon. For example, we were unable to demonstrate exaggerated glucagon secretion in response to a physiological challenge with 6 mM amino acids. This observation is similar to *in vivo* studies of pregnant rats by Saudek *et al.* (1975) in which pharmacological challenges with intravenous alanine also failed to elicit an abnormally high plasma glucagon response. Moreover, mixed meal administration to pregnant women also fails to augment plasma glucagon responses above those found in non-pregnant subjects (Freinkel & Metzger 1975). There was also a trend for greater suppression of glucagon secretion to occur when substrate challenges containing glucose were perifused through pregnancy islets. This, too, resembles *in vivo* data of Daniel *et al.* (1974), Luyckx *et al.* (1975) and Kuhl & Holst (1976) who found exaggerated suppression of plasma glucagon in women in late gestation after oral or intravenous glucose administration.

Our own research has not examined glucagon receptors in pregnancy, nor have we studied degradation rates of glucagon in the pregnant state.

Hull: Have you studied the effect of the peptides and apoproteins on lipoprotein lipase activity in the placenta of the rat?

Kalkhoff: No. We have not studied placental LPL activity and possible effects of apoprotein regulation of the enzyme in this tissue. Perhaps at this time it is worth re-emphasizing problems with the interpretation of *in vitro* LPL assays generally. They cannot distinguish between that portion of the enzyme which is at an active site in the capillary endothelium and that which is in an inactive stored form in the tissue. Moreover, we have shown in Fig. 7 that while the E + P regimen augments adipose tissue LPL activity *in vitro*, serum and serum fractions containing apoproteins from E + P-treated rats inhibit LPL activity of adipose tissue obtained from untreated rats (Figs. 8 and 9). Obviously, to resolve these discrepancies, more *in vivo* studies of circulating triglyceride catabolism and removal of glyceride free fatty acids at various tissue sites are needed before one can rely on *in vitro* LPL assays as true indices of these events.   The potential importance of apoprotein regulation of these enzymes and the influence of sex steroids on circulating apoprotein concentrations also is stressed by Dr Kim and myself (Fig. 10).

Battaglia: You said that if you give oestradiol and progesterone to non-pregnant women, the changes you produce in concentrations of solutes in the blood were in the same direction but not nearly of the same order of magnitude as the changes one sees during 'accelerated starvation' in pregnancy.   What order of magnitude were you referring to?

Kalkhoff: By the 36th hour of fasting, postmenopausal women pretreated with an oestrogen–progestin combination had average total serum ketones of 2157 μmol/l which exceeded control average values (1645 μmol/l) by approximately 30%.   In the studies of human pregnancy by Felig & Lynch (1970), total serum ketone bodies at the 36th hour of fasting were about 2700 μmol/l, or nearly 50% higher than corresponding control values of their non-pregnant women (1380 μmol/l) at the 36th hour.

In our studies of control, sex-steroid-treated and pregnant rats, a similar differential effect of starvation on total serum ketone body concentrations was observed at the 24th hour of total starvation in the three groups.   I would add that accelerated starvation appears to last a finite period.

Freinkel: There are really two components which must be distinguished, i.e. the qualitative and the quantitative aspects.   The metabolic response to dietary deprivation occurs more rapidly in late gestation.   In that sense, it is 'accelerated'.   The non-gravid woman may achieve the *same qualitative* changes but they occur at a slower rate.   It is by no means certain whether she ever achieves changes of the same *quantitative* magnitude.   For example, we have never been able to reduplicate the hyperketonaemia that occurs when the rat is fasted in late gestation with any amount of dietary deprivation or hormone replacement in non-gravid animals.   What we are discussing then is how much of the 'accelerated starvation' of late pregnancy occurs via the enhanced availability of oestrogen, progesterone and somatomammotropin and how much is due to the continuing removal of fuels such as glucose and amino acids which are ordinarily conserved with much more parsimony.   I would suggest that both are contributory.   Pregnancy creates a situation in which the placenta is elaborating sex steroids and somatomammotropin into the maternal circulation in ever-increasing amounts, coincident with the development of the fetus on the other side.   This provides hormones for effecting the maternal fat mobilization, ketogenesis and changes in gluconeogenesis which could compensate for the fetal siphonage (or 'substrate sink'). What is contributed by each component? Our rat studies with differential removal of the products of conception (see above) do not really provide that information and they are further complicated by the surgical trauma to which the animals were subjected. In terms of human pregnancy, the closest analogies might be metabolic studies in women with trophoblastic tumours or mothers who are carrying a dead fetus.

Battaglia: That was exactly the point of my question. Can you give me a quantitative assessment of the contribution of the fetus to these changes? What worries me about the endocrine studies, and I think it worries you too, is that when you introduce the placenta, the rates of production of some of these hormones are very large and are not reflected in the increase in blood levels.

Freinkel: In the present state of knowledge, no one can give you a precise answer. I should add that the limited metabolic observations that have been secured in women with choriocarcinomas or dead babies *in utero* have failed to disclose 'accelerated' hypoglycaemia or fat mobilization during dietary deprivation.

Kalkhoff: There are many questions to be asked about fasting plasma glucose concentrations during pregnancy. In early gestation there may be a significant fall below non-pregnant control levels. This occurs at a time when the fetus is quite small and when fetal extraction of nutrients cannot account for this change. Based on earlier studies by our group (Matute & Kalkhoff 1973), we speculate that the combined action of oestrogens and progesterone facilitate increased hepatic glycogen deposition and suppression of hepatic gluconeogenesis. This could be a factor responsible for the downward trend in fasting plasma glucose concentrations in the early to mid-gestation period. Ultimately, utilization of maternal plasma glucose and amino acids by the growing fetus in late pregnancy may also contribute to the sensitivity of the mother to a fast and the more pronounced hypoglycaemia that ensues.

Shafrir: Is there any evidence that the increased release of triglyceride from the liver of oestradiol-treated rats is the result of recirculation of excessively mobilized FFA or, in part at least, the result of *de novo* fatty acid synthesis? In our studies with glucocorticoid-treated rats, in addition to enhanced mobilization of peripheral fatty acids, a distinct rise in the activity of hepatic enzymes was observed, notably of acetyl-CoA carboxylase, together with an increase in the channelling of precursors into *de novo* fatty acid synthesis (Diamant & Shafrir 1975) and in association with hyperlipidaemia. We have also seen an increase in hepatic fatty acid synthesis as a result of treatment of castrated male and ovariectomized female rats with conjugated oestrogens (unpublished results), and a paper with similar results has recently appeared (Mandour *et al.* 1977).

My second comment relates to the problem of peripheral triglyceride removal. You have shown a decrease in adipose tissue lipoprotein lipase (LPL) activity in oestradiol-treated rats. To my mind a balanced approach is needed since changes in adipose tissue LPL are usually associated with reciprocal changes in muscle LPL, so that total body LPL capacity is redistributed rather than decreased. This appears to occur in fact in rats on glucocorticoid treatment. I would attach much more importance, with regard to triglyceride uptake, to the changes in apolipoprotein composition of VLDL and HDL as demonstrated by the increased content of LPL-inhibitory peptides.

Kalkhoff: We have no evidence that oestrogen treatment results in excessive FFA mobilization by adipose tissue and hypertriglyceridaemia as a consequence of this. In unpublished studies we have observed an increased incorporation of labelled palmitate or α-glycerophosphate into triglyceride (with increased specific activity) in the liver of oestrogen-treated rats.

We have not measured skeletal muscle LPL in our animal model. However, others have reported either no effect of oestradiol treatment on it (Hamosh & Hamosh 1975) or an increase (Wilson *et al.* 1976). Otway & Robinson (1968) report no change in muscle LPL in rat pregnancy.

References

BOURDEL, G. & JACQUOT, R. (1956) Rôle du placenta dans les facultés anabolisantes des rattes gestantes. *C. R. Acad. Sci. 242,* 552–555

CAMPBELL, R. M., INNES, I. R. & KOSTERLITZ, H. W. (1953) Some dietary and hormonal effects on maternal, foetal and placental weights in the rat. *J. Endocrinol. 9,* 68–75

CURRY, D. M. & BEATON, G. H. (1958) Cortisone resistance in pregnant rats. *Endocrinology 63,* 155–161

DANIEL, R. R., METZGER, B. E., FREINKEL, N., FALOONA, G.R. & UNGER, R. H. (1974) Carbohydrate metabolism in pregnancy. XI. Response of plasma glucagon to overnight fast and oral glucose during normal pregnancy and gestational diabetes. *Diabetes 23,* 771–776

DIAMANT, S. & SHAFRIR, E. (1975) Modulation of the activity of insulin-dependent enzymes of lipogenesis by glucocorticoids. *Eur. J. Biochem. 53,* 541–546

FAJANS, S. S. & FLOYD, J. C., JR. (1976) Fasting hypoglycemia in adults. *N. Engl. J. Med. 294,* 766–772

FELIG, P. & LYNCH, V. (1970) Starvation in human pregnancy: hypoglycemia, hypoinsulinemia, and hyperketonemia. *Science (Wash. D. C.) 170,* 990–992

FREINKEL, N. (1965) Effects of the conceptus on maternal metabolism during pregnancy, in *On the Nature and Treatment of Diabetes* (Leibel, B. S. & Wrenshall, G. A., eds.) *(Int. Congr. Ser. 84),* pp. 679–691, Excerpta Medica, Amsterdam

FREINKEL, N. & METZGER, B. E. (1975) Some considerations of fuel economy in the fed state during late human pregnancy, in *Early Diabetes in Early Life* (Camerini-Davalos, R. A. & Cole, H. S., eds.), pp. 289–298, Academic Press, New York

FREINKEL, N., HERRERA, E., KNOPP, R. H. & RUDER, H. J. (1970) Metabolic realignments in late pregnancy: a clue to diabetogenesis? in *Early Diabetes* (Camerini-Davalos, R. A. & Cole, H. S., eds.), pp. 205–219, Academic Press, New York

FREINKEL, N., METZGER, B. E., NITZAN, M., HARE, J. W., SHAMBAUGH, G. E. III, MARSHALL, R. T., SURMACZYNSKA, B. Z. & NAGEL, T. C. (1972) 'Accelerated starvation' and mechanisms for the conservation of maternal nitrogen during pregnancy. *Isr. J. Med. Sci. 8*, 426–439

FREINKEL, N., PHELPS, R. L. & METZGER, B. E. (1979) Intermediary metabolism during normal pregnancy, in *Carbohydrate Metabolism in Pregnancy and the Newborn* (Sutherland, H. W. & Stowers, J. M., eds.) *(2nd Aberdeen Int. Colloq.),* Springer, Berlin

HAMOSH, M. & HAMOSH, P. (1975) The effect of estrogen on the lipoprotein lipase activity of rat adipose tissue. *J. Clin. Invest. 55,* 1132–1135

KNOPP, R. H., SAUDEK, C. D., ARKY, R. A. & O'SULLIVAN, J. B. (1973) Two phases of adipose tissue metabolism in pregnancy: maternal adaptations for fetal growth. *Endocrinology 92,* 984–988

KUHL, C. & HOLST, J. J. (1976) Plasma glucagon and insulin : glucagon ratio in gestational diabetes. *Diabetes 25,* 16–23

LUYCKX, A. S., GERARD, J., GASPARD, U. & LEFEBVRE, P. J. (1975) Plasma glucagon levels in normal women during pregnancy. *Diabetologia 11,* 549–554

MANDOUR, T., KISSEBAH, A. H. & WYNN, V. (1977) Mechanism of oestrogen and progesterone effects on lipid and carbohydrate metabolism: alteration in the insulin: glucagon molar ratio and hepatic enzyme activity. *Eur. J. Clin. Invest. 7,* 181–187

MATUTE, M. L. & KALKHOFF, R. K. (1973) Sex steroid influence on hepatic gluconeogenesis and glycogen formation. *Endocrinology 92,* 762–768

MERIMEE, T.J. & FINEBERG, S. E. (1973) Homeostasis during fasting. II. Hormone substrate differences between men and women. *J. Clin. Endocrinol. Metab. 37,* 698–702

METZGER, B. E., WERNER, H. & FREINKEL, N. (1975) Altered hepatic nitrogen metabolism: a new property of placental lactogen. *57th Annu. Meet., Endocrine Society,* p. 112 (abstr.)

OTWAY, S. & ROBINSON, D. S. (1968) The significance of changes in tissue-clearing factor lipase activity in relation to the lipemia of pregnancy. *Biochem. J. 106,* 677–682

PITKIN, R. M. (1977) Obstetrics and gynaecology, in *Nutritional Support of Medical Practice* (Schneider, H. A. *et al.,* eds.), pp. 407–421, Harper & Row, New York

RAVNIKAR, V., METZGER, B. E. & FREINKEL, N.(1978) Is there a risk of 'accelerated starvation' in normal human pregnancy? *Diabetes 27,* 463 (abstr.)

SAUDEK, C. D., FINKOWSKI, M. & KNOPP, R. H. (1975) Plasma glucagon and insulin in rat pregnancy. Roles in glucose homeostasis. *J. Clin. Invest. 55,* 180–186

SCOW, R.O., CHERNICK, S. S. & BRINLEY, M. S. (1964) Hyperlipemia and ketosis in the pregnant rat. *Am. J. Physiol. 206,* 796–804

SPOONER, P. M., GARRISON, M. M. & SCOW, R. O. (1977) Regulation of mammary gland and adipose tissue lipoprotein lipase and blood triacylglycerol in rats during late pregnancy. Effect of prostaglandins. *J. Clin. Invest. 60,* 702–708

TURTLE, J. R. & KIPNIS, D. M. (1967) The lipolytic action of human placental lactogen on isolated fat cells. *Biochim. Biophys. Acta 144,* 583–592

TYSON, J. E., ANDREASSON, B., HUTH, J., SMITH, B. & ZACUR, H. (1975) Neuroendocrine dysfunction in galactorrhea-amenorrhea after oral contraceptive use. *Obstet. Gynecol. 46,* 1–11

TYSON, J. E., AUSTIN, K., FARINHOLT, J. & FIEDLER, J. (1976) Endocrine-metabolic response to acute starvation in human gestation. *Am. J. Obstet. Gynecol. 125,* 1073–1084

WEINSTEIN, I., SOLER-ARGILAGA, C. & HEIMBERG, M. (1977) Effects of ethinylestradiol on incorporation of $[1-{}^{14}C]$ oleate into triglyceride and ketone bodies by the liver. *Biochem. Pharmacol. 26,* 77–80

WHITELAW, E. & WILLIAMSON, D. H. (1977) Effects of lactation on ketogenesis from oleate and butyrate in rat hepatocytes. *Biochem. J. 164,* 521–528

WILSON, D. E., FLOWERS, C. M., CARLISLE, S. I. & UDALL, K. S. (1976) Estrogen treatment and gonadal function in the regulation of lipoprotein lipase. *Atherosclerosis 24*, 191–199

ZINDER, O., HAMOSH, M., FLECK, T. R. C. & SCOW, R. O. (1974) Effect of prolactin on lipoprotein lipase in mammary gland and adipose tissue of rats. *Am. J. Physiol. 226*, 744–748

Principal substrates of fetal metabolism: fuel and growth requirements of the ovine fetus

FREDERICK C. BATTAGLIA

Department of Pediatrics, University of Colorado Medical Center, Denver, Colorado

Abstract   In those fetuses studied, the glucose uptake by the fetus has been a major source of calories, although in all instances it has been insufficient to account for the total fuel requirements of the fetus.   The glucose/oxygen quotients in different mammalian fetuses vary from about 0.5 to 0.8.   Glucose transport across the placenta has been altered by fetal hyperinsulinaemia and by maternal fasting.   Fetal hypoglycaemia is common to both conditions.   However, umbilical glucose uptake increases with fetal hyperinsulinaemia and decreases with maternal fasting.   During fasting, concomitant with a decrease in fetal glucose supply, there is an increase in amino acid catabolism.   A high rate of placental production of both ammonia and lactate has been demonstrated in several mammalian species.   Umbilical lactate uptake is sufficient to account for about 25% of the oxygen consumption in the ovine fetus.   Ammonia production by the sheep placenta is reflected in increased ammonia concentrations in both the maternal and fetal circulations.   In the ovine fetus, transport of umbilical amino acid has exceeded that required for new tissue growth, supporting the observations of a high urea production rate during fetal life.   Neutral and basic amino acids represent the bulk of the amino acids transported across the placenta.   In contrast there is a net uptake of glutamate from the fetal circulation into the placenta and very little umbilical uptake of aspartic acid.   The umbilical uptake of free fatty acids varies markedly among species.   In some species, such as the sheep and the cow, no umbilical veno-arterial differences for free fatty acids can be demonstrated.

In this paper I have focused on the research carried out with my colleagues in Denver, principally with Dr Giacomo Meschia.   This research has been performed in one mammalian fetus, the fetal lamb.   Unless otherwise specified, all the findings were collected during the last part of gestation, that is, from about 120 to 145 days of gestational age.   The animals were free of operative or anaesthetic stress.   The research has focused on the question: what are the major carbon and nitrogen sources for the developing fetal lamb?   By this I mean the sources for the total carbon and nitrogen requirements, both for fuel and as material for new tissue growth and accretion. The studies described below have attempted to define the quantities of various compounds delivered from the placenta into the fetal circulation. Earlier studies tended to emphasize differences among species as these related to fetal physiology and fetal metabolism. In all probability, these species differences were exaggerated since we could not study fetuses of different species in the same biological state. The impossibility of studying fetal metabolism in smaller mammals free of surgical or anaesthetic stress has been particularly vexing. In recent studies of fetal metabolism certain clues have emerged which suggest that some aspects of fetal metabolism are shared by all mammalian fetuses despite the diversity apparent in adult mammalian biology (Battaglia & Meschia 1978).

VARIABILITY OF SIZE AND OF DIET IN ADULT MAMMALS

Two aspects of adult metabolism are interesting in regard to fetal metabolism. First is the effect of the variability in size of adult mammals on oxygen consumption and glucose entry rate. The second is the enormous variability in diet among mammals. Both oxygen consumption and glucose entry rate follow the $3/4$ power of body weight in adult mammals. Since adult size in eutherian mammals can differ by as much as 10 or 14 millionfold, the range of oxygen consumption and glucose entry per unit body weight is also very large. The primates are no different in this regard from other mammals. The fact that ruminants follow the same relationship between body size and glucose entry rate as other mammals has implications regarding organ metabolism for organs outside the digestive tract. It would appear to make little difference whether the glucose is supplied to organs such as the brain by a high carbohydrate diet or is supplied through gluconeogenesis. The marked differences in diet of adult mammals led to appropriate differences in gastrointestinal function, and particularly in liver function. This may cause us to overlook the similarities in metabolism of organs outside the gastrointestinal tract. If one reviews cerebral or cardiac metabolism among adult mammals, the differences readily apparent among species in studies of liver function are greatly minimized for these other organs. In general, with animals in the fed state and ketoacid concentrations in the blood, the glucose/oxygen quotient across the cerebral circulation is $\simeq 1$. Similarly, the free fatty acid/O_2 quotients across the coronary circulation are equal to 0.6 to 0.8, with glucose making a relatively minor contribution to total carbon uptake by the heart.

Furthermore the differences in adult size must be viewed along with the differences in total fetal mass and gestation length in different species (Leitch *et al.* 1959; Huggett & Widdas 1951). For example, vastly different metabolic demands are placed upon the pregnant bat and the pregnant bear. The bat produces young which may equal 40% of the maternal body weight compared to 0.3% of the maternal weight for the newborn bear. Since the bat is among the smallest of eutherian mammals, it has a high metabolic rate and must continue to fly and forage for food. The diet can be as different as one which is primarily carbohydrate in the fruit-eating bats, to one which is primarily protein in the vampire bats. In some bears, fetal development takes place during hibernation, when the adult bear lives on her body fat while the fetus grows.

FETAL METABOLISM

Studies in metabolism of the fetal lamb were helped by the development of the antipyrine steady-state diffusion technique which permitted simultaneous measurement of umbilical and uterine blood flows. As a constant infusion of antipyrine is given into the fetal circulation one can establish relatively constant arteriovenous differences across the umbilical circulation. A small percentage of the antipyrine infused is metabolized or excreted into the amniotic or allantoic cavities. The bulk of the antipyrine infused diffuses across the placenta into the uterine circulation. Thus, with minor corrections, the rate of infusion equals the rate of transplacental diffusion. By an application of the Fick principle one can then calculate umbilical or uterine blood flows by dividing the rate of transplacental diffusion by the mean umbilical or uterine arteriovenous differences. In addition, one can calculate the transplacental clearance of antipyrine or other compounds expressed as the rate of transplacental diffusion divided by the concentration difference between the two arterial circulations, uterine and umbilical (Meschia *et al.* 1967). Fetal oxygen consumption can be measured through an application of the Fick principle by independent measurements of umbilical blood flow and the mean arterial-venous difference for oxygen content. The measurement of fetal oxygen consumption can be made with considerable precision because the arterial-venous differences across the umbilical circulation are quite large when expressed as a percentage of the arterial oxygen content; the arterial blood changes by about 50% in its oxygen content as it perfuses the placenta. This is not true for many other compounds of importance in fetal metabolism, where the percentage change in the arterial blood as it goes through the placenta may be very small and preclude an application of the Fick principle for the determination of umbilical uptake.

FETAL VERSUS ADULT OXYGEN CONSUMPTIONS

Table 1 compares measurements of fetal oxygen consumption in different

TABLE 1

Oxygen consumption rates per kilogram body weight of adults and fetuses in species of different size: adult values calculated according to Equation 2[a]

Animal	O_2 consumption (ml/min kg)		
	Adult		Fetus
Horse	2.0		7.0
Cattle	2.2		7.4
Sheep	4.0		6-9.4
Rhesus monkey	7.0		7.0
Guinea pig	9.7		8.5
Rat[b]	14.1	23.4[c]	10.4[d]

[a] O_2 consumption in the adult and newborn rat calculated from the data of DeMeyer et al. (1971)
[b] In Battaglia & Meschia (1978)
[c] Forty-eight hours old.
[d] Newborn.

mammalian species with adult oxygen consumption calculated from the three-quarter power of body weight. Fetal oxygen consumption is relatively constant among species, in striking contrast to the different metabolic rates in adult mammals, which reflects the differences in adult size (Battaglia 1978). Thus, the question of whether oxygen consumption of the newborn increases or decreases at birth cannot be answered without reference to the size of the newborn and the adult of that species. In the smaller mammals, oxygen consumption may increase at birth, and in the larger animals it may decrease at birth. The difference reflects the relationship between postnatal oxygen consumption and body size, rather than differences in fetal oxygen consumption.

SUBSTRATES OF FETAL METABOLISM

The glucose/oxygen quotients across the umbilical circulation in the fetal lamb during the last third of gestation were in the order of 0.5, instead of being equal to one; that is, no more than 50% of the oxygen consumption could be accounted for by the umbilical glucose uptake. Furthermore, the glucose/oxygen quotient fell markedly to about 0.2 or less during maternal fasting. Later studies demonstrated that the fall in glucose/oxygen quotient was due to a decrease in umbilical glucose uptake during fasting. The maternal hypoglycaemia which develops during fasting causes a reduction in umbilical glucose uptake leading to fetal hypoglycaemia (Philipps et al. 1977) (Fig. 1). Presumably it is the fetal hypoglycaemia which leads to

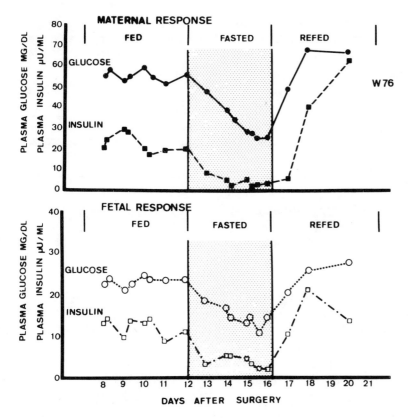

FIG. 1. Changes in maternal and fetal plasma glucose and insulin concentrations in a single pregnant sheep during fed and fasting states (data from Philipps *et al.* 1977).

the decrease in insulin concentrations in fetal plasma with maternal fasting, and hypoinsulinaemia in turn leads to a decrease in fetal glucose utilization. Similar measurements of umbilical glucose/oxygen quotients have been made in the cow, the horse and man. In all cases, these quotients have been less than one.

Thus, for these four species, glucose cannot be considered the sole metabolic fuel of the fetus. In reviewing the literature it is clear that a major reason for hypothesizing that glucose was the sole metabolic fuel of the fetus came from measurements of respiratory quotients (RQ) across the umbilical circulation which were reported as equal to one. However, the RQ cannot be used as a reflection of the kinds of substrates metabolized in a rapidly growing organism since an appreciable percentage of the total carbon coming to the organism would be used for carbon accretion rather than CO_2 production.

In the fetal lamb, for example, only 4.6 of the 7.8 g carbon day^{-1} kg^{-1} that the fetus receives from the umbilical uptake of substrates is excreted as CO_2. It should be emphasized that the umbilical uptake or fetal uptake of substrates refers to the uptake of exogenous substrate. For substances such as glucose which may be produced endogenously, the total utilization rate of glucose, measured as the fetal glucose turnover rate, may be higher than the umbilical uptake since the turnover rate would reflect both the glucose supplied exogenously (i.e. the umbilical glucose uptake) and that supplied endogenously (i.e. gluconeogenesis).

When one turns to metabolizable compounds such as glucose it becomes far more difficult to interpret changes of placental 'clearance', since some of the glucose entering from the uterine circulation would not appear in the umbilical circulation, due to metabolism by the placenta. However, if one compares simultaneous determinations of antipyrine, urea and glucose clearance it is apparent that the glucose clearance across the sheep placenta is much lower than the flow-limited clearance determined by antipyrine (Fig. 2). Glucose clearance is in the order of 10 ml min^{-1} kg^{-1}, a value only 50% of the urea clearance, demonstrating that glucose transport would be primarily determined by placental permeability rather than by uterine or umbilical blood flows (Simmons *et al.* 1974)

To return to the major substrates for the fetus, the fetal lamb requires about 7.8 kg^{-1} day^{-1} of carbon, representing carbon accretion during growth each day and carbon excreted as CO_2 and as urea. An estimate of the urea production rate of the fetus would provide some index of the rate of amino acid catabolism during fetal life. However there is a difficulty in obtaining an estimate of the

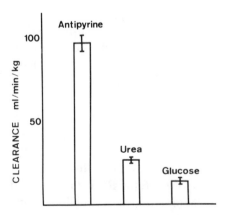

FIG. 2. Mean ± s.e. of placental clearances to antipyrine, urea and glucose in pregnant sheep from 120 days' gestation to term (data from Simmons *et al.* 1974).

urea production rate; namely, the arterial-venous difference of urea across the umbilical circulation is far too small, 0.4 mg/100 ml, to be measured with precision.   Thus, we could not use the Fick principle for determination of the urea production rate.   Measurements of placental clearance were used to circumvent this difficulty.   An infusion of [^{14}C]urea was given into the fetal circulation along with a constant infusion of antipyrine for the measurement of umbilical blood flow.   By the application of the Fick principle the urea clearance for [^{14}C]urea could be determined.   Simultaneously, the concentration difference of urea between the umbilical and uterine arteries was determined.   The arterial concentration difference was 10-fold larger than the umbilical arteriovenous difference.   Thus it could be determined with reasonable precision.   The fetal lamb has a high rate of urea production, sufficient to account for about 25% of the oxygen consumption (Gresham *et al*. 1972).   As part of a search for what might be representing the remaining substrates used as fuel, umbilical arteriovenous differences for fructose, free fatty acids, glycerol, and ketoacids were determined.   None of these compounds had appreciable umbilical arteriovenous differences sufficient to account for more than 1 or 2% of the fetal oxygen consumption.   Several other investigators have also demonstrated that no measurable arteriovenous differences could be found for fructose across the umbilical circulation of other fructogenetic species, including the cow (Silver & Comline 1976) and the pig (Randall & l'Ecuyer 1976).

We next turned to studies of lactate metabolism as a potential fuel for the fetus and were surprised to find that there were large umbilical arteriovenous differences for lactate concentration.   The umbilical uptake of lactate was equal to about 25% of the oxygen consumption (Burd *et al*. 1975).   This is particularly interesting in the light of past ideas in fetal physiology.   At one time the fetus was considered to be developing in an environment of moderate metabolic acidosis.   While it is true that lactate concentrations are high in the fetus compared with the adult, the lactate/pyruvate ratios are normal.   In fact, there is a net uptake of lactate from the placenta to the fetus rather than an excretion of lactate by the fetus into the placenta.   It should be emphasized that lactate production by the placenta under aerobic conditions had been demonstrated for the rat placenta in 1925 and for the human placenta in the 1950s.   In addition, Comline & Silver (1976) reported an appreciable umbilical uptake of lactate in the fetal calf.   Thus, this aspect of placental metabolism is a characteristic shared by at least five different mammalian species.

FUEL AND GROWTH REQUIREMENTS

The oxygen consumption of the fetus serves as a suitable reference point against which to judge the caloric requirements for basal metabolism, since the caloric equivalent of oxygen is about 4.9 kcal (20.58 kJ)/l STP.   If the caloric equivalents for new tissue growth are determined by bomb calorimetry then the total calories required by the fetus for both fuel and growth will be represented by the sum of the two values.   In the sheep fetus during the last third of gestation, the requirements for growth represent almost half of the total caloric requirements of the fetus (Fig. 3).   The proportion of the total caloric requirement of the fetus represented by tissue growth rather than by the oxygen consumption will vary among mammals.   The proportion will be much higher than in the fetal lamb in the smaller mammals where growth is more rapid, and will be much less in man where a newborn of about the same size is produced over a much longer gestation length.   However, the relatively large contribution of tissue growth to the total caloric requirements makes it apparent that a rapidly growing organism can meet a restriction in supply of nutrients by a reduction in its growth rate as well as by a reduction in its basal metabolic rate.

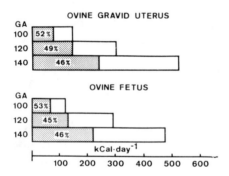

FIG. 3. Estimates of the partition of total caloric requirements in the ovine uterus and fetus.

AMINO ACID METABOLISM

The high rate of urea production in the sheep fetus led us to study the umbilical uptake of individual amino acids in the sheep fetus.   It is well established that the concentrations of most amino acids are much higher in fetal blood of mammals than in maternal blood.   However, such concentration differences tell us nothing about the importance of umbilical uptake of an amino acid relative to its total requirements by the fetus.   The amino acids the fetus must receive from the placenta include all the essential amino acids as well as any amino acid which cannot be synthesized in the fetus at a rate equal to its total utilization rate.   In order to obtain a comparison of umbilical uptake to requirements for growth, amino acid concentrations in whole blood were determined across the umbilical circulation in chronic animal preparations (Lemons *et al.* 1976) (Fig. 4).   The nitrogen requirements of the lamb fetus were estimated to be in the order of 1 g N_2 kg $^{-1}$ day $^{-1}$, representing a requirement for tissue accretion of about 0.65 g and for urea production of about 0.35 g kg^{-1} day $^{-1}$.   For most of the neutral amino acids, large umbilical arteriovenous differences were found.   For the basic amino acids, lysine and histidine, much smaller arteriovenous differences were found.   The acidic amino acids, taurine, aspartic and glutamic acids were not transported to the fetus.   A comparison was made of the amount of each amino acid entering the umbilical circulation with the amount accumulating in the fetal carcass as new tissue growth each day.   This must be regarded as a crude approximation since the only carcass analyses available were those for three newborn calves (Blaxter 1964); i.e. the data were obtained in a different mammalian species and in a newborn rather than during fetal life.   At any rate, within the limits of this approximation, it is clear that most of the neutral amino acids come across in amounts far larger than those required for new tissue growth; this supports the high rate of urea production measured independently in the fetus.   In fact, the total nitrogen coming across as amino acids was equal to about 1.5 g kg^{-1} day^{-1}.   For glutamic acid there was a consistent negative veno-arterial

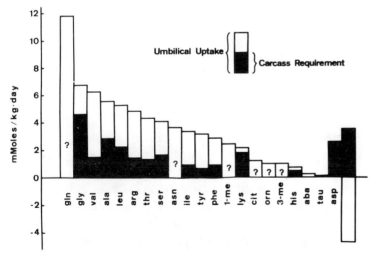

FIG. 4. Mean umbilical uptake of individual amino acids in the fetal lamb during late gestation, compared with estimates of carcass accretion rates.   Reproduced from Lemons *et al.* (1976).

difference; that is, glutamate was consistently taken up from the fetal circulation by the placenta.   This was true despite a much higher glutamate concentration in the fetus than the mother.   I think this points out the fallacy of attempting to interpret fetal–maternal concentration ratios for non-essential amino acids as an index of active transport or even of the direction of amino acid transport.   Amino acid uptake supplied the bulk of the carbon to the fetus, representing about 5.3 g kg^{-1} day^{-1} in contrast to 1.8 g kg^{-1} day^{-1} taken up as glucose and 1.3 g kg^{-1} day^{-1} taken up as lactate.   Since the total amino acid uptake across the umbilical circulation exceeded the total nitrogen requirements of the fetus we turned to look for other excretory forms of nitrogen in the fetus.   This led us to measure ammonia concentrations in fetal blood.   It was a surprise to find that ammonia was not being excreted by the fetus but was being consumed by the fetus.   There was a consistent umbilical uptake of ammonia from the placenta.   Ammonia concentrations were high in fetal blood compared with maternal blood and in pregnant sheep blood compared with non-pregnant sheep blood.   The uterine circulation showed large veno-arterial differences in ammonia concentration, demonstrating that ammonia was being produced in large amounts by the placenta and delivered into both the uterine and umbilical circulations (Holzman et al. 1977).   The ratios of the veno-arterial differences of ammonia and oxygen across the uterine circulation were much larger in early gestation than later, suggesting that ammonia production by the placenta was highest in early gestation and decreased as term approached.   If one compares glutamine, glutamate and ammonia concentrations in the uterine and umbilical circulations, it is clear that far more nitrogen leaves the placenta for the uterine and umbilical circulations as ammonia and far more goes into the umbilical circulation as glutamine than enters the placenta as glutamine from the maternal circulation and enters as glutamate from the fetal circulation (Holzman et al. 1977) (Fig. 5).

FETAL MILK

Thus, in the ovine fetus, the composition of the principal substrates appearing in the umbilical circulation is relatively simple, as they consist primarily of amino acids, glucose and lactate.   If one compares this with milk provided for the newborn animal, the striking difference is the absence of fat.   Among mammals the milk produced by those mammals in which water conservation is important, such as the desert and aquatic mammals, is the highest in fat concentration.   Since water conservation is not a problem for the mother during intrauterine development, it is perhaps not surprising that the uptake of fat is now a major carbon source for the fetal lamb.   This may not be true, of

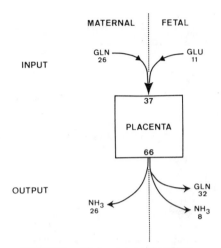

QUANTITIES = μM/min nitrogen equivalents

FIG. 5. Appropriate glutamine (GLN), glutamate (GLU) and ammonia (NH₃) nitrogen flow into and out of the ovine placenta in late gestation (data from Holzman *et al.* 1977).

course, for all mammalian fetuses although it appears to be true for many species. It is clear that amino acids are used both as substrates for fuel and for protein synthesis during fetal development.

ACKNOWLEDGEMENT

These studies were supported by Grants HD-00781 and HD-01866 from NIH.

References

BATTAGLIA, F. C. (1978) Commonality and diversity in fetal development: bridging the inter-species gap. *Pediatr. Res. 12,* 736–745

BATTAGLIA, F. C. & MESCHIA, G. (1978) Principal substrates of fetal metabolism. *Physiol. Rev. 58,* 499–527

BLAXTER, K. L. (1964) Protein metabolism and requirements in pregnancy and lactation, in *Mammalian Protein Metabolism,* vol. 2 (Munro, H.N. & Allison, J. B., eds.), Academic Press, New York

BURD, L. I., JONES, M. D. JR., SIMMONS, M. A., MAKOWSKI, E. L., MESCHIA, G. & BATTAGLIA, F. C. (1975) Placental production and foetal utilization of lactate and pyruvate. *Nature (Lond.) 254,* 710–711

COMLINE, R. S. & SILVER, M. (1976) Some aspects of foetal and utero-placental metabolism in cows with indwelling umbilical uterine vascular catheters. *J. Physiol. (Lond.) 260,* 571–586

DE MEYER, R., GERARD, P. & VERELLEN (1971) Carbohydrate metabolism in the newborn rat, in *Metabolic Processes in the Fetus and Newborn Infant* (Jonxis, J. H. P. *et al.,* eds.), pp. 281–291, Williams & Wilkins, Baltimore

GRESHAM, E. L., JAMES, E. J., RAYE, J. R., BATTAGLIA, F. C., MAKOWSKI, E. L. & MESCHIA, G. (1972) Production and excretion of urea by the fetal lamb. *Pediatrics 50*, 372–379

HOLZMAN, I. R., LEMONS, J. A., MESCHIA, G. & BATTAGLIA, F. C. (1977) Ammonia production by the pregnant uterus. *Proc. Soc. Exp. Biol. Med. 156*, 27–30

HUGGETT, A. ST. G. & WIDDAS, W. F. (1951) The relationship between mammalian foetal weight and conception age. *J. Physiol. (Lond.) 114*, 306–317

LEITCH, I., HYTTEN, F.E. & BILLEWICZ, W. Z. (1959) The maternal and neonatal weights of some mammalia. *Proc. Zool. Soc. Lond. 133*, 11–29

LEMONS, J. A., ADCOCK, E. W. III, JONES, M. D. JR., NAUGHTON, M. A., MESCHIA, G. & BATTAGLIA, F. C. (1976) Umbilical uptake of amino acids in the unstressed fetal lamb. *J. Clin. Invest. 58*, 1428–1434

MESCHIA, G., BATTAGLIA, F. C. & BRUNS, P. D. (1967) Theoretical and experimental study of transplacental diffusion. *J. appl. Physiol. 22*, 1171–1178

PHILIPPS, A. F., CARSON, B. S., MESCHIA, G. & BATTAGLIA, F. C. (1977) Insulin-carbohydrate relationship in the sheep fetus. *Pediatr. Res. 11*, 520 (abstr.)

RANDALL, G. C. B. & l'ECUYER, C. L. (1976) Tissue glycogen and blood glucose and fructose levels in the pig fetus during the second half of gestation. *Biol. Neonate 28*, 74–82

SILVER, M. & COMLINE, R. S. (1976) Fetal and placental O₂ consumption and the uptake of different metabolites in the ruminant and horse during late gestation, in *Oxygen Transport to Tissue II* (*Advances in Experimental Medicine and Biology*, vol. 75) (Grote, J. Jr., et al., eds.), Plenum Press, New York

SIMMONS, M. A., JONES, M. D. JR., BATTAGLIA, F. C., MAKOWSKI, E.L. & MESCHIA, G. (1974) Placental membrane limitation of fetal glucose uptake in sheep. *Gynecol. Invest. 5*, 24 (abstr.)

Discussion

Beard: The human fetus has a higher concentration of blood glucose than does the sheep, so presumably it requires more for energy purposes?

Battaglia: No, one can't make the assumption that differences in substrate concentration in fetal blood reflect differences in metabolic rate of the substrate. For example, fructose concentration is very high in fetal lamb blood, yet under normal circumstances there is very little fructose utilization by the fetus. It is likely that there are some differences in the extent to which various substrates are used to meet the caloric requirements of the fetus in different mammals, including man. However, the urea clearances that we measured in sub-human primates were similar to urea clearances across the placenta in sheep (Battaglia *et al.* 1968). If the arterial urea concentration differences that we and others have measured in man are used for the calculation of the product of the amino acid difference times the placental urea clearance, the resulting estimate of urea production rate in the human fetus is quite high. So if you are asking me whether I think amino acids may play an important role as fuels in the human fetus, as well as being building blocks for protein synthesis, just as they do in the lamb fetus, my answer is yes, I would expect that to be true. The extent to which glucose makes a larger contribution to total energy requirements in humans than in sheep is not settled.   The human placenta, like the rat, sheep, and cow placentas is producing lactate at high rates.

The lactate concentration in the blood doesn't tell us anything about the lactate turnover rate or umbilical uptake of lactate.   Furthermore, lactate produced in the placenta is delivered into both the maternal and fetal circulations, so there is no reason to expect lactate concentration differences in maternal and fetal blood to reflect rates of placental lactate production.   I don't think one could conclude much from the lactate concentrations in the blood.   That is what I was suggesting with glutamate – one couldn't conclude very much from measuring blood levels of glutamate in the baby and mother.

Räihä: It seems an awful waste of amino acids for the fetus to use them as fuel.   Usually nature doesn't waste too much.   Have you any explanation for this?   Could some of the urea produced in the sheep fetus be from the ammonia?

Battaglia: Very little; the bulk of the urea production rate could not be accounted for by the rate of umbilical uptake of ammonia.

Räihä: Have you any information about the enzymes of the urea cycle in the fetal lamb?   In the human, at around the 14th–15th week of gestation urea-cycle enzymes have fairly low activity.   In the fetal rat they are almost absent.   The perfused human fetal liver does not respond to administration of amino acids by increasing urea production very much.   This indicates, at least to me, that the human fetal liver has a very low capacity for increasing urea production when extra amino acids are administered.   This might be different in the sheep.

Battaglia: I want to be very careful about attributing differences to species if we are studying them under quite different conditions.   Were your studies done in late gestation?

Räihä: No.

Battaglia: I studied the sheep at 120–140 days, near term.   If one looked early enough in the fetal lamb I am sure one would find a time in gestation when enzyme activities involved with urea synthesis are absent.   I am not an enzymologist and we have made no measurements of enzyme activity.   If urea is produced, I must assume that enzymes for its synthesis must be there.   You have compared not only different species but also each species at very different gestational ages.   Presumably you studied the liver *in vitro*, while I am presenting *in vivo* data.   I don't want to say that there can't be differences in fetal metabolism in the human and the sheep, but I feel that we have been exaggerating the differences a good bit.

In addition, your teleological objection to a high urea production rate and amino acid uptake worries me.   You say you think it is 'wasteful' for amino acids to be used as a fuel.   Let us look at the alternatives.   If there was a system in which amino acids came across to the fetus in amounts just about equal to the needs for protein synthesis I would say that that is a very unsafe system and would give very little margin of safety to the fetus.   On the other hand, what do you expect the fetus to do if it receives amino acids in excess of its accretion rate?   It may simply catabolize these as fuel.

Räihä: It certainly must depend on when we are studying the animal.   You were studying the sheep at the end of pregnancy and we were studying the rat or the human at an earlier stage of pregnancy.   Urea production is needed immediately after birth, and in the rat the enzymes for urea synthesis appear immediately before birth and continue to rise after birth.   In other words, this system has to be present when the animal is born.   If you study the sheep just before delivery, one would expect it to produce urea.

Battaglia: We are studying it at 120–140 days, not during parturition.

Räihä: It is a question of when the urea cycle enzymes appear.   Early in the fetal period it seems wasteful for the animal to use amino acids as fuel.

Battaglia: Why do you say that?   The alternative is to pump in only the amounts of amino acid needed for protein accretion in the fetus.

Räihä: Smith *et al.* (1977) showed that the lamb fetus takes up the exact amount of amino acid needed for tissue protein synthesis; only glutamate, aspartate and serine seem to be produced by the fetus.

Battaglia: I do not agree with those studies, which incidentally were not carried out in chronic animal experiments.   We have measured arteriovenous differences in a large number of sheep from 120 days onwards and they have a very high amino acid uptake.   That goes with a very high production rate which was measured completely independently.   In the study you have quoted the animals were under surgical and anaesthetic stress and steady-state conditions compatible with continued fetal growth were not defined.   Therefore it is possible, in fact I believe likely, that much of the amino acid transport that Smith *et al.* measured was catabolized rather than used for protein synthesis, since under stress the fetus may not have been growing at a normal rate at all.

Räihä: The amino acids go back, don't they?

Battaglia: Of course the amino acids don't go back to the mother.   The venous–arterial differences are always positive across the umbilical circulation for all the amino acids except glutamate.

Beard: The placenta builds up amino acids and can presumably degrade them.

Battaglia: That is a different question.   I am studying fetal metabolism.   Thus we measure umbilical uptake which represents the amino acids which go to the baby at a certain rate.

Girard: There is the problem of the fuels used by individual tissues of the fetus.   Can you comment on the utilization of amino acids, glucose and lactate by tissues such as the fetal muscle, heart and brain?

Williamson: In this connection, the adult sheep has a very low brain/body weight ratio.   Is that also true of the fetal lamb?

Battaglia: Yes; much lower than primates.

Williamson: But the ratio in the rat is higher than in the sheep.

Battaglia: Yes, but it is much lower than in all primates.   There is every reason to assume approximately the same rate of glucose utilization per 100 grams of brain tissue.   For this reason relatively greater demands are made on the human fetus or newborn infant to meet its cerebral glucose require-ments.   Kipnis's group (Bier *et al.* 1977) showed this nicely with deuterium-labelled glucose turnover rates in the newborn.   Their figure is about 6 or 8 mg kg^{-1} min^{-1}.   That is about what a 400 g brain of a newborn infant weighing 3 kg would consume.   The newborn lamb weighing 3 kg has a 50 g brain.   Therefore, the contribution of cerebral metabolism to total body economy will certainly vary.

Naeye: Is lysine also in critical balance in the human fetus?   There is a major dietary deficiency of lysine in one of the African populations that we have under study.   This population has a different pattern of fetal growth and a slower rate of fetal lung maturation than another African population we have examined that has a more normal dietary content of branched-chain amino acids.

Battaglia: I don't know the answer to that.   Amino acid concentrations in pregnant women have been measured at different stages of gestation.   One group looked at correlations with infant body weight and the only correlation they found between amino acid concentrations in these women and infant body weight was with lysine.   That is suggestive.   Drs Meier, Peterson, Meschia and I are now measuring umbilical uptake of lysine simultaneously with measurements of lysine turnover rate.   Similarly we are attempting to see how much of the [^{14}C]lysine appears as $^{14}CO_2$ and how much is still lysine in the total carcass homogenates.   Perhaps lysine catabolism is relatively insignificant.   In that case, the lysine turnover rate would then give us an instantaneous marker of growth rate in the fetus−something we have needed for metabolic studies in paediatrics.

Young: We have been measuring protein turnover rates of fetal tissues by the continuous infusion of [^{14}C]lysine into the lamb *in utero* (Horn *et al.* 1977).   A considerable amount of the label that we infused as lysine appeared in other metabolites.   The counts associated with lysine were only 25% of the total free tissue counts in brain and heart, 13% in liver and 38% in muscle at the end of a 6-h infusion period.   However, the counts associated with lysine which had been incorporated into protein were 70–80% of the total counts found in protein hydrolysates, suggesting that little transamination had occurred.

Battaglia: That is very interesting.   We do not have sufficient data yet to comment.

Freinkel: To what extent are the short-chain fatty acids derived from the maternal rumen accessible to the fetus?

Battaglia: I don't think the short-chain fatty acids make a big contribution.   Acetate AV differences at the most would equal about 10% of the O_2 consumption, or about 5% of the total carbon requirement.

Freinkel: What about propionic and butyric acid?

Battaglia: The other C_3 and C_4 short-chain fatty acids certainly wouldn't be contributing because they are in extremely low concentrations in the fetus.   They wouldn't be a bulk source of carbon.   In ruminants, it looks as if the peripheral organs (and you might include the fetus as a peripheral organ) 'see' the arterial concentrations in the mother, after the maternal liver has acted on this assortment of substrates that come in through the portal venous stream.

Freinkel: Since it is such a major source of the mother's energy metabolism, is there a limited transplacental flux of short-chain fatty acids?

Battaglia: As I said, it may represent a small but significant source of carbon.   Where is acetate used in the mother other than in the liver?

Freinkel: There has been some recent evidence that acetate can be taken up by the human brain (Juhlin-Dannfelt 1977), and acetate uptake and oxidation by the brain of the herbivore has also been reported (Annison & Lindsay 1961).

Battaglia: There are only two studies that I know of where AV differences for the short-chain fatty acids have been investigated (Pugh & Scarisbrick 1955; Char & Creasy 1976).   The chemical methodology was not entirely satisfactory for measurements of AV differences, and there was not the consistency that is seen with other solutes.   For instance, with lactate a large number of VA differences have been measured in many fetuses yet there is always a VA difference that is positive.   That is not true with acetate.

Freinkel: But is there a meaningful transfer of short-chain fatty acids in the fetal lamb?

Battaglia: I have given you the data for acetate.   The question of whether the transfer is 'meaningful' implies a reference point in metabolism.   For acetate, it represents about 10% of the O_2 consumption, which is about 5% of the total carbon requirement.   That is about 40% of the contribution that lactate makes.   The other short-chain FFA make no contribution.

Young: We have compared umbilical plasma AV differences across the fetal side of the placenta in women at vaginal delivery (Prenton & Young 1969), in the ewe under spinal anaesthesia (Young & McFadyen 1973) and in the guinea-pig with the fetal placenta perfused *in situ* (Hill & Young 1973).   The general pattern of the AV differences for the essential amino acids, both branched-chain neutral and basic, was very similar in all three species to that which you observed using whole blood.   This might be anticipated because the relative amounts of individual amino acids are very similar in the carcasses of growing and adult animals and amongst the species (Southgate 1971).   In both the human and the sheep, the transfer of glutamic acid appeared to be from the fetus into the placenta, as you also observed; this was first observed in the human by Rooth & Nilsson (1964) and confirmed recently (Velasquez *et al.* 1976); this was not found in the guinea-pig, probably due to methodological problems.   Schneider *et al.* (1977) have shown that glutamic acid can be converted into glutamine in the isolated perfused human placenta, and this may account for your large transfer of glutamine from the placenta into the fetal blood.

Battaglia: However, if you asked me what I would find if we measured plasma AV differences of amino acids in the sheep at the time of labour and delivery, I would say I didn't know.   Therefore I can't compare it with the data in the human.   One needs metabolic quotients for VA differences because otherwise one is dependent upon changes in blood flow in relation to body weight among the different species.   Even in studies upon entirely normal women we still found, taking doubly clamped cord samples, an enormous variance in glucose O_2 quotients.   We came up with a mean of about 0.8 but the variance was very large.

Chez: What happens when A is increased or α is decreased in terms of placental transfer?

Battaglia: We have only enough data to tell us that interpreting the change with insulin as an effect on the placenta was incorrect, but I wouldn't go beyond that now.

References

ANNISON, E. F. & LINDSAY, D. B. (1961) Acetate utilization in sheep. *Biochem. J.* 78, 777–785

BATTAGLIA, F. C., BEHRMAN, R. E., MESCHIA, G., SEEDS, A. E. & BRUNS, P. D. (1968) Clearance of inert molecules, Na, and Cl ions across the primate placenta. *Am. J. Obstet. Gynecol.* 102, 1135–1143

BIER, D. M., LEAKE, R. D., HAYMOND, M., ARNOLD, K. J., GRUENKE, L.D., SPERLING, M. A. & KIPNIS, D. M. (1977) Measurement of 'true' glucose production rates in infancy and childhood with 6,6-dideuterglucose. *Diabetes 26*, 1016–1023

CHAR, V. C. & CREASY, R. K. (1976) Acetate as a metabolic substrate in the fetal lamb. *Am. J. Physiol. 230*, 357–361

HILL, P. M. M. & YOUNG, M. (1973) Net placental transfer of free amino acids against varying concentrations. *J. Physiol. (Lond.) 235*, 409–422

HORN, J., SLOAN, I., STERN, M., NOAKES, D. & YOUNG, M. (1977) Effect of insulin on protein turnover in fetal lambs. *Proc. Nutr. Soc. 36*, 118A

JUHLIN-DANNFELT, A. (1977) Ethanol effects of substrate utilization by the human brain. *Scand. J. Clin. Lab. Invest. 37*, 443–449

PRENTON, M. A. & YOUNG, M. (1969) Umbilical vein-artery and uterine-venous plasma amino acid differences. *J. Obstet. Gynecol. 76*, 333–344

PUGH, P. D. S. & SCARISBRICK, R. (1955) Acetate uptake by the foetal sheep. *J. Physiol. (Lond.) 67P.*

ROOTH, G. & NILSSON, I. (1964) Studies on fetal and maternal metabolic acidosis. *Clin. Sci. (Oxf.) 26*, 121–132

SCHNEIDER, H., MÖHLER, K., CHALLIER, J.-C. & DANCIS, J. (1977) Amino acid transfer through the human placenta studied by *in vitro* perfusion. *Gynecol. Invest. 8*, 22–23

SMITH, R. M., JARRETT, I. G., KING, R. A. & RUSSELL, G. R. (1977) Amino acid nutrition in the fetal lamb. *Biol. Neonate 31*, 305–310

SOUTHGATE, D. A. T. (1971) Accumulation of amino acids in the products of conception of the rat and in the young animal after birth. *Biol. Neonate 19*, 272–292

VELASQUEZ, Z. A., ROSADO, A., BERNAL, A., NORIEGA, L. & AREVALO, N. (1976) Amino acid pools in the feto-maternal system. *Biol. Neonate 29*, 28–40

YOUNG, M. & McFADHEN, I. R. (1973) Placental transfer and fetal uptake of amino acids in the pregnant ewe. *J. Perinat. Med. 1*, 174–182

Evidence for fatty acid transfer across the human placenta

D. HULL and M.C. ELPHICK

Department of Child Health, University of Nottingham Medical School, Queen's Medical Centre, Nottingham

Abstract Lipid analysis of blood from umbilical artery and vein, experiments on artificially perfused human placentas, measurements of fetal blood triglyceride concentrations and the relative percentage of essential fatty acids in fetal adipose tissue are all consistent with the view that fatty acids cross the human placenta and that the flow to the fetus is influenced by maternal blood concentrations of free fatty acids and triglycerides.

The placenta, like the other tissues of the body, might obtain fats either directly from the diet, in which case the circulating vehicle would be the triglyceride in chylomicrons, or from the triglyceride stored in maternal adipose tissue, when the circulating vehicle would be albumin-bound free fatty acids (FFA), or from circulating endogenous triglyceride in lipoproteins. The mix of the fatty acids received will vary with the source; for example, the fatty acid composition of triglyceride in chylomicrons reflects that of dietary fat, while the fatty acid composition of the free fatty acids will reflect that of the triglycerides in maternal adipose tissue, part of which will be derived by lipogenesis from excess glucose.

In turn the fetus *may* receive fatty acids from the placenta but it may also *make* them in its own tissues. Indeed there is good evidence from studies *in vitro* and *in vivo* that fetal tissues including placenta have lipogenic capacity (Diamant *et al.* 1975; Sakvrai *et al.* 1969; Jones & Ashton 1976; Coltart 1972; Coltart & Bateman 1975), and they might well be able to make all the fatty acids that the fetus needs, except of course the essential fatty acids, linoleic and linolenic acid and their derivatives. Nevertheless, just because the fetus is capable of making most of its own fatty acids, it does not necessarily follow that it does so. Fatty acids have been shown to cross the placenta and make a sizeable contribution to the fetal lipids in rabbits (Van Duyne *et al.* 1962; Elphick *et al.* 1975), rats (Hummel *et al.* 1974), guinea pigs (Hershfield &

Nemeth 1968) and monkeys (Portman *et al.* 1969) but do not appear to do so to any significant extent in sheep (James *et al.* 1971; Leat *et al.* 1978; Elphick & Hull 1978).   This article is concerned with the evidence relating to the transfer of fatty acids across the human placenta.

EVIDENCE FROM UMBILICAL CORD BLOOD VENOUS-ARTERIAL DIFFERENCES

Free fatty acids to the fetus

   It would be idle to pretend that positive cord venous-arterial (V-A) concentrations measured after vaginal delivery, even if the samples are taken whilst the cord vessels are full and pulsating, represent the situation during pregnancy or even the end of labour.   However, consistent positive values do demonstrate that under certain circumstances fatty acids can be added to the fetal circulation.   There have been a number of reports of cord V-A differences for both free fatty acids and triglyceride (Šabata *et al.* 1968*b*; Tobin *et al.* 1969;

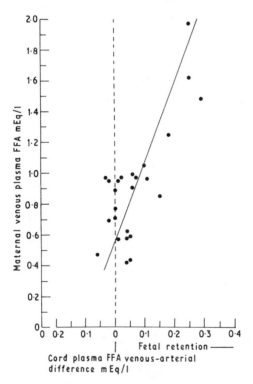

FIG. 1. Relationship between venous-arterial concentration differences in FFA in umbilical cord plasma and maternal concentrations at elective Caesarean section.   (From Elphick *et al.* 1976, by kind permission of the editors of the *British Journal of Obstetrics and Gynaecology.*)

Persson & Tunell 1971; Sheath *et al.* 1972; Elphick *et al.* 1976). Most investigations, but not all, have found significant positive V-A differences in FFA concentrations. If one wishes to calculate net flows it would appear more reasonable to use values obtained during elective Caesarean section. From our own studies (Elphick *et al.* 1976) (Fig. 1) on blood taken before delivery by Caesarean section, it was found that cord V-A difference was directly related to the concentration of the FFA in the maternal circulation. Some of the maternal levels were high, a response to be expected with surgery; similar levels are found during labour. The high fetal V-A difference with which they were associated would indicate high flows of fatty acid to the fetus. However, during normal pregnancy (Persson & Lunell 1975; Gillmer *et al.* 1977), peaks of this order would rarely occur and would not be maintained. Assuming a placental flow of say 200 ml/kg fetus, calculations suggest that a low V-A FFA concentration difference of around 0.05 mM would meet most of the fetal requirements for storage and structure.

One would expect the relationship indicated by the line in Fig. 1 to vary with controlling factors. In rabbits it was found to move to the left after a glucose infusion (unpublished data). Also the V-A differences of fatty acids might be influenced by changes in alternative placental supplies of fatty acids, for example circulating triglyceride. In rabbits after infusion of 'artificial chylomicrons' in the form of Intralipid (KabiVitrium, London), the cord V-A difference of free fatty acids was greater, particularly of those fatty acids found in the Intralipid (Elphick & Hull 1977). Similarly, infusions in women before delivery by Caesarean section also led to the appearance of a large fraction of Intralipid fatty acids (18:1, 18:2) in the FFA compartment of cord venous blood (Elphick *et al.* 1978*a*).

Cord blood samples collected for a study of placental metabolism of arachidonic acid by Filshie & Anstey (1978), with additional samples from further elective Caesarean sections, permitted us to analyse by gas chromatography the individual FFAs which were added to the fetal circulation. The concentrations of individual fatty acids in maternal plasma FFA and their V-A concentration differences in the umbilical cord are shown in Fig. 2. The V-A difference for each fatty acid was positive and related significantly to the mean maternal levels ($r = 0.969; P < 0.001$). Nevertheless, for each fatty acid and for their combined total, the difference of the venous level from the arterial level did not reach statistical significance on paired Student's t test analysis. Measurement of small V-A differences by gas chromatography is technically difficult. With larger numbers of patients the differences might well become significant. These findings would argue against selective transfer of fatty acids.

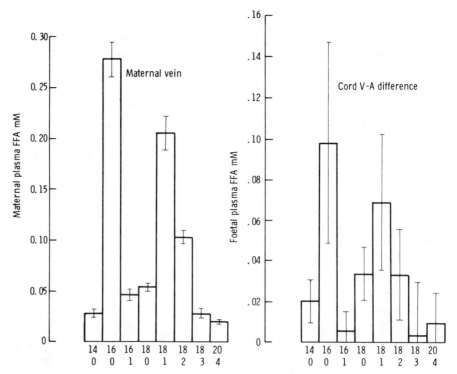

FIG. 2. Plasma concentrations of different fatty acids in the FFAs of maternal venous blood and their venous-arterial concentration differences in umbilical cord. Fatty acids are shown in shorthand notation (number of carbon atoms over number of double bonds). Each value represents the mean ± S.E. found in 18 patients undergoing elective and emergency Caesarean section. Data kindly supplied by G.M. Filshie and M.D. Anstey.

In summary, this evidence would seem to indicate that, in humans, fatty acids do cross the placenta and enter the fetal circulation as FFA, that they *might* be a major source of supply to the fetus, and that they *might* be derived from either maternal circulating FFA or triglyceride.

Triglycerides to the fetus

Triglycerides are found in the fetal circulation. Presumably, as in the adult, these (endogenous) triglycerides are derived mainly from the liver. Their biological role in the fetus is not clear. It has been observed that their levels rise after increases in FFA concentrations, so they may be a vehicle by which these fatty acids are discharged back to adipose tissue stores. Endogenous triglycerides appear to be cleared from the circulation in a similar manner to chylomicra.

Concentrations of triglycerides in umbilical blood were measured before FFA were thought of!   As long ago as 1935 Boyd & Wilson found significant V-A differences of triglyceride in cord blood and they put forward the hypothesis that as lipid concentrations in the maternal bloodstream increase, the placenta passes more of these substances on to the umbilical blood, from whence they are absorbed in increasing amounts by the fetus.

We measured concentrations of total triglyceride in cord blood taken at elective Caesarean section and found that the V-A difference varied widely.   The mean value did not differ significantly from zero but in a number of paired samples the V-A difference was of a magnitude which was well outside the range of technical error, a variability suggesting that in some infants triglycerides were entering the fetal circulation from the placenta.

Some obstetricians use intravenous nutrition in the expectation that it will provide calories for the mother and also for her unborn child (Chang *et al.* 1977).   When Intralipid infusions were given before delivery by elective Caesarean section there was a highly significant cord V-A difference in triglyceride concentrations, and the fatty acid profile of the difference reflected that of the maternal triglyceride, which itself had been distorted by the large percentages of oleic (18:1) and linoleic (18:2) acids in Intralipid (Elphick *et al.* 1978*a*).   From this it would appear that triglyceride *can* be discharged into the fetal circulation.   Whether it is, and to what degree under normal conditions, remains to be demonstrated.

EVIDENCE FROM PLACENTAL PERFUSION STUDIES

The problems inherent in studying placental transfer in humans have led to a number of attempts to set up perfusion systems on the isolated placenta.   Using a method similar to that described by Krantz *et al.* (1962) in which the whole placenta is perfused, Szabo *et al.* (1969) estimated a transfer rate of 15–50 μmoles palmitic acid/hour.   More control and relatively higher flow rates can be achieved by perfusing individual cotyledons (Schneider *et al.* 1972).   Using this technique Dancis *et al.* (1973) calculated the palmitate and linoleate transfer rates to be some fivefold greater than the figure given by Szabo *et al.* (1969); even so Dancis *et al.* (1973) estimated that the rates they found could supply only 20% of the fat laid in the last month of pregnancy.   To make these calculations a number of assumptions have to be made for which unfortunately there is little supporting evidence.   Dancis *et al.* (1973) compared the transfer rates of fatty acids with antipyrine.   The rates varied with the chain length of the fatty acid.   However, on the basis of further investigations, they considered that the decreasing placental transfer with increasing chain length could be related to the binding characteristics of the various fatty acids to albumin (Dancis *et al.* 1974).

We wondered whether the concentration of FFA on the maternal side influenced the net transfer rates observed in the placenta. Using a modification of the cotyledon technique described by Schneider *et al.* (1972), we measured the effect of increasing the fatty acid concentration in the perfusate on the maternal side on the transfer of labelled palmitate into the circuit on the fetal side in seven term placentas within 5 minutes of delivery. Increasing the concentration of palmitate on the maternal side from a mean of 0.3 mM to 1.3 mM increased the net transfer rate tenfold (Elphick *et al.* 1978*b*).

It might be concluded from these studies that fatty acids do cross the placental membranes, that there is little evidence for selective transfer of the different fatty acids, and that the net transfer from mother to fetus is sensitive to the FFA concentration on the maternal side.

EVIDENCE FROM FETAL TRIGLYCERIDE CONCENTRATIONS

Triglyceride concentrations have been measured in cord blood in studies of placental transfer (Boyd & Wilson 1935; Senn & McNamara 1937; Rafstedt & Swahn 1954; Van Duyne & Havel 1960; Brody & Carlson 1962; Wille & Phillips 1971); in studies of fetal metabolism (Melichar *et al.* 1964; Šabata & Štembera 1967; Šabata *et al.* 1968*a*; Fosbrooke & Wharton 1973; Harris 1974); and as a screening procedure for inherited disorders of lipid metabolism (Glueck *et al.* 1971; Glueck *et al.* 1972; Kwiterovich *et al.* 1973; Goldstein *et al.* 1973). In later studies hyperlipidaemic states were found to be associated with fetal distress and complications of pregnancy (Tsang *et al.* 1974; Andersen & Friis-Hansen 1976; Cress *et al.* 1977).

Our interest in triglyceride concentration in cord blood arose out of a simple experimental study on pregnant rabbits near term (Edson *et al.* 1975). If food but not fluid was withheld for 48 hours towards the end of term then the total fat stores of the fetus increased nearly 100% and in particular the fat content of the liver increased fourfold. As the liver responds to excess fat loads by increasing the production of endogenous triglyceride, it was perhaps not surprising to find that the mean concentration of triglyceride in fetal blood of unfed does was high; the average was 2.5 mM compared with the usual concentration of 1.4 mM (Edson & Hull 1977). In this situation, as food was withheld from the mother, the maternal concentration of glucose and chylomicron triglyceride would be low and fatty acid would be mobilized from maternal adipose stores. It would seem that by far the most likely explanation was that the extra fatty acid in the fetus was derived from the free fatty acids in the maternal circulation.

Theoretically cord triglycerides may be increased if triglycerides are released by the placenta or if the fetal liver produces more endogenous triglyceride in response to excess fatty acid load. Again, theoretically, this excess load of fatty acid may be derived from the placenta, from fetal adipose tissue or excess fatty acid manufactured by the fetal tissues, particularly the liver. In the reports on cord triglyceride concentration no information on maternal food intake before birth is given. As the experimental studies on rabbits suggest that this could be important, we measured triglyceride concentration in cord blood obtained during normal births and related it, amongst other things, to maternal food intake over the previous two or three days. It is known that fasting produces a larger increase in maternal FFA levels in pregnant than in non-pregnant women (Kim & Felig 1972), while the rise in FFA concentration which occurs during labour is smaller in mothers who take food during this time (Šabata et al. 1963). It was found that four women had not eaten for more than 24 hours before delivery. In all four the triglyceride concentration in the cord blood was above 1.5 standard deviations of the mean of the group ($n = 120$) (Elphick et al. 1978c). The suggested association of high triglyceride concentrations in cord blood with maternal food intake immediately before delivery obviously needs confirmation from a larger group. The evidence as it stands, however, is consistent with the findings in rabbits, where it has been demonstrated that stores of fetal lipids vary with the state of maternal nutrition, and that under certain circumstances major fractions of the fatty acids stored in the fetus are derived from the mother.

EVIDENCE FROM ESSENTIAL FATTY ACIDS IN THE FETUS

The presence of linoleic (18:2) and linolenic (18:3) acids and their derivatives, arachidonic acid (20:4) and the longer chain polyunsaturated acids in fetal tissues not only demonstrates that some fatty acids must cross the placenta but also gives an indication of the size of the maternal contribution.

This is illustrated by comparing the transfer of fatty acids in rabbits and sheep from the maternal circulating FFA to the fetal circulating FFA compartment and on to the fetal adipose tissue stores (Fig. 3). In anaesthetized rabbits fatty acids rapidly cross the placenta, the net transfer is related to the maternal circulating concentration and the relationship is similar for palmitic and linoleic acids (Elphick & Hull 1977). Selective transfer did not appear to occur. In fetal adipose tissue linoleic acid forms 20% of the stored triglyceride. Linoleic acid forms a similar percentage of the V-A differences in free fatty acids in cord blood and of the free fatty acids in the maternal blood. If there is no selective transfer of fatty acids across the placenta, this would

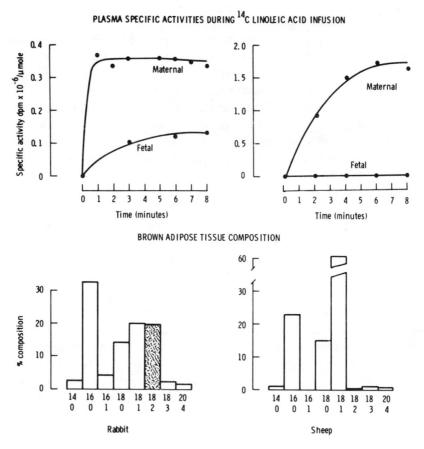

FIG. 3. Relationship between the specific activity of linoleic acid in maternal and fetal plasma FFA and the fetal adipose tissue content of linoleic acid. [^{14}C]linoleic acid was given by constant intravenous infusion over 8-10 min to a pregnant rabbit and sheep.   The fetal plasma radioactivity was measured.   Note the extremely low activity of [^{14}C]linoleic acid in fetal lamb blood and low tissue content of linoleic acid.   Fatty acids identified as in Fig. 2. (Linoleic acid is shown shaded.)

suggest that in rabbits most of the stored triglycerides are derived from the mother.   In contrast, in sheep very little free fatty acid enters the fetal circulation from the placenta.   After injection of labelled linoleic acid into the sheep maternal bloodstream, only trivial amounts of labelled linoleate were detected (Elphick & Hull 1978).   Activity was only just detectable by the most sensitive methods we were able to use.   The specific activity was certainly less than 1% of that in the mother.   No cord V-A differences were found.   The fetal stores of adipose tissue contained only minute amounts of linoleic acid.

In man there are a number of studies on the fatty acid composition of adipose tissue at birth.   From the data published by Baker *et al.* (1964), in which linoleic acid formed 2.4% of the fatty acid stores in adipose tissue, it can be calculated that if there is no selective transfer of FFA then *at least* 15% of the fetal stores were derived from the maternal circulation.   The calculation *assumes* that selective transfer does not occur to any marked degree and there is some experimental evidence to support this assumption.   However 15% is probably an underestimate, for the adipose stores contain those fatty acids which the fetus does not use for structure.   The rapidly growing fetus requires essential fatty acids to form phospholipids for cellular and intracellular structures, particularly in nervous tissue, so these essential fatty acids will be selectively removed.

The fatty acid composition of adipose tissue from fetuses of women in the UK changes in the last trimester: the linoleic acid fraction falls.   In adipose tissue from fetuses of Dutch women whose diet contains more unsaturated fats, the fall is far less marked (E.M. Widdowson, personal communication).   This observation also suggests that under normal circumstances a major proportion of fetal fatty acids is supplied directly from the mother.

The fatty acid composition of triglyceride in fetal adipose tissue differs from that of fetal plasma FFAs, which are poorer in palmitic but richer in linoleic acids.   Studies of fetal adipose tissue in rabbits *in vitro* suggest that it rapidly incorporates fatty acids as it grows and lipolysis and mobilization are probably slight (Hudson & Hull 1977).   In man the fatty acid pattern of fetal circulating FFA reflects, at least in part, the contribution of FFA from the mother.   After birth there is a large increase in lipid mobilization associated with a rise in plasma FFA concentrations.   The fatty acid composition of circulating free fatty acids after birth will move towards that of its adipose tissue.   Chen *et al.* (1965) found a sharp postnatal fall in the percentage of free linoleic acid and a rise in free palmitic acid in the circulating FFA of the newborn.   At 24 hours after birth the plasma FFA composition becomes very like that of the adipose tissue.   Chen *et al.* (1965) attributed these changes to a change in the source of FFA.

In conclusion, in humans as in certain other species, the mother supplies her fetus with fatty acids.   What fraction of the fatty acids in the fetus is derived from the mother and what fraction is made locally may well vary with a number of factors, including the state of maternal nutrition.   It is possible that under normal conditions the fetus derives most of its fatty acids from the mother.

References

ANDERSEN, G. E. & FRIIS-HANSEN, B. (1976) Neonatal hypertriglyceridemia: a new index of antepartum-intrapartum fetal stress. *Acta Paediatr. Scand. 65,* 369–374

BAKER, L., PODHIPLEUX, P. & WILLIAMS, M. L. (1964) Fatty acid composition of subcutaneous fat in premature and full term infants. *Soc. Pediatr. Res. 34th Annu. Meet.* Seattle, Washington, abstr., p. 127

BOYD, E. M. & WILSON, K. M. (1935) The exchange of lipids in the umbilical circulation at birth. *J. Clin. Invest. 14,* 7–15

BRODY, S. & CARLSON, L. A. (1962) Plasma lipid concentrations in the newborn with special reference to the distribution of the different lipid fractions. *Clin. Chim. Acta 7,* 694-699

CHANG, A., ABELL, D., BEISCHER, N. & WOOD, C. (1977) Trial of intravenous therapy in women with low urinary estriol excretion. *Am. J. Obstet. Gynecol. 127,* 793–797

CHEN, C. H., ADAM, P. A. J., LASKOWSKI, D. E., McCANN, M. L. & SCHWARTZ, R. (1965) The plasma free fatty acid composition and blood glucose of normal and diabetic pregnant women and of their newborns. *Pediatrics 36,* 843–855

COLTART, T. M. (1972) Effect on fetal liver lipids of ^{14}C glucose administered intravenously to the mother. *J. Obstet. Gynaecol. Br. Commonw. 79,* 639–643

COLTART, T. M. & BATEMAN, C. (1975) Carbohydrate-induced lipogenesis in the human placenta of normal and diabetic pregnancies. *Br. J. Obstet. Gynaecol. 82,* 471–475

CRESS, H. R., SHAHER, R. M., LAFFIN, R. & KARPOWICZ, K. (1977) Cord blood hyperlipoproteinemia and perinatal stress. *Pediatr. Res. 11,* 19-23

DANCIS, J., JANSEN, V., KAYDEN, H. J., SCHNEIDER, H. & LEVITZ, M. (1973) Transfer across perfused human placenta II. Free fatty acids. *Pediatr. Res. 7,* 192–197

DANCIS, J., JANSEN, V., KAYDEN, H.J., BJORNSON, L. & LEVITZ, M. (1974) Transfer across perfused human placenta III. Effect of chain length on transfer of free fatty acids. *Pediatr. Res. 8,* 796–799

DIAMANT, Y. Z., MAYOREK, N., NEUMAN, S. & SHAFRIR, E. (1975) Enzymes of glucose and fatty acid metabolism in early and term human placenta. *Am. J. Obstet. Gynecol. 121,* 58–61

EDSON, J. L. & HULL. D. (1977) Effect of maternal starvation on metabolic response to cold of newborn rabbit. *Pediatr. Res. 11,* 793–795

EDSON, J. L., HUDSON, D. G. & HULL. D. (1975) Evidence for increased fatty acid transfer across the placenta during a maternal fast in rabbits. *Biol. Neonate 27,* 50–55

ELPHICK, M. C. & HULL, D. (1977) Rabbit placental clearing-factor lipase activity and the passage across the placenta of fatty acids derived from triglycerides injected into the circulation of the mother. *J. Physiol. (Lond.) 273,* 475–487

ELPHICK, M. C. & HULL, D. (1978) The transfer of fatty acids across the sheep placenta. *J. Physiol. (Lond.), 276,* 56P

ELPHICK, M. C., HUDSON, D. G. & HULL, D. (1975) Transfer of fatty acids across the rabbit placenta. *J. Physiol. (Lond.) 252,* 29-42

ELPHICK, M. C., HULL, D. & SANDERS, R. R. (1976) Concentrations of free fatty acids in maternal and umbilical cord blood during elective Caesarean section. *Br. J. Obstet. Gynaecol. 83,* 539–544

ELPHICK, M. C., FILSHIE, G. M. & HULL, D. (1978*a*) The passage of fat emulsion across the human placenta. *Br. J. Obstet. Gynaecol. 85,* 610-618

ELPHICK, M. C., EDSON, J. L & HULL, D. (1978*b*) *Biol. Neonate,* in press

ELPHICK, M. C., HARRISON, A. T., LAWLOR, J. P. & HULL, D. (1978*c*) Cord blood hypertriglyceridaemia as an index of foetal stress; use of a simple screening test and results of further biochemical analysis. *Br. J. Obstet. Gynaecol., 85,* 303-311

FILSHIE, G.M. & ANSTEY, M. D. (1978) The distribution of arachidonic acid in plasma and tissue of patients near term undergoing elective or emergency Caesarean section. *Br. J. Obstet, Gynaecol., 85,* 119-123

FOSBROOKE, A. S. & WHARTON, B.A. (1973) Plasma lipids in umbilical cord blood from infants of normal and low birth weight. *Biol. Neonate 23*, 330–338

GILLMER, M. D. G., BEARD, R. W., OAKLEY, N. W., BROOKE, F. M., ELPHICK, M. C. & HULL, D. (1977) Diurnal plasma free fatty acid profiles in normal and diabetic pregnancies. *Br. Med. J. 2*, 670–673

GLUECK, C. J., HECKMAN, F., SCHOENFIELD, M., SEINER, P. & PEARCE, W. (1971) Neonatal familial type II hyperlipoproteinemia; cord blood cholesterol in 1800 births. *Metabolism 20*, 597–608

GLUECK, C. J., TSANG, R., FALLAT, R., FORD, S., EVANS, G., BECKETT, D. & STEINER, P. (1972) Pediatric familial type IV hyperlipoproteinemia. *Trans. Assoc. Am. Phys. 85*, 139–150

GOLDSTEIN, J. L., ALBERS, J. J., HAZZARD, W. R., SCHROTT, H. R., BIERMAN, E. L. & MOTULSKY, A. G. (1973) Genetic and medical significance of neonatal hyperlipidemia. *J. Clin. Invest. 52*, 35a (abstr. 27)

HARRIS, R. J. (1974) Plasma nonesterified fatty acids and blood glucose in healthy and hypoxemic newborn infants. *J. Pediatr. 84*, 578–584

HERSHFIELD, M. S. & NEMETH, A. M. (1968) Placental transport of free palmitic and linoleic acids in the guinea pig. *J. Lipid Res. 9*, 460–468

HUDSON, D. G. & HULL, D. (1977) Uptake and metabolism of C^{14} palmitate by fetal rabbit tissue. *Biol. Neonate 31*, 316–323

HUMMEL, L., SCHIRRMEISTER, N., ZIMMERMANN, T. & WAGNER, H. (1974) Studies of the lipid metabolism using ^{14}C-1-palmitate in fetal rats. *Biol. Neonate 24*, 298–305

JAMES, E., MESCHIA, G. & BATTAGLIA, F. C. (1971) A-V differences of free fatty acids and glycerol in the ovine umbilical circulation. *Proc. Soc. Exp. Biol. Med. 138*, 823–826

JONES, C. T. & ASHTON, I. K. (1976) Lipid biosynthesis in liver slices of the foetal guinea-pig. *Biochem. J. 154*, 149–158

KIM, Y. J. & FELIG, P. (1972) Maternal and amniotic fluid substrate levels during caloric deprivation in human pregnancy. *Metabolism 21*, 507–512

KRANTZ, K. E., PANOS, T. C. & EVANS, J. (1962) Physiology of maternal-fetal relationship through the extracorporeal circulation of the human placenta. *Am. J. Obstet. Gynecol. 83*, 1214–1228

KWITEROVICH, P.O., LEVY, R. I. & FREDRICKSON, D.S. (1973) Neonatal diagnosis of familial type-II hyperlipoproteinaemia. *Lancet 1*, 118–122

LEAT, W. M. F., HARRISON, F. A. & JUDGE, S. R. (1978) Transfer of linoleic acid to the foetal and neonatal sheep. *Proc. Nutr. Soc., 37*, 52A

MELICHAR, V., NOVÁK, M., HAHN, P. & KOLDOVSKY, O. (1964) Free fatty acid and glucose in the blood of various groups of newborns. Preliminary report. *Acta Paediatr. Scand. 53*, 343–344

PERSSON, N. & LUNELL, N. O. (1975) Metabolic control in diabetic pregnancy. *Am. J. Obstet. Gynecol. 122*, 737–745

PERSSON, B. & TUNELL, R. (1971) Influence of environmental temperature and acidosis on lipid mobilization in the human infant during the first two hours after birth. *Acta Paediatr. Scand. 60*, 385–398

PORTMAN, O.W., BEHRMAN, R.E. & SOLTYS, P. (1969) Transfer of free fatty acids across the primate placenta. *Am. J. Physiol. 216*, 143–147

RAFSTEDT, S. & SWAHN, B. (1954) Studies on lipids, proteins and lipoproteins in serum from newborn infants. *Acta Paediatr. 43*, 221–234

ŠABATA, V. & ŠTEMBERA, Z. K. (1967) Parameters of glucose and lipid metabolism in deliveries of hypotrophic newborns, in *Intrauterine Dangers to the Foetus (Excerpta Med. Monogr.)* pp. 561-566, Excerpta Medica, Amsterdam

ŠABATA, V., NOVÁK, M. & MELICHAR, V. (1963) Ovlivněni hladin lipidů a glykémie příjmem potravy za porodu a v prvých dneck šestinedělí. *Česk Gynekol. 28*, 152–156

ŠABATA, V., ŠTEMBERA, Z.K. & NOVÁK, M. (1968a) Levels of unesterified and esterified fatty acids in umbilical blood of hypoxic fetuses. *Biol. Neonat. 12*, 194–200

ŠABATA, V., WOLF, H. & LAUSMANN, S. (1968b) The role of free fatty acids, glycerol, ketone bodies and glucose in the energy metabolism of the mother and fetus during delivery. *Biol. Neonat. 13*, 7–17

SAKVRAI, T., TAKAGI, H. & HOSOYA, N. (1969) Metabolic pathways of glucose in human placenta. Changes with gestation and with added 17-beta-estradiol. *Am. J. Obstet. Gynecol. 105*, 1044–1054

SCHNEIDER, H., PANIGEL, M. & DANCIS, J. (1972) Transfer across the perfused human placenta of antipyrine, sodium and leucine. *Am. J. Obstet. Gynecol. 114*, 822–828

SENN, M.J. & MCNAMARA, H. (1937) Lipids of blood plasma in neonatal period. *Am. J. Dis. Child. 53*, 445–454

SHEATH, J., GRIMWADE, J., WALDRON, K., BICKLEY, M., TAFT, P. & WOOD, C. (1972) Arteriovenous nonesterified fatty acids and glycerol differences in the umbilical cord at term and their relationship to fetal metabolism. *Am. J. Obstet. Gynecol. 113*, 358–362

SZABO, A. J., GRIMALDI, R.D. & JUNG, W.F. (1969) Palmitate transport across perfused human placenta. *Metabolism 18, 406–415*

TOBIN, J. D., ROUX, J.F. & SOELDNER, J. S. (1969) Human fetal insulin response after acute maternal glucose administration during labor. *Pediatrics 44*, 668–671

TSANG, R., GLUECK, C., EVANS, G. & STEINER, P.M. (1974) Cord blood hypertriglyceridemia. *Am. J. Dis. Child. 127*, 78–82

VAN DUYNE, C. M. & HAVEL, R. J. (1960) The plasma lipids in pregnancy and in the newborn. *Clin. Obstet. Gynecol. 3*, 326

VAN DUYNE, C. M., HAVEL, R. J. & FELTS, J. M. (1962) Placental transfer of palmitic acid -1-C^{14} in rabbits. *Am. J. Obstet. Gynecol. 84*, 1069–1074

WILLE, L. E. & PHILLIPS, G. B. (1971) Lipoprotein and lipid composition of neonatal serum. *Clin. Chim. Acta 34*, 457-462

Discussion

Williamson: When you infused Intralipid did you check the maternal free fatty acid concentrations? Studies at Northwick Park (R.S. Elkeles, personal communication) would suggest a big rise.

Hull: The maternal free fatty acid profile was altered but not the actual concentration.

Williamson: I was just wondering if this might explain your results.

Battaglia: What does the 15–20% figure for the linoleic contribution mean?

Hull: If linoleic acid forms 20% of the lipids in the mother's circulation, and if they are the sole source of fatty acids available to the fetus, then the fetal stores, if the fetus does not take up fatty acids selectively, should contain 20% linoleic acid. If fetal stores only contain a quarter of that (5% linoleic acid), then one can deduce that at least 25% of the fat has come from the maternal circulation.

Battaglia: I gather that the normal range of FFA concentrations fluctuates during the day and at different times of gestation. Based on the normal range at the time of delivery you should be able to estimate from the plot what the VA difference for FFA is in the cord at that maternal concentration. What does that convert into, either as the oxygen equivalent in the fetus or as a percentage of total carbon required in the fetus?

Hull: Theoretically one could argue that on an accepted fetal blood/placental blood flow a venous–arterial difference of the order of 0.05 mmol is needed to supply the fatty acids for structure and for triglyceride formation in adipose tissue stores. That is the same sort of figure that Bengt Persson and others got in VA differences from cord blood taken at term after vaginal delivery. We got the same figures, on average, at elective Caesarean section.

Battaglia: So that AV difference is for building the body fat stores in the fetus, not for the total carbon requirement? That is, it refers to the carbon accretion in lipid stores alone?

Hull: Yes.

Shafrir: The mechanism of the transport of fatty acids across the placenta is a difficult question. Long-chain fatty acids have a very high association constant with albumin, of the order of 10^7 or 10^8, which means that, under physiological conditions, only one in ten million molecules to maybe one in hundred million molecules is an unbound free fatty acid. Maternal albumin does not pass into the fetal circulation. It is very difficult to visualize, then, how molecules that are so tightly bound to their carrier can rapidly cross into the fetal circulation. Therefore the word transport should not be understood as a direct transfer of molecules across a semi-permeable membrane. It is possible that an intermediate carrier protein is there to facilitate FFA exchange but this seems unlikely to me. In most cells strong FFA binding occurs to mitochondria and microsomes, whereas cytoplasmic proteins show a very low affinity to FFA (Shafrir & Ruderman 1974).

When placental tissue is incubated in *in vitro* experiments with albumin-bound fatty acids, the first very rapid step is esterification of fatty acids, not transfer. I wish to emphasize that the fatty acid does not penetrate into the cell as a free molecule but almost simultaneously with the entry it is esterified into triglyceride and phospholipid components. To effect the release of fatty acids to the fetal side the presence of a potent lipolytic activity would be required. As you have very neatly pointed out, Professor Hull, there are distinct species differences in the transport of fatty acids. In sheep and rat there is very little direct transport of fatty acids, whereas in the rabbit, guinea-pig and human an appreciable transport has been reported. In my opinion the mechanism should be related to the lipolytic activities of the placenta, of which we know very little. There might be some activity of a lipoprotein lipase and of an intracellular lipase in the placenta but these activities in the different species have not been explored, as far as I know. The purpose of my comment is to turn us away from looking on the passage of fatty acid molecules across the placenta as a simple diffusion.

Hull: I agree, and here I was discussing mainly what comes through on the other side of the placenta. We have measured lipoprotein lipase activity in human and in rabbit placentas. On the standard method for measuring lipoprotein lipase it seems to have a high activity in the rabbit, and intracellular lipase activity seems high too. We have been less successful in finding lipoprotein lipase activity in human placentas. If triglyceride is taken up, lipoprotein lipase activity must be there and in most tissues it is argued that it is in the capillary. Only a few species have placentas with maternal capillaries and the human isn't one of them, and neither is the rabbit, so it is interesting to know where that lipoprotein lipase is situated in the placenta.

The fatty acid label is very quickly taken up into phospholipids, as well as triglyceride, when it is injected into the maternal or fetal circulations in the rabbit. What happens in the phospholipids may well influence some of the fatty acids which come across, particularly arachidonic acid.

Beard: Have you any evidence to explain the marked species differences in enzyme composition in the placenta?

Hull: No. I am more surprised that the sheep stops transport than that the others let it through.

Kalkhoff: It is most intriguing that with glucose infusion there is more free fatty acid transfer and when the sheep is starved more lipid is found on the other side. This goes back to what has been said about increased substrate availability. Have you extrapolated this to a diabetic animal where the concentrations of glucose and free fatty acids are higher than usual? The model lends itself well to what we are all vitally interested in.

Hull: I must confess that I wasn't thinking about the diabetic situation very much until I was invited to this meeting, but I now have one or two questions to which the rabbit might provide the answers.

Kalkhoff: Is the lipoprotein lipase heparin-sensitive?

Hull: We have demonstrated that it is heparin-sensitive *in vitro*, but *in vivo* it is a different question. In our studies we avoid heparin. We haven't deliberately perfused heparin and studied its effects in the placenta.

Kalkhoff: The controlling mechanism might be prostaglandins too, since the mechanism might be involved in the parturition process. Other people have implicated prostaglandins.

Battaglia: Silver & Comline (1976), for instance, were also unable to find any AV differences in free fatty acids in cows and horses and I think that has been shown in the pig as well. The rabbit and the human must be much more fatty than the sheep fetus at birth. Perhaps where the fat content of the fetal body is very low, the carbon sources of the fetus would not include fat. Even in the rabbit, where there is a good deal of fatty acid transfer, you did not find an excess of fats transported across the placenta beyond that required for the fat stores.   This raises the question, if we take it back to lean body mass is there a common denominator among the mammals in terms of how carbon balance is attained?

Hull: The rabbit is probably not much more 'fatty' at birth, in your sense, than the lamb.   More fatty acids may cross the placenta when fat is being laid down in adipose tissue because that lowers umbilical artery concentration.   The observation that the fat content may be doubled in fetuses of starved does when a large percentage of the extra fat is initially in the liver and a smaller percentage in adipose tissue doesn't support your argument.   The fetus has to take, in one sense, what is coming to it.   My view is that the fetus is in metabolic balance with the mother, and when the mother's metabolism changes then the balance changes in the fetus.

Gillmer: How much subcutaneous adipose tissue does the fetus of a sheep or rabbit possess?   Are these species analogous to the human in this respect?

Hull: I don't know that the percentage of body weight is too informative in this way.   The figure varies from lamb to lamb.

Gillmer: A characteristic feature of the growth-retarded human fetus is its relative lack of subcutaneous fat.   Is this also true of the rabbit fetus?

Hull: The amount of fat in the human at birth averages 10% of total weight but there is a wide variation.   Some organs, for example the heart and the kidney, have a fairly constant relationship to body weight and variations from the mean are relatively small.   On the other hand, adipose tissue, wet weight and fat content may vary widely.

Shafrir: The characteristics of the newborn should not be related only to the transport of preformed fatty acids.   The fetus has a capacity for *de novo* synthesis of fat from glucose.   The species that do not transport significant amounts of fatty acids may have ample capacity to convert carbohydrate to lipid.

Hull: The lamb must make a large percentage of its own fats by lipogenesis.   What interests me is where it gets its essential fatty acids from for brain development.

Naismith: There is some evidence that the major source of the long-chain polyunsaturated fatty acids is phosphoglyceride in the maternal plasma, rather than the free fatty acids.

Hull: In my paper I did not discuss the possible role of phospholipids in the maternal circulation as a possible supply for the placenta.   Some of the essential fatty acids, particularly the long-chain ones, might be derived from the phospholipids.

Naismith: It has been suggested that phosphoglycerides cross unchanged, with no breakdown in transfer. We have evidence that suggests that the placenta desaturates linoleic acid (D.J. Naismith & T.A.B. Sanders, unpublished work 1978) but I don't know whether it is split off from the phosphoglycerides in the process.

Hull: In the profile for rabbits and humans, the one fatty acid that doesn't fit in is arachidonic acid. We infused it into rabbits and its specific activity is much lower than linoleic acid and palmitic acid, suggesting that the fatty acid that is coming from the placenta into the fetal circulation is from a source other than free fatty acids and triglycerides.

Freinkel: The phosphoglyceride and triglyceride metabolism of the placenta appear to be mediated separately. We have found that placental neutral fats increase markedly, without commensurate changes in the phospholipids whenever there is fat mobilization *in vivo* (Herrera & Freinkel 1975) or increased availability of fatty acids *in vitro* (Freinkel 1965; Diamant *et al.* 1977*a,b*). We have been particularly interested in this phenomenon because we have felt that placental lipids might be implicated in placental ageing (Freinkel 1965) and that they might serve as the essential fatty acid donors for prostaglandin biosynthesis (Wilson *et al.* 1977). To date, we have not found a correlation between the steatosis of the placenta after fat mobilization *in vivo* and subsequent placental biosynthesis of prostaglandins *in vitro* (Wilson *et al.* 1977).

Hull: The relationship between the placenta's own lipid metabolism and what it releases into the fetal circulation may be separate too. In the sheep fatty acids are taken up by the placenta but none gets through into the fetal circulation.

References

DIAMANT, S., DIAMANT, Y. Z. & FREINKEL, N. (1977*a*) Placental phospholipid metabolism. *Proc. 2nd Int. Congr. Human Reprod.,* Tel Aviv, Israel

DIAMANT, Y. Z., DIAMANT, S. & FREINKEL, N. (1977*b*) Ageing of the placenta and changes in its triglyceride metabolism. *Proc. 2nd Int. Congr. Human Reprod.,* Tel Aviv, Israel

FREINKEL, N. (1965) Effects of the conceptus on maternal metabolism during pregnancy, in *On the Nature and Treatment of Diabetes* (Leibel, B. S. & Wrenshall, G. A., eds.), pp. 679–691, *Int. Congr. Series 84,* Excerpta Medica, Amsterdam

HERRERA, E. & FREINKEL, N. (1975) Metabolites in the liver, brain and placenta of fed or fasted mothers and fetal rats. *Horm. Metab. Res. 7,* 247

SHAFRIR, E. & RUDERMAN, N. B. (1974) Enzymes of carbohydrate and fat metabolism in anti-insulin serum diabetes: inactivation by free fatty acids and the protective effect of cellular protein. *Diabetologia 10,* 731–742

Silver, M. & Comline, R. S. (1976) Fetal and placental O_2 consumption and the uptake of different metabolites in the ruminant and horse during late gestation, in *Oxygen Transport to Tissue – II* (Reneau, D.D. & Grote, J. eds.), pp. 731-736, Plenum, New York

Wilson, L., Diamant, Y., Diamant, S. & Freinkel, N. (1977) Effects of aging and steatosis on rat placental content and production of prostaglandins (PG).   *10th Annu. Meet. Soc. Study Reprod.,* pp. 64–65 (abstr. 105)

Metabolism during normal and diabetic pregnancy and its effect on neonatal outcome

M.D.G. GILLMER* and BENGT PERSSON †

* Department of Obstetrics and Gynaecology, St Mary's Hospital Medical School, London and
† Department of Obstetrics and Gynaecology, Sabbatsberg Hospital, and Department of Paediatrics, St Goran's Hospital, Karolinska Institutet, Stockholm

Abstract   Diurnal profile studies have been used to define the fetal carbohydrate and lipid substrate environment in normal and diabetic women during late pregnancy.   In women with normal glucose tolerance the diurnal plasma glucose concentration was maintained within close limits (mean ± S.D., 4.70 ± 0.38 mmol/l) but in chemical and insulin-dependent diabetics there was a marked increase in both the mean diurnal glucose value and in the variability of the plasma glucose levels observed through the day (mean ± S.D., 5.61 ± 1.03 and 6.02 ± 1.26 mmol/l respectively, $P < 0.01$).   No difference was observed between the peripheral insulin activity of the normal and chemical diabetic women, and the impaired glucose tolerance of the latter group was due to a deficient insulin response to glucose.   The diurnal glucose variability, expressed as the standard deviation of the mean, was found to be inversely correlated with the residual C-peptide response in insulin-requiring diabetics.

The mean diurnal plasma free fatty acid (FFA) concentration was slightly raised in chemical diabetic subjects compared to normal women (mean ± S.D. 0.77 ± 0.34 and 0.68 ± 0.20 mmol/l respectively) but this difference was not significant.   Insulin treatment produced a marked reduction in circulating FFA concentration, with a mean value in the insulin-dependent diabetic group of 0.45 ± 0.11 mmol/l ($P < 0.001$).

Neonatal glucose assimilation during the first two hours of life correlated strongly with several functions of maternal carbohydrate tolerance.   This was associated with higher plasma insulin concentrations at birth, and a marked tendency to hypoglycaemia in the infants of untreated chemical diabetic women.   Impaired mobilization of triglyceride stores was also observed during the two hours after birth in the infants of diabetic women.   This, however, appears to be due not to impaired lipolysis but to rapid re-esterification of FFA.

These findings all indicate a state of functional hyperinsulinism in the infant of the diabetic woman secondary to maternal hyperglycaemia.

Although women with clinical diabetes mellitus rarely became pregnant in the pre-insulin era, the fact that pregnancy itself could be diabetogenic was first recognized nearly a century ago (Matthews-Duncan 1883).   In those women

who became pregnant the perinatal mortality was high (in excess of 50%) and
the maternal mortality approached 25% (Williams 1909).   After the advent
of insulin in the early 1920s, a dramatic decline in maternal mortality to 1% or
less was achieved but the perinatal mortality remained well in excess of 20%
until the early 1950s (Essex et al. 1973; Pedersen 1977).

In recent years many centres have reported a major improvement in the
perinatal outcome and a reduction in both obstetric (Pedersen 1967; Peel
1972; Brudenell 1975) and neonatal complications (Karlsson & Kjellmer
1972; Persson et al. 1975), and it has been suggested that this has been due to
improved metabolic control.   The excessive fetal size, characteristic of this
condition, also appears to have declined as the pregnancy outcome has improved (Oakley 1965; Pedersen 1977).

The changes in carbohydrate metabolism which occur during normal pregnancy have been intensively investigated in the last 20 years (for review, see
Pedersen 1977).   Most studies have relied on 'stress' tests, in which either a
glucose load has been administered to the mother, orally or intravenously (for
review, see Hadden 1975), or the changes in glucose and insulin or other
metabolites and hormones have been monitored after she has fasted for a
prolonged period (Felig & Lynch 1970; Kim & Felig 1972).   Little attention
has, however, been directed to the physiological changes in carbohydrate and
lipid metabolism which occur in response to normal diet and activity in human
pregnancy.   In addition, the effects of carbohydrate restriction and insulin
therapy on metabolic control in chemical and insulin-dependent diabetic
women and the changes in fetal substrate availability which these therapeutic
measures produce are poorly defined.

We have studied carbohydrate and lipid metabolism in normal and diabetic
pregnancies (Gillmer et al. 1975a,b, 1977; Persson et al. 1973, 1975, 1976)
and endeavoured to relate the maternal findings obtained in treated and
untreated patients to those of the neonate both by means of an intravenous
glucose tolerance test two hours after delivery and by following the spontaneous changes in carbohydrate metabolism which occur during the first two
hours after birth.   The advantage of this physiological approach is that it has
provided both an 'index of normality' and indicated the goal one should aim at
in attempting to achieve an 'ideal' therapeutic result.

DIURNAL PLASMA GLUCOSE AND INSULIN PROFILES IN NORMAL AND
DIABETIC PREGNANCY

The diurnal plasma glucose and insulin findings in nine normal women who
were studied in both early and late pregnancy are shown in Fig. 1.   A total
daily carbohydrate intake of 180 g was provided, with main meals containing

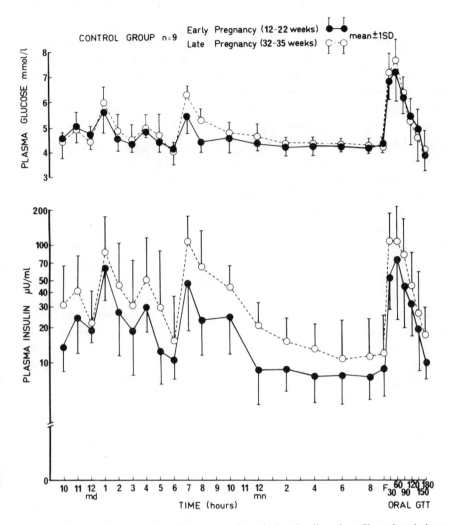

FIG. 1. Plasma glucose and insulin concentrations during the diurnal profile and oral glucose tolerance test (GTT) in nine normal women studied in the second and third trimester of pregnancy (based on Gillmer *et al.* 1975*a*). md: mid-day; mn: midnight.

40 g at noon and 6 p.m., and snacks containing 20 g at 10 a.m., 3 p.m., and 9 p.m.; 40 g was consumed at home before the study as part of the patient's breakfast. During the day all the patients were encouraged to be active, but between 10 p.m. and 7 a.m. they were asleep. At the conclusion of the diurnal study a 50-g oral glucose tolerance test (GTT) with half-hourly sampling was performed between 9 a.m. and noon with the patient recumbent.

The mean plasma glucose remained below 5.6 mmol/l, except during the hour after a meal, with an overall mean diurnal plasma glucose value (from 10 a.m. to 8 a.m. the following morning) of 4.53 mmol/l in early pregnancy and an increase of only 0.22 mmol/l in late pregnancy. These early and late pregnancy profiles closely resemble those reported in normal healthy men and non-pregnant women when continuous (Service *et al.* 1970) or intermittent sampling was used (Loreti *et al.* 1974; Alberti *et al.* 1975). Contrary to some reports (Burt 1962; Lind *et al.* 1973), no significant alteration in glucose tolerance was observed after the 50-g 3-hour oral glucose tolerance test.

The pre-prandial plasma glucose concentrations were generally lower in late pregnancy, a finding in keeping with the reduced fasting levels reported by several workers (Bleicher *et al.* 1964; Tyson *et al.* 1969; Lind *et al.* 1973; Victor 1974), while the post-prandial values were higher. As a result the diurnal plasma glucose range was greater in late pregnancy with a mean value of 2.56 ± s.d. 0.38 mmol/l compared with 2.05 ± s.d. 0.43 mmol/l.

It is apparent from the diurnal insulin profiles that to maintain this degree of normoglycaemia in late pregnancy a greatly increased insulin response to glucose was required throughout the day and night. Analysis of the insulin response to glucose during the oral GTT, using the technique described by Sluiter and co-workers (1976 *a,b;* see Fig. 2), reveals a significant increase in the corrected insulin response (CIR), and a significant decrease in the approximate peripheral insulin activity (A) without any overall change in glucose tolerance. These findings confirm that there is an increase in peripheral resistance to insulin during late pregnancy (Burt 1960; Yen 1973), and may in part explain the increased diurnal plasma glucose fluctuation observed at this time.

Obesity is also associated with insulin resistance and, like pregnancy, may be diabetogenic in certain individuals. The role of obesity as a factor contributing to insulin resistance in pregnancy has not, however, been previously defined. Twenty-four women with normal glucose tolerance in late pregnancy were assigned to two groups on the basis of their percentage ideal body weight (IBW) before pregnancy. Those in whom the percentage IBW was less than 110 were considered non-obese (14 patients) and those in whom it exceeded this value were considered to be obese (10 patients). The mean value for the non-obese group was 93.7 ± s.d. 8.1.% and for the obese group 126.9 ± s.d. 23.1%. The mean plasma glucose and insulin concentrations during the diurnal study in the obese and non-obese women are shown in Fig. 3. The pre-prandial (10 a.m. and 6 p.m.) and nocturnal fasting plasma glucose concentrations of the obese subjects were significantly higher than those of the non-obese ($P < 0.05$). The mean diurnal plasma glucose con-

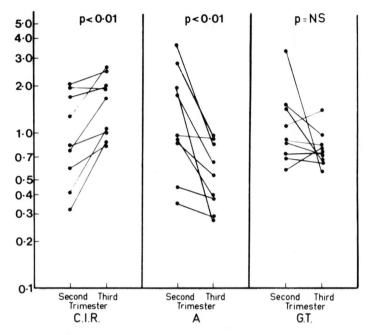

FIG. 2.   Corrected insulin response (CIR), approximate peripheral insulin activity (A) and glucose tolerance index (GT) (calculated according to Sluiter *et al.* 1976*a*,*b*) in nine normal women studied in the second and third trimester of pregnancy.

centration was also slightly higher in the obese group, but this difference was not statistically significant.   The diurnal plasma glucose range, on the other hand, was much lower in the obese group ($P = 0.033$; see Table 1).   The plasma insulin response to glucose in this group was, however, much greater than that of the non-obese women, suggesting that the insulin resistance associated with obesity is superimposed on that which is specific to pregnancy.   This observation may help to explain the higher incidence of diabetes arising *de novo* during pregnancy in obese women.   These findings also provide a rational basis for the use of dietary restriction in the management of obese pregnant chemical diabetic patients (Sutherland & Stowers 1975).

The diurnal plasma glucose and insulin profiles of 13 chemical diabetic women (White class A; total glucose tolerance area 43 mmol/l units) and 24 normal women of similar height and weight, who were studied in late pregnancy, are shown in Fig. 4.   The plasma glucose concentration of the chemical diabetic women ($5.61 \pm$ s.d. 1.03 mmol/l) was significantly higher than that of the normal women ($4.70 \pm$ s.d. 0.38 mmol/l; $P<0.01$).   Despite the consist-

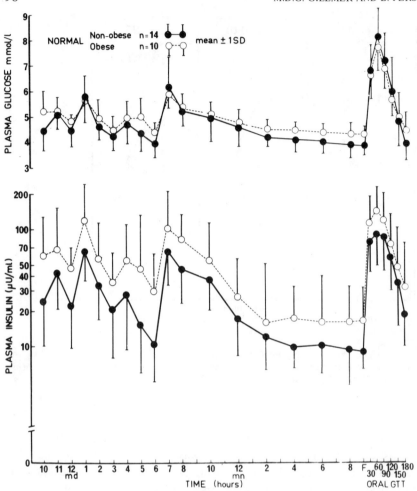

FIG. 3.   Plasma glucose and insulin concentrations during the diurnal profile and oral GTT in 14 non-obese and 10 obese women with normal glucose tolerance studied in the third trimester of pregnancy. md: mid-day ; mn: midnight.

TABLE 1

The mean diurnal plasma glucose value and diurnal plasma glucose range in 14 non-obese and 10 obese women with normal glucose tolerance (mean ± s.d.).

	No.	Mean diurnal plasma glucose value (mmol/l)	Diurnal plasma glucose range (mmol/l)
Non-obese	14	4.59 ± 0.34	2.92 ± 1.14
Obese	10	4.86 ± 0.37	2.10 ± 0.58

ently raised mean plasma glucose levels of the chemical diabetic women, their mean plasma insulin levels ($\log_{10}$ transformed data) were similar to those of the control group.   The concentrations at 8 p.m. and 10 p.m. were, however, significantly lower in the chemical diabetic patients ($P < 0.02$).   In addition, the chemical diabetic group displayed a reduced insulin response to

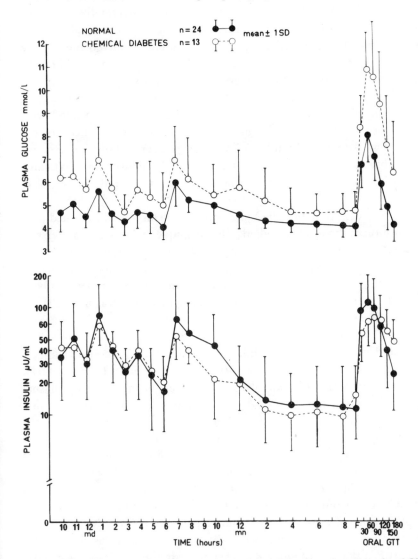

FIG. 4.   Plasma glucose and insulin concentrations during the diurnal profile and oral GTT in 24 normal women and 13 chemical diabetics studied during the third trimester of pregnancy (based on Gillmer *et al.* 1975*a*). md: mid-day; mn: midnight.

the glucose challenge, with a delayed peak and significantly lower mean insulin concentrations 30 and 60 min after the glucose load. The approximate peripheral insulin activity, calculated using the method of Sluiter and co-workers (1976a,b), was similar in the normal and chemical diabetic groups but the corrected insulin response was significantly reduced in the chemical diabetic group (see Fig. 5). The insulin response to meals was relatively greater than that after the glucose load in both the normal and chemical diabetic women and it seems likely that the protein content of mixed meals may augment the pancreatic β-cell response either directly as amino acid or indirectly through gastrointestinal secretagogues, a process which may compensate, at least in part, for the poor insulin secretion in chemical diabetics.

Whether chemical diabetes arising during pregnancy is associated with hyperinsulinaemia or hypoinsulinaemia has long been a matter of controversy. Several workers have found a delayed but exaggerated insulin response to oral glucose and meals (Kalkhoff et al. 1964; Carrington & McWilliams 1966; Persson & Lunell 1975), while others have reported a reduced response to an intravenous glucose challenge (Yen et al. 1971; Spellacy 1975). The differences between these findings may, however, be largely due to the differing composition of the groups studied. For example, in the study of Persson & Lunell (1975), the chemical diabetic group were on average 1 cm shorter and 5 kg heavier than the control group. It therefore seems likely that in some studies the chemical diabetic group may include a number of obese women with a relatively exaggerated insulin response which is nevertheless inadequate to maintain normoglycaemia. This may also explain why Persson & Lunell (1975) found a strong positive correlation between the mean values of glucose and insulin during an 8-h diurnal sampling period in control subjects and gestational diabetic patients ($r = 0.91$ and 0.83 respectively; $P < 0.001$), whereas a positive correlation was observed between the mean diurnal plasma glucose concentration and the total diurnal insulin area only in the 24 normal women ($r = 0.61$; $P < 0.001$), and not in the chemical diabetic group ($r = 0.046$; not significant) whose results are described above.

The usefulness of the glucose tolerance test, both as a diagnostic tool for detecting chemical diabetes during pregnancy, and for providing an indication of the prevailing plasma glucose concentrations during a normal day, has been confirmed by the strong positive correlation obtained between several of the indices of the oral GTT and the mean diurnal plasma glucose value (see Table 2). A strong negative correlation ($r = -0.880$; $P < 0.001$) was also demonstrated between the rate of glucose assimilation after an intravenous glucose load (K_t) and the mean 8-h diurnal glucose concentration in the study of Persson & Lunell (1975).

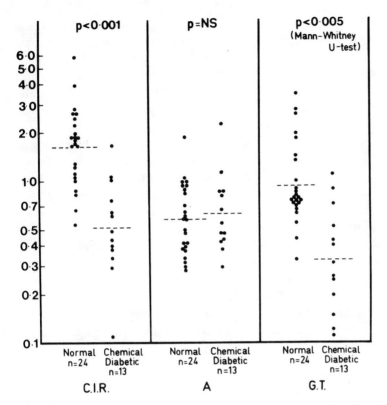

FIG. 5. Corrected insulin response (CIR), approximate peripheral insulin activity (A) and glucose tolerance (GT) (calculated according to Sluiter *et al.* 1976*a,b*) in 24 normal women and 13 chemical diabetics studied in the third trimester of pregnancy.

TABLE 2

Pearson correlation coefficient (*r*) between the oral GTT (glucose tolerance test) and diurnal indices of carbohydrate tolerance in 24 normal and 13 chemical diabetic women (from Gillmer *et al.* 1975*a*).

	Mean diurnal plasma glucose	Maximum diurnal plasma glucose	Diurnal plasma glucose range
Oral GTT total area	0.827[a]	0.781[a]	0.568[b]
Oral GTT incremental area	0.687[a]	0.754[a]	0.667[a]
Oral GTT 2-h plasma glucose	0.760[a]	0.737[a]	0.581[a]

[a] $P < 0.0001$ [b] $P < 0.001$

The diurnal plasma glucose concentrations in 13 insulin-dependent diabetics (White classes B, C and D) and the 24 normal women studied in the last
trimester of pregnancy are shown in Fig. 6. These patients had all been
hospital inpatients for at least two weeks and were treated with a mixture of
short and intermediate-acting insulins given before breakfast (8 a.m.) and
again before supper (6 p.m.). In addition, they were all judged to be well
controlled from the routine blood sugar estimations performed during the
week preceding the diurnal profile study. It is apparent that the mean diurnal
plasma glucose in this group (5.88 ± s.d. 1.19 mmol/l) was, however, much
higher than that of the control patients. Diurnal fluctuation was also greatly
increased, due mainly to the marked hyperglycaemia which occurred after
breakfast and the strong tendency to hypoglycaemia during the night which
resulted in a diurnal plasma glucose range of 6.95 ± s.d. 2.04 mmol/l. The
plasma glucose concentrations achieved, although excellent when compared
with those obtained in some non-pregnant diabetic patients (Service *et al.*
1970; Alberti 1973), bear little resemblance to those of normal women and
reflect the practical difficulties encountered when one tries to achieve a
balance between carbohydrate consumed and the insulin administered to
juvenile-onset diabetics. Thus in the insulin-dependent diabetic women the
mean plasma glucose concentration during the day (6.47 ± s.d. 1.75 mmol/l)

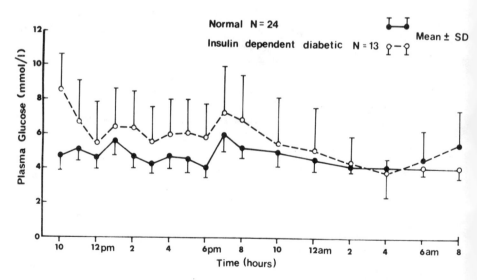

FIG. 6. Plasma glucose concentrations during the diurnal profile in 24 normal women and 13
insulin-dependent diabetics studied in the third trimester of pregnancy (based on Gillmer *et al.*
1975*a)*.

was greatly in excess of that observed in normal women (4.89 ± s.d. 0.43; $P < 0.01$), while at night hypoglycaemia developed in several patients and the mean for the lowest nocturnal glucose concentration was only 2.99 ± s.d. 0.66 mmol/l, compared to 3.73 ± s.d. 0.49 mmol/l in the normal group ($P < 0.005$).

The significance of these findings requires careful consideration, for although control may be judged to be satisfactory as far as the health of the mother is concerned, the possible effects of such an unstable glucose environment on the developing fetus are far-reaching. Thus it has been suggested that poor diabetic control during the first trimester may be responsible for abnormal embryogenesis (see Gabbe 1977 for review). In addition, Reid (1970) has suggested that some fetal cells may be particularly sensitive to changes in the plasma glucose concentration and that marked fluctuations may carry a greater risk of fetal deformity than persistent hyperglycaemia. It therefore seems preferable to avoid extreme fluctuations of the maternal plasma glucose concentrations whenever possible, although this is an ideal which is not easy to achieve in practice. The hyperglycaemia observed after breakfast, which also occurs in non-pregnant insulin-dependent diabetics (Jersild 1967), is particularly difficult to control. It probably represents a 'Somogyi effect' (Campbell 1976) and could possibly be eliminated if the patient took additional food after midnight or if the evening intermediate-acting insulin was replaced with divided doses of soluble insulin; both of these modifications to routine therapy, however, tend to be unacceptable in clinical practice.

Several recent studies, in which C-peptide measurements were used to assess endogenous insulin secretion, have shown that the degree of control which can be achieved in insulin-treated diabetics is greatly improved even if there is only minimal residual β-cell function (Faber & Binder 1977; Shima et al. 1977; Yue et al. 1978). In addition, Hendriksen and co-workers (1977) noted that most of the diabetics in their study who displayed residual C-peptide secretion (36 out of 83) had been diabetics for less than five years. In an investigation of seven insulin-treated diabetics in late pregnancy, Lewis et al. (1976) detected C-peptide in three patients who received insulin for the first time during pregnancy but not in four juvenile-onset diabetics. Similar results have been obtained in 12 insulin-treated diabetics (six chemical and six insulin-requiring, ketosis-prone patients) by B. Persson and co-workers (work in progress). Plasma C-peptide immunoreactivity and glucose concentrations were measured in these patients and a control group at frequent intervals during a so-called 8-h profile (7.30 a.m. to 4 p.m.) in late pregnancy (mean 36 weeks). All the women studied were encouraged to be active in the ward and received prefabricated meals at 8 a.m., 11.30 a.m. and 3 p.m.; these contained 380, 550 and 190 kcal (1600, 2300 and 800 kJ), respectively, and each consisted of 45% carbohydrate, 27% fat and 28% protein.   C-peptide and glucose values were closely correlated in the non-diabetic controls and insulin-treated gestational diabetics, but only half of the insulin-requiring diabetics had detectable C-peptide levels.   The relation between glucose and C-peptide from the 8-h profile in three individuals – one control, one chemical diabetic and one insulin-requiring diabetic – is shown in Fig. 7.   Indices of the regulatory stability of blood glucose, such as the individual values for the mean amplitude of glycaemic excursions (MAGE; Service *et al.* 1970) and the standard deviation (s.d.) of all glucose values during the 8-h profile, tended to be inversely correlated to the total area under the 8-h C-peptide curve.   However, in accordance with the data reported by Lewis and co-workers (1976) it was found to be possible to achieve low glucose variability (as measured by MAGE or s.d.) in insulin-requiring diabetics with no detectable C-peptide levels in late pregnancy.   This observation is also in agreement with the well-recognized clinical experience that regulation of the blood glucose level in the diabetic becomes easier as gestation progresses (Persson 1974; Lev-Ran & Goldman 1977).   In a larger series of 41 insulin-treated pregnant diabetics Persson and co-workers have also determined the fasting levels of C-peptide on several occasions (an average of eight times) during the last trimester of gestation.   The average C-peptide level from each subject displayed a significant inverse correlation with both the mean of daily difference in paired blood glucose values

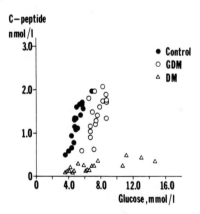

FIG. 7.   Relation between plasma concentrations of C-peptide and glucose in one control subject, one insulin-treated gestational diabetic (GDM), and one insulin-dependent diabetic (DM) during an 8-h period in the third trimester of pregnancy.

(MODD) determined at 10 a.m. (an index of day-to-day glucose variations) and the standard deviation of all fasting glucose values determined during the last trimester of pregnancy ($r = -0.63$ and $r = -0.65$ respectively; $P <$ 0.001). These results confirm recently published findings in non-pregnant subjects (Shima *et al.* 1977; Hendriksen *et al.* 1977; Faber & Binder 1977; Yue *et al.* 1978) and clearly indicate that the degree of diabetic instability is inversely correlated with the residual β-cell secretory function. It is of interest in this context that morphological changes in the diabetic placenta such as villous branching, syncytial knots and vasculo-syncytial membranes are associated with the degree of maternal blood glucose stability. These placental changes become more common with increasing instability of blood glucose control (expressed as MODD-values) calculated for the period 12–30 weeks of pregnancy (Björk & Persson 1978).

The cause of the sudden unexpected death of the macrosomic diabetic fetus in late pregnancy remains uncertain and although two theories have been proposed both link death to diabetic control by inference alone. Thus Shelley and co-workers (1975) observed a close positive correlation between maternal hyperglycaemia and fetal hyperlactataemia in the fetal lamb when a rise in the plasma lactate concentration was induced by making the ewe breathe a mixture of 9% oxygen, 3% carbon dioxide and 88% nitrogen. They therefore suggested that fetal death may occur when maternal hyperglycaemia complicates a pregnancy in which there is relative fetal hypoxia due to placental insufficiency. Oakley *et al.* (1972), on the other hand, observed relatively lower plasma glucose and higher plasma insulin concentrations in the fetus of the diabetic mother compared to that of the normal woman and suggested that inappropriate fetal hyperinsulinism during asymptomatic episodes of nocturnal hypoglycaemia may result in cerebral damage or even fetal death. Little is known, however, about the effect of maternal hypoglycaemia on the human fetus in late pregnancy. The acute effects of insulin-induced hypoglycaemia on the concentration of other circulating substrates and hormones and on fetal heart activity have therefore been studied by Persson and co-workers (work in progress) in five subjects (two insulin-treated chemical diabetics and three insulin-requiring ketosis-prone diabetics). All the women received their usual insulin treatment in the morning and approximately two hours after lunch they were given an intravenous injection of fast-acting insulin (0.1 i.u./kg body weight). Venous blood samples were taken before and at frequent intervals after the insulin administration. These were analysed for glucose, lactate, free fatty acids (FFA), glycerol, 3-hydroxybutyrate, C-peptide, cyclic AMP and amino acids. Four of the five diabetics had detectable levels of C-peptide and these declined in parallel with the plasma glucose concentration after the insulin injection (Fig. 8). This ability to 'shut off' insulin secretion during hypoglycaemia was also observed by Shima *et al.* (1977) in diabetic subjects with residual β-cell function and is an important mechanism in blood glucose regulation.   Plasma FFA and 3-hydroxybutyrate concentrations also fell after the insulin injection, suggesting decreased lipid mobilization (Figs. 9 and 10).   The essentially unchanged glycerol concentrations during the first 15 min after the insulin injection (Fig. 9) were unexpected and suggest that there was no measurable decrease in lipolysis during this period.   A progressive increase in the glycerol and lactate concentrations was observed about 20 min after insulin administration.   This can probably be attributed to enhanced catecholamine secretion induced by glycopenia (Christensen *et al.* 1975), an explanation which is supported by the fact that a similar increase in cyclic AMP was observed about 20 min after the insulin injection and was followed at about 30 min by mild adrenergic symptoms in all the subjects studied.

There was no change in the fetal heart rate during the period of hypoglycaemia but there was a marked decline in baseline variability.   This returned to normal after intravenous glucose administration or the spontaneous rise in the plasma glucose concentration.

It has previously been shown that insulin administration lowers the concentration of the amino acids isoleucine, leucine, tyrosine, phenylalanine and valine (Crofford *et al.* 1964).   No significant change in the plasma concentration of free amino acids was, however, observed during the insulin-induced hypoglycaemia in the five pregnant diabetics in this study (Table 3, p. 108).

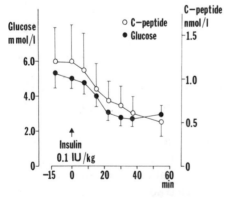

FIG. 8.   The effect of intravenous insulin administration on plasma C-peptide (n = 4) and glucose concentrations in five insulin-treated diabetics in the third trimester of pregnancy (mean ± S.E.M.).

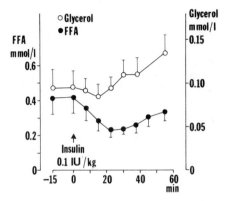

FIG. 9.   The effect of insulin-induced hypoglycaemia on the plasma free fatty acid (FFA) and glycerol concentrations in five insulin-treated diabetics in the third trimester of pregnancy (mean ± S.E.M.).

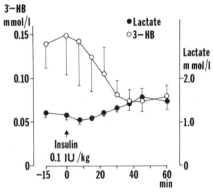

FIG. 10.   The effect of insulin-induced hypoglycaemia on the plasma 3-hydroxybutyrate (3-HB) and blood lactate concentrations in five insulin-treated diabetics in the third trimester of pregnancy (mean ± S.E.M.).

DIURNAL PLASMA FREE FATTY ACID PROFILES IN NORMAL AND DIABETIC PREGNANT WOMEN

Although it is widely accepted that late pregnancy is characterized by a state of accelerated starvation (Bleicher *et al.* 1964), there is considerable controversy whether the plasma FFA concentration after an overnight fast rises with advancing gestation.   Treharne *et al.* (1977), who have recently reviewed this subject, found that most recent studies including their own and those of Persson & Lunell (1975) have failed to demonstrate a significant increase in plasma FFA concentration in late pregnancy.   This may, however, be due to

TABLE 3

The effect of insulin-induced hypoglycaemia on venous plasma free amino acid concentrations in five diabetic women in late pregnancy (B. Persson *et al.,* work in progress) (mean ± S.E.M.)

Amino acid (μmol/l)	Before insulin [a]	After insulin [b]
Alanine	397 ± 57	392 ± 51
Valine	184 ± 27	186 ± 36
Proline	263 ± 17	260 ± 17
Lysine	212 ± 31	211 ± 25
Glycine	146 ± 23	142 ± 22
Histidine	106 ± 16	107 ± 11
Leucine	102 ± 16	103 ± 21
Glutamic acid	60 ± 9	56 ± 8
Phenylalanine	46 ± 5	46 ± 5
Isoleucine	60 ± 11	62 ± 13
Arginine	45 ± 8	46 ± 7
Tyrosine	43 ± 6	42 ± 7
Methionine	31 ± 7	34 ± 8
Aspartic acid	6 ± 1	6 ± 1

[a] = Insulin given as described in the text.
[b] = 55 min after the insulin injection.

differences in the length of the overnight fast. Treharne and co-workers also found similar levels of plasma FFA and glucose after an overnight fast in obese and non-obese women in early and late pregnancy.

Short-term changes in circulating plasma FFA, glycerol and 3-hydroxybutyrate, have been measured by Persson & Lunell (1975) over an 8-h period (as described above) in five control subjects, eight chemical diabetics (White Class A) and seven insulin-dependent diabetics. These profiles are shown in Figs. 11, 12 and 13. Higher overnight fasting values of all three substrates were observed in the chemical and insulin-dependent diabetic patients but these differences were not significant. After breakfast there was a rapid fall in the level of all three substrates in the control and chemical diabetic patients, reaching a nadir after about $1^1/_2$ hours, but with much lower FFA and 3-hydroxybutyrate concentrations in the control group. The levels of all three substrates gradually rose, in parallel, to near fasting values before lunch at 11.30 a.m., after which the concentrations again fell. In the insulin-dependent diabetics a mixture of lente and semi-lente insulin was given at 7.30 a.m., followed by the standardized breakfast at 8 a.m. The plasma FFA, glycerol and 3-hydroxybutyrate concentrations subsequently fell to levels similar to those seen in the control and chemical diabetic women but thereafter remained at low concentrations for the remaining 6 h of the study. Significant positive correlations were found between the paired FFA and glycerol levels in the control, chemical diabetic and insulin-dependent diabetic patients (r = 0.64, 0.73 and 0.87 respectively; $P < 0.001$). A significant inverse correlation between the plasma FFA and glucose concentrations was found

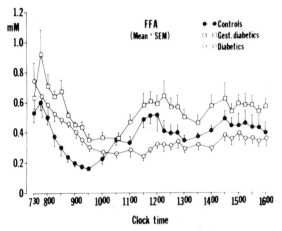

FIG. 11. Plasma free fatty acid (FFA) concentrations in five control subjects, eight gestational diabetics and seven insulin-dependent diabetics during an 8-h profile in the third trimester of pregnancy (from Persson, B. & Lunell, N.O. (1975) Metabolic control in diabetic pregnancy. *Am. J. Obstet. Gynecol. 122,* 737–745).

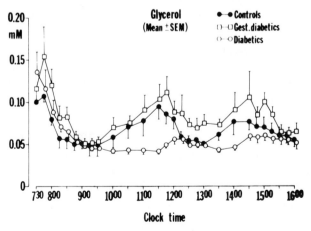

FIG. 12. Plasma glycerol concentrations in five control subjects, eight gestational diabetics and seven insulin-dependent diabetics during an 8-h profile in the third trimester of pregnancy (from Persson, B. & Lunell, N.O. (1975) Metabolic control in diabetic pregnancy. *Am. J. Obstet. Gynecol. 122,* 737–745).

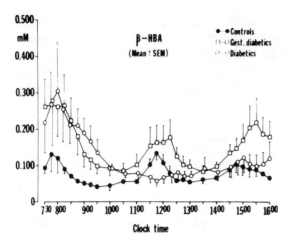

FIG. 13. Plasma 3-hydroxybutyrate (β-HBA) concentrations in five control subjects, eight gestational diabetics and seven insulin-dependent diabetics during an 8-h profile in the third trimester of pregnancy (from Persson, B. & Lunell, N.O. (1975) Metabolic control in diabetic pregnancy. *Am. J. Obstet. Gynecol. 122*, 737–745).

only in the control group ($r = 0.32$; $P < 0.001$). The reduced plasma FFA concentration of the insulin-treated diabetic women may be ascribed to the effect of exogenous insulin, which by inhibiting lipolysis and enhancing lipogenesis overcomes the state of accelerated starvation which characterizes late pregnancy. The observation that plasma FFA concentrations are depressed in the insulin-dependent diabetic patients despite the marked hyperglycaemia which they display may be explained by the differential action of exogenous insulin during late pregnancy this was not true of its antilipolytic effects. The absence of any correlation between plasma glucose and FFA and the raised that although there was marked resistance to the hypoglycaemic actions of insulin during late pregnancy this was not true of its antilipolytic effects. The absence of any correlation between plasma glucose and FFA and the raised levels of both substrates in chemical diabetics can be ascribed to insulin deficiency. The observation that there is a weak positive correlation ($r = 0.375$; $P = 0.048$) between the total glucose tolerance area and fasting 3-hydroxybutyrate concentration in normal women and untreated chemical diabetic patients would appear to support this concept (M.D.G. Gillmer *et al.*, unpublished observations).

NEONATAL OUTCOME

The infants delivered by diabetic women, especially those of White Class A

(Pedersen 1977), have a greater birth weight and birth length than expected for their gestational age and sex. They are also endowed with increased body fat and glycogen reserves (Osler 1961), but despite this they are more prone to develop neonatal hypoglycaemia (McCann et al. 1966).

In view of the differing carbohydrate and lipid environments provided for the developing fetus by the control, chemical diabetic, and insulin dependent diabetic woman described in the preceding sections it would appear to be appropriate to consider whether these metabolic aberrations could explain the characteristic fetal overgrowth and neonatal behaviour of the infant of the diabetic mother.

Neonatal hypoglycaemia

According to the hypothesis proposed by Pedersen (1952), maternal hyperglycaemia leads to fetal hyperglycaemia and subsequent hyperinsulinism. He demonstrated that the mean maternal glucose concentration during the last two months of pregnancy and the maternal glucose concentration at delivery were both inversely correlated with the mean glucose level in the infant during the first 24 h after birth. Evidence in support of this concept was provided by the finding that a variety of indices, derived from the maternal diurnal glucose profiles and oral glucose tolerance tests of the control and chemical diabetic women as described in the first section above, displayed a highly significant negative correlation with the absolute plasma glucose concentration of the neonate two hours after delivery (Gillmer et al. 1975b; see Table 4) and a positive correlation with the rate of glucose utilization during

TABLE 4

Pearson correlation coefficient (r) between maternal and neonatal indices of carbohydrate tolerance (from Gillmer et al. 1975b).

	Neonatal incremental K	Neonatal plasma glucose (at 2 h)
Oral GTT total area	0.678[a]	−0.690[a]
Oral GTT 2-h plasma glucose	0.593[a]	−0.620[a]
Oral GTT incremental area	0.571[a]	−0.591[a]
Mean diurnal plasma glucose	0.456[b]	−0.409[c]
Mean daytime plasma glucose	0.473[b]	−0.451[b]
Maximum diurnal plasma glucose	0.502[b]	−0.513[b]
Diurnal plasma glucose range	0.444[c]	−0.471[b]

[a] $P < 0.001$ [b] $P < 0.005$ [c] $P < 0.05$

the first two hours after birth (expressed as the 'neonatal incremental K value'). In addition, the plasma insulin concentration was higher, two hours after delivery, in the infants of the chemical diabetic patients than in those of the normal women, while the plasma glucose concentration was much lower (see Table 5). These findings have not been confirmed in more recent studies (Martin *et al.* 1975; Persson *et al.* 1976; Hall *et al.* 1977) but it must be emphasized that the 10 chemical diabetics whose infants were included in the present analysis were all *untreated*. Of the 13 patients originally studied, three required diet and insulin and were therefore excluded from the analyses, whereas in most other studies patients in whom strict diet or insulin therapy was used to normalize the maternal plasma glucose profile have not been excluded. This may have resulted in a different feto-maternal relationship.

It is also of interest that the diurnal index which displayed the strongest correlation with the 'neonatal incremental K value' was the maximum (or peak) diurnal plasma glucose and the best single GTT index was the 1-h (or peak) value. Persson and co-workers (1976) also found a positive correlation between the so-called mean of the daily differences in paired blood glucose values at 10 a.m. in the mothers (MODD) and the 2-h K_t values of the infants. Wide fluctuations in the blood glucose concentration during pregnancy thus seem to be of importance in provoking hyperinsulinism in the fetus and neonate. This is in keeping with the findings of Grasso and co-workers (1975), who showed that when an intravenous glucose infusion is given to premature neonates so that the plasma glucose concentration is raised to about 6 mmol/l (the level which probably occurs after meals in the fetus of the chemical diabetic woman) this sensitizes the pancreatic β-cell so that a subse-

TABLE 5

Neonatal plasma glucose and insulin values at birth and two hours later (mean ± S.D.) (number in brackets). (From Gillmer *et al.* 1975*b*.)

	Neonatal glucose (mmol/l)		Neonatal insulin (mU/l)	
	Birth	*At 2 h*	*Birth*	*At 2 h*
Normal women	4.70 ± 0.89 (21)	2.39 ± 0.39 (21)	0.71 ± 0.59 (21)	0.27 ± 0.23 (20)
Chemical diabetics	4.93 ± 1.07 (10)	1.59 ± 0.58 (10)	1.19 ± 0.69 (8)	0.48 ± 0.18 (9)
$P <$	N.S.	0.002	N.S.	0.02

quent glucose infusion results in a greatly enhanced insulin response. These observations emphasize the need for strict control of maternal plasma glucose concentrations throughout pregnancy and labour in diabetic women.

Other factors which have been reported to predispose the infant of the diabetic mother to neonatal hypoglycaemia include deficient catecholamine (Stern et al. 1968) and glucagon secretion (Bloom & Johnston 1972) after delivery. No significant difference in the glucagon response during the first two hours after delivery was observed by Gillmer and co-workers (unpublished observations) in the infants of 20 normal and 9 untreated chemical diabetic women.

The mature human fetus has about 35 g glycogen and more than 500 g fat (Wolf et al. 1974). At birth the hepatic glycogen reserve diminishes rapidly and mobilization of triglyceride stores for energy production becomes essential as protein breakdown appears to be minimal during this period (Kraus et al. 1974). High plasma levels of free fatty acid and glycerol have been demonstrated in the immediate postnatal period in newborn infants (Novak et al. 1964; Persson & Gentz 1966; Wolf et al. 1974), indicating a rapid increase in lipolysis, and samples of subcutaneous fat from the gluteal region of newborn babies have also shown a high rate of glycerol release (Novak & Monkus 1970).

Reduced plasma free fatty acid concentrations have, however, been reported in the infants of diabetic mothers during this period despite their greatly increased adipose stores (Chen et al. 1965; Joassin et al. 1967; King et al. 1969; Mølsted-Pedersen et al. 1972), suggesting that lipolysis is inhibited as a result of the state of functional hyperinsulinism in these infants. Persson and co-workers (1973) confirmed these findings (Fig. 14) but reported that the mean plasma glycerol concentrations of the infants of control, chemical diabetic, and insulin-dependent diabetic women rose in parallel during the first two hours after birth. These observations suggest that although there is a comparable increase in postnatal lipolysis in all three groups, rapid re-esterification of FFA must occur in the infants of the insulin-dependent diabetic women and to a lesser extent in the infants of chemical diabetic women. These findings provide additional indirect evidence of a state of functional hyperinsulinism in the infants of diabetic mothers. Finally, although the asymptomatic hypoglycaemia observed during the immediate neonatal period provides a convenient marker of the effect of maternal glucose intolerance on fetal and neonatal carbohydrate metabolism, it does not appear to be of great practical importance as there is no evidence that it has any long-term effect on intellectual performance (Persson et al. 1978). This implies either that the circulating plasma glucose concentration does not

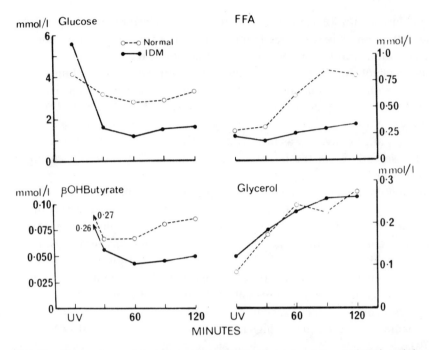

FIG. 14.   Plasma glucose, 3-hydroxybutyrate (βOHbutyrate), free fatty acid (FFA), and glycerol concentrations in control infants and infants of insulin-dependent diabetic mothers (IDM) in the umbilical venous blood at birth (UV) and during the first 2 h after delivery (drawn from data in Persson *et al.* 1973).

represent that available in the tissues, or alternatively that the neonatal brain uses other fuels.   Certainly the human fetal brain has the enzymes necessary to use ketones as an energy source (Williamson 1975) and 3-hydroxybutyrate utilization has been demonstrated, using the isolated perfused fetal head in mid-gestation.   In addition, Persson and co-workers (1978) have recently suggested that energy for the human brain in the immediate neonatal period may be derived not only from circulating glucose (Adam *et al.* 1975) but also from the glycogen stores in the medulla and spinal cord, a hypothesis which is based on the observation that newborn cats and dogs have glycogen stores in these tissues which are three to four times higher than those of the adult animal.

Fetal size at birth

A positive correlation between infant birth weight and the umbilical vein plasma insulin at birth has been found in several studies (Shima *et al.* 1966;

Thomas *et al.* 1967; Spellacy *et al.* 1973). This has been confirmed by M.D.G. Gillmer *et al.* (unpublished work) in an investigation of 23 normal infants and 10 infants delivered by untreated chemical diabetic women ($P <$ 0.05). A significant positive correlation between the mean diurnal plasma glucose and the total oral GTT area of the mother and the infant birth weight and plasma insulin concentration at delivery was also found in this study ($P <$ 0.05). The existence of a tripartite association between maternal carbohydrate tolerance, infant birth weight and neonatal plasma insulin concentration in these patients does not of course prove a causal relationship between the three factors but does appear to provide additional support for the Pedersen hypothesis (1952). In addition Whitelaw (1977) has reported a significant positive correlation between fasting plasma glucose values in pregnant diabetics and both the total skinfold thickness and mean gluteal adipose cell diameter of their offspring.

Szabo & Szabo (1974) have, however, questioned the concept that the excess adipose tissue mass of the infants born to diabetic mothers results from the transplacental transfer of excessive amounts of glucose. They have suggested that glucose is not the major precursor of fetal triglyceride fatty acids but only of the α-glycerophosphate necessary for triglyceride formation and that the higher FFA concentration in pregnant diabetics results in increased transfer of FFA to the fetus. Their views are supported by the demonstration in various species (Van Duyne *et al.* 1960, 1962; Hershfield & Nemeth 1968; Portman *et al.* 1969; Hull 1975) of placental transfer of FFA from the mother to fetus *in vitro* (Szabo *et al.* 1969; Dancis *et al.* 1973) and *in vivo* (Šabata *et al.* 1968; Sheath *et al.* 1972: Elphick *et al.* 1976). Further evidence that this transfer occurs in man may be derived from the observation that there is an average umbilical vein–artery FFA concentration difference of about 0.06 mmol/l which is positively correlated with the maternal FFA concentration at delivery (Šabata *et al.* 1968; Sheath *et al.* 1972; Elphick *et al.* 1976). The Szabos also supported their hypothesis by showing that the fasting maternal plasma FFA concentration is positively correlated with birth weight (Szabo *et al.* 1975). This finding has not, however, been confirmed in two recent studies (Gillmer *et al.* 1977; Treharne *et al.* 1977) in which a positive correlation was found between the fasting and mean diurnal plasma glucose concentration and infant percentile birth weight only ($r = 0.347$ and 0.311 respectively; $P < 0.05$). It is, however, of interest that in the study of Gillmer *et al.* (1977), similar mean percentile birth weights were observed in the untreated chemical diabetic and insulin-dependent diabetic patients (59 ± s.d. 22 and 61 ± s.d. 27) despite the differences in the mean diurnal plasma glucose and FFA concentrations in these two groups (Table 6). The extent to which the fetus

TABLE 6

Mean (± s.d.) diurnal plasma glucose and FFA (free fatty acid) concentrations in normal subjects and diabetics (from Gillmer *et al.* 1977).

	No. of patients	Mean diurnal plasma glucose (mmol/l)	Mean diurnal plasma FFA (mmol/l)
Normal subjects	23	4.70 ± 0.38	0.68 ± 0.20
Chemical diabetics	13	5.61 ± 1.03	0.77 ± 0.34
Insulin-dependent diabetics	11	6.02 ± 1.26	0.45 ± 0.11

uses the various substrates available to it is difficult to determine but as the FFA concentrations in the umbilical blood of the babies of normal and diabetic women are not significantly different (Sheath *et al.* 1972; Chen *et al.* 1965), it seems reasonable to assume that materno-fetal transfer will depend on the maternal concentration in the two groups.   It is thus possible that while the fetus of the chemical diabetic is exposed to both raised glucose and FFA concentrations, the rather higher plasma glucose levels of the insulin-dependent diabetics are offset by their greatly reduced plasma FFA concentration.   Fetal size may thus be influenced more by the total amount of available substrate crossing the placenta rather than by the maternal concentrations of glucose or FFA alone.

Only a few measurements of amino acid concentrations in the infants of diabetic mothers have been published (Butterfield & O'Brien 1963; Ghadimi & Pecora 1964; Cockburn *et al.* 1971; Reisner *et al.* 1973; Vejtorp *et al.* 1977).   Cockburn and co-workers found no difference in the total maternal or fetal amino acids in normal and diabetic pregnancies, whereas Vejtorp and co-workers found lower amino acid concentrations in the infants of the diabetic mothers than those of normal women and also a significantly reduced feto-maternal ratio in the diabetic group.   This could be a consequence of fetal hyperinsulinaemia with enhanced amino acid uptake, or alternatively there may be impaired placental transfer of amino acids.   The difference between the findings of these two studies is difficult to explain but the fact that the mean birth weight in the study of Cockburn *et al.* (1971) was 1 kg higher than that in the study of Vejtorp *et al.* (1977) may be a major factor.   The latter group have suggested that the progressive fall in mean infant birth weight through the White classes (Pedersen 1977) may in part result from impaired placental amino acid transfer.   Further research is, however, necessary to confirm or refute this hypothesis.

ACKNOWLEDGEMENTS

Bengt Persson was supported by grants from the Swedish Medical Research Council, projects 19P-4106 and 19X-3787 and the Tielmans Fund for Pediatric Research.

References

ADAM, P. A. J., RÄIHÄ, N., RAHIALA, E. L. & KEKOMÄKI, M. (1975) Oxidation of glucose and D-B-OH butyrate by the early human fetal brain. *Acta Paediatr. Scand. 64*, 17–24

ALBERTI, K. G. M. M. (1973) Blood metabolites in the diagnosis and treatment of diabetes mellitus. *Postgrad. Med. J. Suppl. (7) 49*, 955–963

ALBERTI, K. G. M. M., DORNHORST, A. & ROWE, A.S. (1975) Metabolic rhythms in normal and diabetic man. Studies in insulin treated diabetics. *Isr. J. Med. Sci. 11*, 571–580

BJÖRK, O. & PERSSON, B. (1978) Placental morphology in maternal diabetes mellitus. *Abstr. Clin. Res. 26*, 189

BLEICHER, S. J., O'SULLIVAN, J. B. & FREINKEL, N. (1964) Carbohydrate metabolism in pregnancy V. The interrelationships of glucose, insulin and free fatty acids in late pregnancy and postpartum. *N. Engl. J. Med. 271*, 866–872

BLOOM, S. R. & JOHNSTON, D. I. (1972) Failure of glucagon release in infants of diabetic mothers. *Br. Med. J. 4*, 453–454

BRUDENELL, M. (1975) Care of the clinical diabetic woman in pregnancy and labour, in *Carbohydrate Metabolism in Pregnancy and the Newborn* (Sutherland, H. W. & Stowers, J. M., eds.), pp. 221–225, Churchill Livingstone, Edinburgh

BURT, R. L. (1960) Plasma nonesterified fatty acids in pregnancy II. Experimental modification. *Am. J. Obstet. Gynecol. 80*, 965–971

BURT, R. L. (1962) Glucose tolerance in pregnancy. *Diabetes 11*, 227–228

BUTTERFIELD, L. J. & O'BRIEN, D. (1963) The effect of maternal toxaemia and diabetes on transplacental gradients of free amino acids. *Arch. Dis. Child. 38*, 326–327

CAMPBELL, I. W. (1976) The Somogyi phenomenon. A short review. *Acta Diabetol. Lat. 13*, 68–73

CARRINGTON, E. R. & McWILLIAMS, N. B. (1966) Investigation of serum insulin activity during pregnancy in normal and subclinically diabetic mothers. *Am. J. Obstet. Gynecol. 96*, 922–927

CHEN, C. H., ADAM, P. A. J., LASKOWSKI, D. E., McCANN, M. L. & SCHWARTZ, R. (1965) Plasma free fatty acid composition and blood glucose of normal and diabetic pregnant women and their newborns. *Pediatrics 36*, 843–855

CHRISTENSEN, N. J., ALBERTI, K. G. M. M. & BRANDSBORG, O. (1975) Plasma catecholamines and blood substrate concentrations: studies in insulin induced hypoglycaemia and after adrenaline infusions. *Eur. J. Clin. Invest. 5*, 415–423

COCKBURN, F., BLAGDEN, A., MICHIE, E. A. & FORFAR, J. O. (1971) The influence of pre-eclampsia and diabetes mellitus on plasma free amino acids in maternal, umbilical vein and infant blood. *J. Obstet. Gynaecol. Br. Commonw. 78*, 215–231

CROFFORD, O. B., FELTZ, P. W. & LACY, W.W. (1964) Effect of glucose infusions on the individual plasma free amino acids in man. *Proc. Soc. Exp. Biol. Med. 117*, 11–14

DANCIS, J., JANSEN, V., KAYDEN, H. J., SCHNEIDER, J. & LEVITZ, M. (1973) Transfer across perfused human placenta II. Free fatty acids. *Pediatr. Res. 7*, 192–197

ELPHICK, M. G., HULL, D. & SANDERS, R. R. (1976) Concentrations of free fatty acids in maternal and umbilical cord blood during Caesarean section. *Br. J. Obstet. Gynaecol. 83*, 539–544

ESSEX, N. L., PYKE, D. A., WATKINS, P. J., BRUDENELL, J. M. & GAMSU, H. R. (1973) Diabetic pregnancy. *Br. Med. J. 4*, 89–93

FABER, O. K. & BINDER, C. (1977) B-cell function and blood glucose control in insulin dependent diabetics within the first month of insulin treatment. *Diabetologia 13,* 263–268

FELIG, P. & LYNCH, V. (1970) Starvation in human pregnancy: hypoglycemia, hypoinsulinemia and hyperketonemia. *Science (Wash. D.C.) 170,* 990–992

GABBE, S. G. (1977) Congenital malformations in infants of diabetic mothers. *Obstet. Gynecol. Surv. 32,* 125–132

GHADIMI, H. & PECORA, P. (1964) Free amino acids of cord plasma as compared with maternal plasma during pregnancy. *Pediatrics 34,* 182–191

GILLMER, M. D. G., BEARD, R. W., BROOKE, F. M. & OAKLEY, N. W. (1975*a*) Carbohydrate metabolism in pregnancy. Part I. Diurnal plasma glucose profile in normal and diabetic women. *Br. Med. J. 3,* 399–402

GILLMER, M. D. G., BEARD, R. W., BROOKE, F. M. & OAKLEY, N. W. (1975*b*) Carbohydrate metabolism in pregnancy. Part II. Relation between maternal glucose tolerance and glucose metabolism in the newborn. *Br. Med. J. 3,* 402–404

GILLMER, M. D. G., BEARD, R. W., OAKLEY, N. W., BROOKE, F. M., ELPHICK, M. C. & HULL, D. (1977) Diurnal plasma free fatty acid profiles in normal and diabetic pregnancies. *Br. Med. J. 2,* 670–673

GRASSO, S., DISTEFANO, G., MESSINA, A., VIGO, R. & REITANO, G. (1975) Effect of glucose priming on insulin response in the premature infant. *Diabetes 24,* 291–294

HADDEN, D. R. (1975) Glucose tolerance test in pregnancy, in *Carbohydrate Metabolism in Pregnancy and the Newborn* (Sutherland, H. W. & Stowers, J. M., eds.), pp. 19–41, Churchill Livingstone, Edinburgh

HALL, R. T., RHODES, P. G., FERNANDES, F. & GRUNT, J. (1977) Glucose disappearance in infants of diabetic mothers. I. Relation to maternal glucose tolerance and insulin production. *Early Hum. Dev. 1,* 247–256

HENDRIKSEN, C., FABER, O. K., DREJER, J. & BINDER, C. (1977) Prevalence of residual B-cell function in insulin-treated diabetics evaluated by the plasma C-peptide response to intravenous glucagon. *Diabetologia 13,* 615–619

HERSHFIELD, M. S. & NEMETH, A. M. (1968) Placental transport of free palmitic and linoleic acids in the guinea pig. *J. Lipid Res. 9,* 460–468

HULL, D. (1975) Storage and supply of free fatty acids before and after birth. *Br. Med. Bull. 31,* 32–36

JERSILD, M. (1967) Postprandial blood sugar rise in diabetics. *Acta Med. Scand. Suppl. 476,* 101–107

JOASSIN, G., PARKER, M. L., PILDES, R. S. & CORNBLATH, M. (1967) Infants of diabetic mothers. *Diabetes 16,* 306–311

KALKHOFF, R., SCHACH, D. S., WALKER, J. L., BECK, P., KIPNIS, D. M. & DAUGHADAY, W. H. (1964) Diabetogenic factors associated with pregnancy. *Trans. Assoc. Am. Phys. 77,* 270–280

KARLSSON, K. & KJELLMER, I. (1972) The outcome of diabetic pregnancies in relation to the mother's blood sugar level. *Am. J. Obstet. Gynecol. 112,* 213–220

KIM, Y. J. & FELIG, P. (1972) Maternal and amniotic fluid substrate levels during caloric deprivation in human pregnancy. *Metabolism 21,* 507–512

KING, K. C., ADAM, P. A. J., CLEMENTE, G. A. & SCHWARTZ, R. (1969) Infants of diabetic mothers attenuated glucose uptake without hyperinsulinemia during continuous glucose infusion. *Pediatrics 44,* 381–392

KRAUS, H. S., SCHLENKER S. & SCHWEDESKY, D. (1974) Developmental changes of cerebral ketone body utilisation in human infants. *Hoppe-Seyler's Z. Physiol. Chem. 355,* 164–170

LEV-RAN, A. & GOLDMAN, J. A. (1977) Brittle diabetes in pregnancy. *Diabetes 26,* 926–930

LEWIS, S. B., WALLIN, J. D., KUZUYA, H., MURRAY, W. K., COUSTAN, D. R., DAANE, T. A. & RUBENSTEIN, A.H. (1976) Circadian variation of serum glucose, C-peptide immunoreactivity and free insulin in normal and insulin-treated diabetic pregnant subjects. *Diabetologia 12,* 343–350

LIND, T., BILLEWICZ, W. Z. & BROWN, G. (1973) A serial study of changes occurring in the oral glucose tolerance test during pregnancy. *J. Obstet. Gynaecol. Br. Commonw. 80*, 1033–1039

LORETI, L., SUGASE, T. & FOA, P.P. (1974) Diurnal variations of serum insulin, total glucagon, cortisol, glucose and free fatty acids in normal and diabetic subjects before and after treatment with chlorpropamide. *Horm. Res. (Basel) 5*, 278–292

MARTIN, F. I. R., KAHLENBURG, G. W., FUSSEL, J. & JEFFERY, P. (1975) Neonatal hypoglycaemia in infants of insulin-dependent diabetics. *Arch. Dis. Child. 50*, 472–476

MATTHEWS-DUNCAN, J. (1883) On puerperal diabetes. *Trans. Obstet. Soc. Lond. 24*, 256–285

MCCANN, M. L., CHEN, C. H., KATIGBAK, E. B., LOTCHEN, J. M., LIKLY, B. F. & SCHWARTZ, R. (1966) Effects of fructose on hypoglucosemia in infants of diabetic mothers. *N. Engl. J. Med. 275*, 1–7

MØLSTED-PEDERSEN, L., WAGNER, L., KLEBE, J. G. & PEDERSEN, J. (1972) Aspects of carbohydrate metabolism in newborn infants of diabetic mothers IV. Neonatal changes in plasma free fatty acid concentration. *Acta Endocrinol. 71*, 338–345

NOVAK, M. & MONKUS, E. (1970) Determination of the oxygen consumption of isolated adipose tissue cells obtained by needle trocar puncture. *Anal. Biochem. 36*, 454–463

NOVAK, M., MELICHAR, V. & HAHN, P. (1964) Postnatal changes in the blood serum content of glycerol and fatty acids in human infants. *Biol. Neonat. 7*, 179–194

OAKLEY, W. G. (1965) The treatment of pregnancy in diabetes mellitus, in *On the Nature and Treatment of Diabetes Mellitus* (Leibel, B.S. & Wrenshall, G. A., eds.), pp. 673–678, Int. Congr. Series 84, Excerpta Medica, Amsterdam

OAKLEY, N. W., BEARD, R. W. & TURNER, R. C. (1972) Effect of sustained maternal hyperglycaemia on the fetus in normal and diabetic pregnancies. *Br. Med. J. 1*, 466–469

OSLER, M. (1961) *Body Composition of Newborn Infants of Diabetic Mothers.* Thesis, Copenhagen

PEDERSEN, J. (1952) *Diabetes and Pregnancy. Blood Sugar of Newborn Infants.* Thesis, Danish Science Press, Copenhagen

PEDERSEN, J. (1967) *The Pregnant Diabetic and her Newborn. Problems and Management,* 1st edn., Munksgaard, Copenhagen

PEDERSEN, J. (1977) *The Pregnant Diabetic and her Newborn. Problems and Management,* 2nd edn., Munksgaard, Copenhagen

PEEL, J. P. (1972) A historical review of diabetes and pregnancy. *J. Obstet. Gynaecol. Br. Commonw. 79*, 385–395

PERSSON, B. (1974) Assessment of metabolic control in diabetic pregnancy, in *Size at Birth (Ciba Found. Symp. 27),* pp. 247–273, Elsevier/Excerpta Medica/North-Holland, Amsterdam

PERSSON, B. & GENTZ, J. (1966) The pattern of blood lipids, glycerol and ketone bodies during the neonatal period, infancy and childhood. *Acta Paediatr. Scand. 55*, 353–362

PERSSON, B. & LUNELL, N. O. (1975) Metabolic control in diabetic pregnancy. *Am. J. Obstet. Gynecol. 122*, 737–741

PERSSON, B., GENTZ, J. & KELLUM, M. (1973) Metabolic observations in infants of strictly controlled diabetic mothers I. *Acta Paediatr. Scand. 62*, 465–473

PERSSON, B., FEYCHTING, H. & GENTZ, S. (1975) Management of the infant of the diabetic mother, in *Carbohydrate Metabolism in Pregnancy and the Newborn* (Sutherland, H. W. & Stowers, J. M., eds.) pp. 232–248, Churchill Livingstone, Edinburgh

PERSSON, B., GENTZ, J., KELLUM, M. & THORELL, J. (1976) Metabolic observations in strictly controlled diabetic mothers II. *Acta Paediatr. Scand. 65*, 1–9

PERSSON, B., GENTZ, J. & LUNELL, N. O. (1978) Diabetes in pregnancy, in *Reviews in Perinatal Medicine,* vol. 2 (Scarpelli, E. M. & Cosmi, E.V., eds.), pp. 1–55, Raven Press, New York

PORTMAN, O. W., BEHRMAN, R. E. & SOLTYS, O. (1969) Transfer of free fatty acids across the primate placenta. *Am. J. Physiol. 216*, 143–147

REID, R.A. (1970) Diabetes and congenital abnormalities. *Lancet 1*, 1030–1031

REISNER, S. H., ARANDA, J. V., COLLE, E., PAPAGEORGIO, A., SCHIFF, D., SCRIVER, O. R. & STERN, L. (1973) The effect of intravenous glucagon on plasma amino acids in the newborn. *Pediatr. Res. 7*, 184–191

ŠABATA, V., WOLF, H. & LAUSMANN, S. (1968) The role of free fatty acids, glycerol, ketone bodies, and glucose in the energy metabolism of the mother and fetus during delivery. *Biol. Neonat. 13,* 7–17

SERVICE, F. J., MOLNAR, G. D., ROSEVEAR, J. W., ACKERMAN, E., GATEWOOD, L. C. & TAYLOR, W. F. (1970) Mean amplitude of glycemic excursions a measure of diabetic instability. *Diabetes 19,* 644–655

SHEATH, J., GRIMWADE, J., WALDRON, K., BICKLEY, M., TAFT, P. & WOOD, C. (1972) Arteriovenous nonesterified fatty acids and glycerol differences in the umbilical cord at term and their relationship to fetal metabolism. *Am. J. Obstet. Gynecol. 113,* 358–362

SHELLEY, H. J., BASSETT, J. M. & MILNER, R. O. G. (1975) Control of carbohydrate metabolism in the fetus and the newborn. *Br. Med. Bull 31,* 37–43

SHIMA, K., PRICE, S. & FOA, P. P. (1966) Serum insulin concentration and birthweight in human infants. *Proc. Soc. Exp. Biol. Med. 121,* 55–59

SHIMA, K., TANAKA, R., MORISHITA, S., TARUI, S., KUMAHARA, Y., & NISHIKAWA, M. (1977) Studies on the etiology of 'Brittle Diabetes'. Relationship between diabetic instability and insulinogenic reserve. *Diabetes 26,* 717–725

SLUITER, W. J., ERKELENS, D. W., REITSMA, W. D. & DOORENBOS, H. (1976*a*) Glucose tolerance and insulin release, a mathematical approach I. Assay of the beta-cell response after oral glucose loading. *Diabetes 25,* 241–244

SLUITER, W. J., ERKELENS, D. W., TERPSTRA, P., REITSMA, W. D. & DOORENBOS, H. (1976*b*) Glucose tolerance and insulin release, a mathematical approach. Approximation of the peripheral insulin resistance after oral glucose loading. *Diabetes 25,* 245–249

SPELLACY, W. N. (1975) Maternal and fetal metabolic interrelationships, in *Carbohydrate Metabolism in Pregnancy and the Newborn* (Sutherland, H. W. & Stowers, J. M., eds.), pp. 45–57, Churchill Livingstone, Edinburgh

SPELLACY, W. N., BUHI, W. C., BRADLEY, B. & HOLSINGER, K. K. (1973) Maternal, fetal and amniotic fluid levels of glucose, insulin and growth hormone. *Obstet. Gynecol. 41,* 323–331

STERN, L. S., RAMOS, A. & LEDUC, J. (1968) Urinary catecholamine excretion in infants of diabetic mothers. *Pediatrics 42,* 598–605

SUTHERLAND, H. W. & STOWERS, J. M. (1975) The detection of chemical diabetes during pregnancy using the intravenous glucose tolerance test, in *Carbohydrate Metabolism in Pregnancy and the Newborn* (Sutherland, H. W. & Stowers, J. M., eds.), pp. 153-166, Churchill Livingstone, Edinburgh

SZABO, A. J. & SZABO, O. (1974) Placental free fatty acid transfer and adipose tissue development: an explanation of fetal adiposity in infants of diabetic mothers. *Lancet 2,* 498–499

SZABO, A. J., GRIMALDI, R. D. & JUNG, W. F. (1969) Palmitate transport across perfused human placenta. *Metabolism 18,* 406–415

SZABO, A. J., OPPERMAN, W., HANOVER, B., GUGUUCCI, C. & SZABO, O. (1975) Fetal adipose tissue development: relationship to maternal free fatty acid levels, in *Early Diabetes in Early Life* (Camerini-Davalos, R. A. & Cole, J. S., eds.), Academic Press, New York

THOMAS, K., DE GASPARO, K. & HOET, J. J. (1967) Insulin levels in umbilical artery and vein of newborn of normal and untreated latent diabetic mothers. *Diabetologia 3,* 299–305

TREHARNE, I. A. L., SUTHERLAND, H. W., STOWERS, J. M. & ROSS, I. S. (1977) Maternal plasma glucose and free fatty acid concentrations related to infant birthweight. *Br. J. Obstet. Gynaecol. 84,* 272–280

TYSON, J. E., RABINOWITZ, D., MERIMEE, T. J. & FRIESEN, H. (1969) Response of plasma insulin and growth hormone to arginine in pregnant and postpartum females *Am. J. Obstet. Gynecol. 103,* 313–319

VAN DUYNE, C. M., PARKER, H. R., HAVEL, R. J. & HOLM, L. W. (1960) Free fatty acid metabolism in fetal and newborn sheep. *Am. J. Physiol. 199,* 987–990

VAN DUYNE, C. M., HAVEL, R. J. & FELLS, J. M. (1962) Placental transfer of palmitic acid-1-C^{14} in rabbits. *Am. J. Obstet. Gynecol. 84,* 1069–1074

VEJTORP, M., PEDERSEN, J., KLEBBE, J. G. & LUND, E. (1977) Low concentrations of plasma amino acids in newborn babies of diabetic mothers. *Acta Paediatr. Scand. 66,* 53–58

VICTOR, A. (1974) Normal blood sugar variation during pregnancy. *Acta Obstet. Gynaecol. Scand. 53,* 37–40

WHITELAW, A. (1977) Subcutaneous fat in newborn infants of diabetic mothers: an indication of quality of diabetic control. *Lancet 1,* 15–18

WILLIAMS, J. W. (1909) The clinical significance of glycosuria in pregnant women. *Am. J. Med. Sci. 137,* 1–26

WILLIAMSON, O. H. (1975) Regulation of the utilisation of glucose and ketone bodies by the brain in the perinatal period, in *Early Diabetes in Early Life* (Camerini-Davalos, R.A. & Cole, J.S., eds.), pp. 195–202, Academic Press, New York

WOLF, H., STAVE, U., NOVAK, M. & MONKUS, E. F. (1974) Recent investigations on neonatal fat metabolism. *J. Perinat. Med. 2,* 75–87

YEN, S. S. C. (1973) Endocrine regulations of metabolic homeostasis during pregnancy. *Clin. Obstet Gynecol. 16,* 130–147

YEN, S. S. C., TSAI, C. C. & VELA, P. (1971) Gestational diabetogenesis. Quantitative analyses of glucose insulin interrelationships between normal pregnancy and pregnancy with gestational diabetes. *Am. J. Obstet. Gynecol. 111,* 792–800

YUE, D. K., BAXTER, R. C. & TURTLE, J. R. (1978) C-peptide secretion and insulin as determinants of stability in diabetes mellitus. *Metabolism 27,* 35–44

Discussion

Pedersen: I agree with most of what you said, but I thought it was generally agreed that in diabetic pregnancy there is no correlation between congenital malformations and hypoglycaemic shock, or, if there is, it is rather an inverse correlation. There have been up to 30 instances of insulin coma during the first trimester without any congenital malformations (Mølsted-Pedersen *et al.* 1964) and a series of 44 cases from Birmingham gave similar results (J. Malins, personal communication 1978). Next, there is a positive correlation with White's classifications. Cases classed as D and F had the highest rate of congenital malformations. The metabolic state of these women is much more severe than in women of classes B and C.

Gillmer: I would agree that most published reports show a higher incidence of congenital malformations with increasing severity of diabetes. In his review of this subject, however, Gabbe (1977) mentions a report of congenital malformations in infants of women treated with hypoglycaemic shock therapy.

Chez: Impastato *et al.* (1964) reported that 6 of 19 patients receiving insulin coma therapy sustained fetal damage. Five of these began their therapy before the 10th week of pregnancy. After the first trimester I think we are talking about the normal incidence of anomalies. This particular instance seems to be an all-or-none phenomenon. An insulinoma in pregnancy has been reported by Rubens *et al.* (1977). The patient had recurrent and severe hypoglycaemia with no abortion or congenital anomaly.   Rubens refers to one other similar patient.

Gillmer: In previous studies relating congenital malformation rates to the severity of diabetes, hypoglycaemic episodes may not have been recognized. Our diurnal profile studies (Gillmer *et al.* 1975) clearly demonstrated a high incidence of hitherto unrecognized nocturnal hypoglycaemia in insulin-dependent pregnant diabetics.   This probably occurs more frequently in the severe brittle diabetic, and an analysis of congenital malformation rates in brittle and stable diabetics would therefore be of interest.

Beard: We are talking about two separate things.   One is the acute episode of hypoglycaemia after insulin shock.   A lot of things are occurring there, not only metabolic changes but probably circulatory too, so it is difficult to draw any real conclusions.   What we are more concerned about is the prolonged hypoglycaemia in the insulin-dependent diabetic which is sometimes seen at night, which might be quite a different story.

Brudenell: I would be surprised if symptomatic hypoglycaemia in early pregnancy was associated with an increased incidence of congenital abnormalities.   In the first three months of pregnancy symptomatic hypoglycaemia in insulin-dependent diabetics is relatively uncommon.   The well-controlled non-pregnant diabetic woman is usually kept at a slightly hyperglycaemic level to avoid hypoglycaemia, which most diabetics fear.   This situation persists into the first trimester unless the woman has hyperemesis.

Pedersen: Hypoglycaemia after 8–10 weeks is characteristic in pregnant diabetic women.   Thus insulin coma peaks at about that time (Pedersen 1977).

Gillmer: The hypoglycaemic action of insulin has also been shown to be slightly enhanced during the first trimester compared to that observed during later pregnancy and in non-pregnant women (Yen 1973).

Garrow: Dr Gillmer, you mentioned that about half the chemical diabetics were also obese and that dietary treatment might be appropriate.   What dietary treatment do you suggest?   Were any of the women whose glucose and insulin profiles you showed on the diet?

Gillmer: Any suggestion of dietary restriction during pregnancy is greeted with raised eyebrows because of the association between ketonuria in pregnancy and intellectual impairment in the offspring reported by Churchill *et al.* (1969) and more recently by Stebhens *et al.* (1977).   I, however, think that it is reasonable to use, in the obese chemical diabetic patient, a form of carbohydrate restriction which aims to reduce fasting glucose levels to the normal range; this causes the patient to break down her triglyceride stores and use these for energy purposes, but stops short of fasting ketonuria.   We have achieved this in some chemical diabetic women but I am not sure whether it is possible in all obese patients.   We are now studying the effect of diet in obese women with normal glucose tolerance.   The effect of diet in obese chemical diabetics may be different.

Chez: I can't understand how a single episode can be the variable that makes the significant difference in a large group of patients.   When Lind & Hytten (1972) asked normal women to examine their urine daily or once a week throughout gestation, there was a high frequency of glycosuria.   No one that I know of has done the same thing for acetonuria in normal women, testing every urine passed on one day a week throughout 40 weeks of gestation.   Since a large number of patients vomit during the first trimester, and have diets that are for various reasons inadequate or inappropriate, acetonuria must be a common phenomenon throughout normal pregnancy.   The only information we have is from that one study where it was looked at during a prenatal clinic and was therefore identified as a statistical variable.   We should be suspicious and cautious in our interpretations.

Gillmer: We have measured the blood D-β-hydroxybutyrate concentrations in two women with normal glucose tolerance noted to have fasting ketonuria in late pregnancy despite a normal diet.   Their blood D-β-hydroxybutyrate concentrations were the same as those of non-ketonuric women during the last trimester of pregnancy.   As far as I am aware, very little is known about the relationship between urinary and blood ketones in normal women in late pregnancy.

I should also mention that the mean birth weight of the six obese women that we have studied so far is not different from that of a control group of comparable height.

Kalkhoff: How many calories are you talking about?

Gillmer: The diet of each obese patient is tailored according to her percentage ideal body weight.   Each diet contains between 120 and 150 grams of carbohydrate.   This is not a vast reduction from the 180 to 200 grams taken by normal women but it appears to be sufficient to mobilize stored triglyceride.   The total calorie content is approximately 1500 kilocalories (6300 kJ).

Chez: The amount of protein per kilogram of body weight is important in designing diets for pregnant women.   The present US standards urge at least 1.0 if not 1.3 g protein/kg per day.

Gillmer: We are using carbohydrate restriction as opposed to total dietary restriction.   We are not altering protein intake – simply the carbohydrate.

Freinkel: I believe that it will be very important to define your objectives and your end-point in this type of treatment.   In my presentation (this volume), I made a plea for more rigorous terminology for gestational diabetes.   The published papers in this area are very confusing because there is no uniformity in terminology.   Some workers call the patients gestational diabetics; others refer to them as chemical diabetics; some make the diagnosis retrospectively, others prospectively; etc.   I should like to make a plea for a classification along the lines that we have discussed in our manuscript.   As I mentioned, we designate diabetes discovered during pregnancy (using the oral glucose tolerance criteria of O'Sullivan & Mahan 1964) as A_1 when fasting plasma glucose is less than 105 mg/dl (5.83 mmol/l); as A_2 when fasting plasma glucose ranges from 105 to 130 mg/dl; and as B when fasting plasma glucose exceeds 130 mg/dl (7.2 mmol/l).   On a pathophysiological basis, we assume that the A_1 patient elaborates enough insulin to restrain catabolism in the fasted state and displays abnormalities only after eating.   In other words, she only manifests 'underutilization'.   On the other hand, the A_2 patient not only exhibits 'underutilization' in the fed state but also has some 'overproduction' as evidenced by the increase in fasting plasma glucose.   I tried to emphasize in my presentation that these considerations do not apply only to glucose but obtain equally for all the components in the dietary mixture that are also influenced by insulin action, such as amino acids and fats.   On a theoretical basis, one would assume that the abnormalities in the fasted state should be rectifiable by the administration of long-acting exogenous insulin.   On the other hand, the abnormalities in the A_1 patients reflect some limitation in insulin release in the acute phase.   Such abnormalities are difficult to rectify with current modalities for the delivery of insulin.   We have been making some efforts by more liberal administration of regular insulin with meals, but it is almost impossible to replicate endogenous acute insulin secretion.

In essence, what I am trying to say is that the evaluation of any therapeutic intervention will require prior rigorous classification of categories of patients and correspondingly precise establishment of therapeutic end-points.   We have been studying experimental weight reduction in Class A_1 gestational diabetics in our Diabetes in Pregnancy Center at Northwestern University in order to see whether this can offset the insulin resistance of obesity and enable adequate insulin secretion to supervene in the acute phase.   We are monitoring the fate of all ingested nutrients in this endeavour to evaluate whether the desired effects on 'acute' insulin secretion are not vitiated by an exaggeration of 'accelerated starvation'.   We have not been studying obese gestational diabetics classified as A_2 in comparable fashion because we infer, on the basis of their raised fasting plasma glucose levels, that the endogenous basal elaboration of insulin is insufficient to restrain catabolism even in the fasted state and that therapy with exogenous insulin is clearly indicated.

Gillmer: We would agree that the pregnant woman with a fasting venous plasma glucose in excess of 5.8 mmol/l requires insulin therapy.

Freinkel: I do not mean to assign inappropriate emphasis to ketones nor to extrapolate beyond the existing data in this regard. What is more important is that every single component in the ingested dietary mixture may be subjected to compromised anabolism because of inadequate acute insulin action. Thus, what one is truly trying to evaluate with the weight restriction programme is whether adequate acute anabolism and acute insulin secretion can be restored in such patients. Unless this is clearly articulated as an end-point, it will be difficult to assess the efficacy of your programme.

Gillmer: Would you not agree that weight reduction is a reasonable first step to achieving fasting normoglycaemia in the obese chemical diabetic? It is after all standard practice in the obese maturity-onset diabetic. Insulin therapy in obese pregnant chemical diabetics will produce normal fasting glucose values but it will also change the total substrate availability.

Freinkel: One can also establish some measurable parameters in patients requiring therapy with exogenous insulin. Although it may be impossible to normalize the immediate postprandial state in such subjects, one should be able to attain normalization after overnight fast and I would emphasize again that this should also apply to insulin-responsive nutrients other than glucose, e.g. amino acids, free fatty acids, esterified glycerides and ketones.

Gillmer: In our earlier studies (Gillmer *et al.* 1975) we used the neonatal plasma glucose concentration two hours after delivery as an index of the effect of maternal hyperglycaemia on the fetus. Approximately half of the infants delivered by the Class A_1 diabetics whom we studied displayed hypoglycaemia (plasma glucose ≤ 1.7 mmol/l). These were women who had a basal plasma glucose concentration of less than 5.8 mmol/l and, by your definition, normal basal insulin production.

The primary aim of treatment is to reduce the fasting glucose concentrations, not to improve pancreatic insulin production. This latter aim is achieved more slowly, as we know from studies in non-pregnant obese chemical diabetics.

Freinkel: I am afraid that there are very few data along these lines even in non-gravid subjects. For example, normalization of acute-phase insulin secretion was not examined in some of the best studies showing reversion of most metabolic abnormalities after weight reduction in non-gravid obese subjects (Kalkhoff *et al.* 1971).

Beard: It seems that we may have been overlooking the endogenous insulin response in our decisions on how and when to treat patients with insulin.

Freinkel: That is precisely what I have been trying to say. In other words, the nature of the acute insulin secretory response and the acute disposition of ingested nutrients may be the important variables in influencing our approaches.

Chez: What is the end-point for 'good'?   Clinically, diabetics who are getting insulin two or three times a day produce normal infants.

Freinkel: Our clinical approach since 1970 has been based on these considerations.   We have been treating most of our Class B diabetics with three injections of regular insulin with meals, in addition to the more traditional administration of intermediate-acting insulins.   The former have been designed to mimic 'acute' insulin release and the latter to provide adequate basal insulinization in the fasted state.

References

CHURCHILL, J. A., BERENDES, H. W. & NEMORE, J. (1969) Neuropsychological deficits in children of diabetic mothers.   *Am. J. Obstet. Gynecol. 105,* 257–268

GABBE, S. G. (1977) Congenital malformations in infants of diabetic mothers.   *Obstet. Gynecol. Surv. 32,* 125–132

GILLMER, M. D. G., BEARD, R. W., BROOKE, F. M. & OAKLEY, N. W. (1975) Carbohydrate metabolism in pregnancy.   Part I, Diurnal plasma glucose profile in normal and diabetic women.   *Br. Med. J. 3,* 399–402

GILLMER, M. D. G., BEARD, R. W., BROOKE, F. M. & OAKLEY, N. W. (1975) Carbohydrate metabolism in pregnancy.   Part II, Relation between maternal glucose tolerance and glucose metabolism in the newborn.   *Br. Med. J. 3,* 402–404

IMPASTATO, D. J., GABRIEL, A. R. & LARDARO, H. H. (1964) Electric and insulin shock therapy during pregnancy.   *Dis. Nerv. Syst. 25,* 542–546

KALKHOFF, R. K., KIM, H. J., CERLETTY, J. & FERROU, C. A. (1971) Metabolic effects of weight loss in obese subjects: Changes in plasma substrate levels, insulin and growth hormone responses.   *Diabetes 20,* 83–91

LIND, T. & HYTTEN, F. E. (1972) The excretion of glucose during normal pregnancy.   *J. Obstet. Gynaecol. Br. Commonw. 78,* 961–965

O'SULLIVAN, J. B. & MAHAN, C. H. (1964) Criteria for the oral glucose tolerance test in pregnancy.   *Diabetes 13,* 278–285

MØLSTED-PEDERSEN, L., TYGSTRUP, I. & PEDERSEN, J. (1964) Congenital malformations in newborn infants of diabetic women.   *Lancet 1,* 1124–1126

PEDERSEN, J. (1977) *The Pregnant Diabetic and Her Newborn,* 2nd edn., pp. 191-197, Munksgaard, Copenhagen

RUBENS, R., CARLIER, A., THIERY, M. & VERMEULEN, A. (1977) Pregnancy complicated by insulinoma.   *Br. J. Obstet. Gynaecol. 84,* 543–547

STEBHENS, J. A., BAKER, G. L. & KITCHELL, M. (1977) Outcome at 1, 3 and 5 years of children born to diabetic women.   *Am. J. Obstet. Gynecol. 127,* 408–413

YEN, S. S. C. (1973) Endocrine regulation of metabolic homeostasis during pregnancy.   *Clin. Obstet. Gynecol. 16,* 130–141

General Discussion II

Brudenell: Real-time ultrasound allows one to see what is actually happening to the fetus throughout a 24-hour period, if the patient can bear to be screened for that period. Seona Stubbs at Kings College Hospital has recently looked at fetal movement and breathing in some of our insulin-dependent diabetics. Although it is a preliminary observation, there is a correlation between the level of blood glucose and fetal breathing activity. When the blood glucose level falls fetal breathing movements diminish, and as the blood glucose level goes up again so fetal breathing movements increase. This seems to be true, too, for lactate, pyruvate and alanine, which Seona Stubbs also looked at on a 24-hour profile basis, with the patient under the real-time ultrasound scanner every three hours. It looks as though what is happening in the diabetic mother in metabolic terms has a direct effect on the fetus. Whether fetal breathing is a direct measure of fetal well-being is perhaps debatable but there is certainly an effect on the fetus. Over a long period of time this might be deleterious.

Beard: Have you done simultaneous continuous recordings of fetal heart rate?

Brudenell: In a patient who is having hourly blood glucose samples and is being wakened every three hours for scans, it is very difficult to do the heart rate as well. For the moment we are concentrating on the breathing.

Chez: John Patrick in London, Ontario, has been sharing some unpublished data with a number of people. The hours from midnight to 6.0 or 7.0 a.m. when there is gradual maternal hypoglycaemia are the exact time when fetal breathing movements increase. It is the opposite to what one sees during the day, when there is postprandial hyperglycaemia with an increased rate of fetal breathing movements.

Can we expand this particular topic into the question of hydramnios in diabetes? The amniotic cavity is another anatomical compartment which we have not talked about much and I am wondering whether there is any exchange of substrate with that compartment.   In terms of substrate concentration there, as well as turnover, the amniotic cavity might be an important place for some of the measuring that is being done.   I perceive the exchange as an intake–output type of thing.   Because of volumes, especially in primates, it may be an important place that we have to add on as a sink – or even a reservoir – for some future need.

For instance, here is a theory.   If there is a relationship between hyperglycaemia and fetal breathing, and if there is a relationship between fetal breathing and net tracheal/bronchial outflow from the lungs (and we know that there is a specific contribution of lung fluid to amniotic fluid volume), relative hyperglycaemia for 24 hours will enhance relative fetal hyperpnoea.   This could result in an enhancement of net fluid outflow and therefore hydramnios on that basis.   Also, what does that increased fluid do to the balance sheets we have been creating today for substrates?

Beard: That is a fascinating concept.

Brudenell: In our experience fetal breathing movements follow the blood glucose level fairly closely in most women.   As they become hypoglycaemic in the small hours of the morning, fetal breathing diminishes, in contrast to what Dr Chez has just reported.

Beard: Do fetal breathing movements diminish in the early hours of the morning in non-diabetics?

Brudenell: Yes, in general they do.

Gillmer: Fetal movement generally increases at night, compared to the day, in non-diabetics, but I am not sure about breathing movements.

Naeye: What is the significance of fetal breathing?   There are great variations between presumably normal human fetuses.

Brudenell: Fetal breathing may well turn out to be yet another disappointment in terms of precise evaluation of fetal well-being.   But if we thought a fetus was not breathing we would be very worried about it and we wouldn't be happy to let it go on unless there was other clear evidence that it was undamaged.   Sustained diminution in fetal breathing, like profound changes in fetal movements generally, are significant but it is very difficult to apply this to every individual case.

Beard: That is why I have argued consistently that continuous fetal heart rate records are at least as valid.   At present information on the fetal heart rate is easier to obtain and more reliable than fetal breathing.

Battaglia: Jean Girard mentioned individual organ metabolism in the discussion of my paper (p. 70).   There is good evidence from the studies of Breuer *et al.* (1967) that the heart of the newborn puppy is burning glucose, not free fatty acids.   The switch to free fatty acids as fuel for the heart occurs at some time postnatally.   I don't know of studies in fetuses but the clinical reports of congestive heart failure in the newborn, associated with severe hypoglycaemia, together with the studies on puppies, at least suggest that the fetal and newborn heart may be an obligatory carbohydrate consumer.   Therefore changes in fetal heart rate may still be very important, as Professor Beard suggests. The heart rate changes may be one more index that this organ's metabolic profile is different in the fetal and the immediate neonatal period from later in postnatal life.

Chez: Downing's work (Downing *et al.* 1977) suggests that the fetal heart in sheep has a component of non-esterified fatty acid for fuel as well as glucose.   But in the presence of persistent hyperglycaemia the mitochondria lose their need for, and no longer utilize, non-esterified fatty acids.   The mitochondria become entirely glucose-dependent.   Downing has also told me that if insulin is added to an isolated system using cardiac tissue from piglets and kittens, the heart loses its sensitivity to catechols and cannot respond with its normal alacrity.   We also know that there is a widened maternal–fetal plasma glucose gradient in the presence of maternal hyperglycaemia or hyperinsulinaemia with the fetal blood glucose closer to some magic level of hypoglycaemia.

Another fact we know is that when the fetus that is already anaerobic becomes hypoglycaemic its pH plummets.   This all adds up to a clinical set-up in which there is combined hypoglycaemia in the presence of hypoxia and a totally glucose-dependent heart which is not responsive to catechols under stress.   This fetal heart may then enter a state of synchrony leading to unexplained fetal death without the presence of maternal metabolic acidosis.   I can see a biochemical linkage that way, using three different species.

Beard: That is extending the concept of metabolic death with a sort of terminal hypoxia in these babies.

Pedersen: Although I felt that hypoglycaemia in congenital malformations was not important, I certainly agree that hypoglycaemia can be seen in the fetus.   This has a practical aspect for monitoring just before delivery.   Abnormalities may be due to fetal hypoglycaemia.   If the people who monitor are not well trained, they might go on to deliver instead of giving the mother more glucose.

Beard: You are suggesting that before delivery of the baby one should try to restore its blood sugar level?

Pedersen: Yes.

Brudenell: In general terms, the only stress to the fetus that produces regular fetal heart changes is anoxia.   Are metabolic changes in the diabetic mother therefore being mediated through anoxia, with some mild hypoxia plus hyperglycaemia making acidosis more severe?

Beard: I don't think we can agree with what you are suggesting. It is not only hypoxia that produces fetal heart changes. We have described tachycardia in the fetus of a mild diabetic mother who developed hypoglycaemia, almost certainly due to endogenous catecholamine release. This is in the absence of hypoxia. It can be successfully treated simply by giving the mother intravenous glucose (Roversi *et al.* 1977).

Naeye: The hearts of newborn infants of diabetic mothers are often abnormal. Many such neonates who die have cardiac hypertrophy, presumably due to increased cardiac work before birth.

Beard: Couldn't that be myocardial hypertrophy associated with the generalized macrosomia which is probably an insulin effect?

Naeye: It is often out of proportion to body weight.

Milner: I am becoming progressively more confused. The phrase 'generalized macrosomia' has just been used about infants of diabetic mothers. Fifteen years ago I thought that infants of diabetic mothers were bigger than normal because insulin was an anabolic hormone. I then read the work of Osler (1965) and realized that the infants were bigger than normal because they were heavier than normal but that they had an appropriate lean body mass for gestational age. Then I learnt that there was a small increase in lean body mass in morphometric terms (Naeye 1965), the increase being both in cell size and number in the heart, kidney and liver. So for years I disciplined myself to dissociate this weakest anthropometric index of growth–body weight–into two compartments, storage fat and lean body mass. Yet today my colleagues have been talking about growth and size and body weight as though they are synonymous. Could the people who did the original work sharpen the definitions for us?

Beard: That depends on the particular study to which you are referring.

Milner: I look upon insulin in the human fetus as having a permissive effect on fetal growth, not an overall controlling effect. In the last 10 weeks of gestation, insulin may control the filling of adipocytes with lipids that are going to make white adipose tissue. We think of the infant with transient neonatal diabetes mellitus as the clinical example *par excellence* of the converse of this hypothesis: a fetus that is insulinopenic born with little adipose tissue (Gentz & Cornblath 1969). Yet the infant with transient diabetes mellitus may have a normal lean body mass. It is possible that insulin can produce no more than a 5–10% modulation of lean body mass, while having the potential to underfill or overfill the white adipose cells. What is not clear is whether insulin can cause hyperplasia of white adipocytes. Does anyone dispute this?

Beard: Are you really asking what are our current concepts about the effect of hyperinsulinism on the various body compartments of the fetus?

Milner: My statements are based on a wide variety of contributions to studies of the human fetus.   There is morphometric work, work on DNA/protein ratios, anthropometric work, radiological studies, carcass analysis and so on.   When one puts all these together, this is the way it seems to me at the end.   But I am confused because my colleagues seem to look upon it rather differently.

Pedersen: We would certainly like to know the answers to all your questions.   But you seem to forget the inhomogeneity of the infants of diabetic mothers.   There is a wide variation both between and within White's classes, so the answers are not easy.   I would advise you to calculate what we call the overweight, not the birth weight.   That is, by determination of the subcutaneous fat you can calculate from the birth weight and the gestation time what the relative fat mass is.

Milner: I understand you perfectly.   I have no problems in accepting that point of view.   One has to take weight as a function of gestational age.   One also has the problem of placental function in any woman, diabetic or non-diabetic.   I don't think these variables are too complicated to permutate into the concepts I was talking about, and which I regard as the more fundamental pathophysiology: diabetic pregnancy as seen from the fetal point of view.

Naeye: Cell size is increased in most organs of newborns of diabetic mothers.   However, their brains do not appear to be affected.

Chez: Do brain and kidney participate in the organomegaly?

Naeye: The renal findings are complicated.   In addition to cellular hypertrophy, the glomeruli often become enlarged, perhaps due to an increased blood volume in the fetus.

Chez: If you take away extramedullary erythropoiesis from the liver, do you think the liver is still enlarged?

Naeye: Yes, excessive extramedullary haematopoiesis will not explain all of the enlargement.   The hepatic parenchymal cells are enlarged.

Gillmer: Is it possible to link the observation that the brain of the fetus of the diabetic mother is smaller than normal with the finding that plasma free fatty acid concentrations are reduced during insulin therapy (Table 6, p.116) and the fact that essential fatty acids are required for brain growth?   In other words could there be a reduction in the availability of essential fatty acids which interferes with brain development in these pregnancies?

Beard: We have heard of the different fuels that the fetus is presented with.   The impression I get is that there is a lot of fuel spilling over into the fetus and the fetus grows at a regulated rate.   What is imposing that regulation? If it is the fetus itself, what are the factors that are influencing that regulation? Or is it mainly maternally dominated? The diabetic model is interesting because, with even a marginally increased 24-hour glucose profile and slightly higher free fatty acids, the mother produces a baby that becomes hyperinsulinaemic, possibly in an attempt to control its own internal milieu for glucose. Can anyone put forward proposals about whether the fetus is regulating its own milieu and what the mechanisms are?

Battaglia: There are many ways, either in clinical states or in experimental animals, in which one could change substrate flow to the fetus. That is, the umbilical uptake of nutrients could be reduced by placental pathology, by reductions in blood flow or by changes in substrate concentration in the mother. So the first question might be whether there is any evidence that there is reduced substrate flow to the baby. The next question is, how does the baby respond to that? Certainly the fetus makes a very appropriate defence against starvation. It develops hypoinsulinaemia, thus it reduces its glucose utilization rate, and it slows its rate of growth. All these steps are appropriate in terms of surviving a restriction in nutrient supply. We don't see any change in metabolic rate, which would be the adult's response to starvation, so that might be a more fixed biological parameter, if you like. If one asks whether chronic hyperinsulinaemia can produce true growth of fat-free or lean body mass of the fetus, I think it is very possible, depending on when it is done and how long it is sustained. It might be partly a function of whether the fetus has the potential to put down large amounts of body fat. At least it is possible that insulin might change true lean body mass if it is sustained for long enough in a mammalian fetus. The discussion gets jumbled if we move from changes in blood flow in the fetal side of the placenta, to uterine blood flow, to poor placentation and building smaller placentas, to starving the mother and changing substrate concentrations in her blood. It is not easy to come to grips with these questions if too many things are changing at the same time. At least it is possible today to define what the fetus receives and this should be viewed in the context of its requirements. How much does the fetus of a particular mammalian species need for growth, and how much does it need for fuel to meet its oxygen consumption, whether it is from fat, protein or carbohydrate? If one finds that it is 10% of the total need or 70% of the total need, then one has a yardstick. As we jump in the discussion between different species growing at different rates, with different gestation lengths and different body compositions, I have trouble knowing whether we are all using the same reference points.

Blázquez: In the rat fetus I think insulin is probably the most important factor for growth. This assumption is supported by the fact that insulin receptors in liver appear early in development (Blázquez *et al.* 1976) and insulin stimulates DNA and protein synthesis by fetal hepatocytes in culture (Leffert 1974).

Chez: I believe that the fetus has constraints against excess growth. In a non-polytocous species such as the human, which already has a relatively close relationship between the fetal head and the maternal internal pelvis, it would make sense to me for there to be such constraints if there is to be vaginal delivery. Clinically there are women who gain an excess amount of weight and whose glucose tolerance is normal, yet in whom there is a specific levelling off of fetal growth. It seems to me that there is still a fetal weight plateau regardless of pre-pregnant weight and weight gain in pregnancy, at about 14 kg total weight gain. One does not see fetal–newborn weight continuing to go up in a linear fashion. For me, at least, this confirms my concept of constraint. Therefore I perceive insulin in terms of its basal levels as just that: a requirement for normal growth. When a fetal β-cell is prematurely induced by hyperglycaemia or even hyperaminoacidaemia (which we haven't so far talked much about), that constraint has been removed, to the detriment of the fetus. There is a possibility that the fetus will die unless delivery is induced. In nature it could not be delivered. In that case, everything we are talking about in terms of fetal hyperinsulinaemia is pathology by itself. When fetal hyperinsulinaemia occurs, which I believe is not until the last six or eight weeks in a human pregnancy, it is the source of the macrosomia that we see.

On the question about hyperinsulinaemia by itself, without substrate, R. Schwartz (unpublished work, 1978) can infuse insulin into third-trimester monkey fetuses for over 21 days with a subcutaneously placed minipump and obtain hyperinsulinaemic levels. In the presence of what we would consider normoglycaemia on the maternal side, although we do not know the levels on the fetal side, he gets animals that are four standard deviations in body weight above the control weight for the population. They are characterized by gross adipose tissue obesity, cardiomegaly and hepatomegaly, but the brain and the kidney do not participate in the organomegaly. Schwartz has not done the more specific tissue compositions yet. It seems to me that in the monkey, at least, we have evidence that hyperinsulinaemia all by itself is the growth factor, without any need for excess substrate.

Hoet: Was there any insulin in fetal urine? Were the kidneys, or was the glomerulus, increased in size, as in the infants of diabetic mothers?

Chez: My impression is that they have not yet looked critically at the components of the kidney but rather at the total weight of the organ.

Hoet: The infant of the diabetic mother must have a major glycosuria. We found in the rat that as soon as the blood sugar of the mother rat is increased by 50–100 ml (2.8–5.5 mmol/l), there is definite fetal glycosuria within about 40 min.   The bladder easily contains 100 mg/100 ml of glucose (Hoet & Reusens 1976).   The increase in the weight of the liver and heart may be due to the anabolic effect of insulin.   However, the increased size of the glomeruli of infants of diabetic mothers observed by Dr Naeye, for example, may be due to an adaption to the greater glucose load to the kidneys.   It might be a consequence of the adaptive function of the kidney to an unusual fetal glycosuria.

Battaglia: We haven't done any long-term insulin infusions to attempt to alter fetal growth rate.   Earlier I presented some data in which insulin had been infused into the fetus over a few hours and an increased glucose uptake in the baby could be demonstrated.   We were interested in whether this insulin effect could be sustained with infusions over some days.   With infusions lasting three days we found that the increased umbilical glucose uptake was sustained (B.S. Carson *et al.,* in preparation, 1978).   We didn't find any evidence of an adaptation over this period of time.   What surprised us was that the fetal arterial O_2 contents during insulin infusion were as low as we have seen with a surviving fetus.   The O_2 content was reduced as low as 1 mmol/l, which is the concentration one would observe in the fetus at an altitude of 4300 m.   The O_2 content increases again when the insulin infusion is stopped.   We are attempting to describe a dose-response curve but at high dosing levels the fetus has died, not surprisingly.   If twin fetuses are catheterized and insulin is given first to one fetus there is a fall in O_2 content; when insulin is given to the second fetus there is again a fall in O_2 content.   All I can tell you at present is that we are quite surprised that fairly severe hyperinsulinaemia produces marked changes in oxygenation over three days.   Glucose concentration of itself does not explain the fetal death *in utero.*

Kalkhoff: Might that not be due to the acuity of the glucose fall rather than to the magnitude?   In other words, one can certainly see changes like this in someone who has horrendous hypoglycaemia.

Battaglia: That is not the case.   When we infused insulin into the fetus for a few hours and glucose levels fell very quickly, there were no changes in oxygenation.

Räihä: The question of hyperinsulinaemia in the fetus and in the infant of the diabetic mother is a complex one.   We have seen from many of the studies shown here that it changes substrate levels.   I will show later that it very dramatically affects the adaptation of specific enzyme development in the perinatal period.   Even from a purely biochemical point of view, the effect of hyperinsulinaemia may be very dramatic.

Beard: The importance of the work that Fred Battaglia has described is that it demonstrates how well the fetus can withstand hypoglycaemia.   However, it looks as though insulin may well be implicated in one of the processes that lead to death of the fetus of the diabetic.   It is, I think, a useful step forward in our understanding of the problem.

Girard: About 10 years ago Picon (1967) did experiments in the rat, a species in which the fetus has no white adipose tissue.   He showed that by injecting insulin during the last four days of gestation one can increase both the body weight and the accumulation of nitrogen in the carcass.   This suggests that in the presence of high insulin levels one can increase retention of nitrogen and body weight.   I think this is one piece of evidence that insulin affects fetal growth.

Hoet: Was the placenta changed too?

Girard: This was not measured.

Beard: It is unfortunate that the placenta has been excluded from these discussions because we have so little information on it.

Hoet: I agree that the placenta has to come into the picture.

Young: How much insulin did you infuse to get those results, Dr Battaglia?

Battaglia: I don't remember the dose per kilogram.   We gave a bolus injection followed by a constant infusion.   The plasma concentration of insulin ranged from 50 to 1000 μU/ml among the different animals.

Young: We have also infused insulin into the lamb *in utero*, between 126 and 136 days of gestation, in order to determine its influence on tissue protein synthetic rates (Horn *et al.* 1977).   A fivefold increase in fetal plasma insulin, from 18 μU/ml to about 100 μU/ml during six hours, did not influence either the level of free amino acids in the placental tissue or the protein synthetic rate in this organ; this suggests that the hormone does not influence placental nitrogen metabolism from the fetal circulation.   (The influence of insulin on protein synthetic rate in the other fetal organs is described on p. 199.)

Battaglia: The levels we achieved were as high as 1000 μU/ml but we saw the changes in glucose/O_2 quotients at 50 μU/ml.   I can't say what the changes in oxygenation are at concentrations between 50 and 1000 μU/ml.

References

BLÁZQUEZ, E., RUBALCAVA, B., MONTESANO, R., ORCI, L. & UNGER, R. (1976) Development of insulin and glucagon binding and the adenylate cyclase response in liver membranes of the prenatal, postnatal and adult rat: evidence of glucagon 'resistance'. *Endocrinology 98*, 1014–1023

BREUER, E., BARTA, E., PAPPOVA, E. & ZLATOS, L. (1967) Developmental changes of myocardial metabolism.   I.   Peculiarities of cardiac carbohydrate metabolism in the early post-natal period in dogs. *Biol. Neonat. 11*, 367–377

DOWNING, S. E., LEE, J. C. & RIEKER, R. P. (1977) Mechanical and metabolic effects of insulin on newborn lamb myocardium. *Am. J. Obstet. Gynecol. 127,* 649–656

GENTZ, J. C. H. & CORNBLATH, M. (1969) Transient diabetes of the newborn. *Adv. Pediatr. 16,* 345–363

HOET, J. J. & REUSENS, B. (1976) Etude de l'autonomie du pancréas foetal et de ses implications cliniques. *Bull. Mém. Acad. R. Méd. Belg. 131,* 193–203

HORN, J., SLOAN, I., STERN, M., NOAKES, D. & YOUNG, M. (1977) Effect of insulin on protein turnover in fetal lambs. *Proc. Nutr. Soc. 36,* 118A

LEFFERT, H. L. (1974) Growth control of differentiated fetal rat hepatocytes in primary mono-layer culture. VII. Hormonal control of DNA synthesis and its possible significance to the problem of liver regeneration. *J. Cell Biol. 62,* 792–801

NAEYE, R. L. (1965) Infants of diabetic mothers. A quantitative morphologic study. *Pediatrics 35,* 980–988

OSLER, M. (1965) Structural and chemical changes in infants of diabetic and pre-diabetic mothers, in *On the Nature and Treatment of Diabetes* (Leibel, B. S. & Wrenshall, G. A., eds.), p. 692, Int. Congr. Series 84, Excerpta Medica, Amsterdam

PICON, L. (1967) Effect of insulin on growth and biochemical composition of the rat fetus. *Endocrinology 81,* 1419–1421

ROVERSI, G. D., GORGIULO, M., NICOLINI, U., PEDRETTI, E. & CANDIANI, G. (1977) Diabète de la mère et risque péri-natal. *Rev. Méd. Suisse 97,* 401

Hormonal regulation of perinatal enzyme differentiation in the mammalian liver

NIELS C.R. RÄIHÄ

Department of Obstetrics & Gynecology and Pediatrics, University Central Hospital, Helsinki

Abstract   The adaptation of newborn mammals to extrauterine life depends in large part on the maturation of biochemical and physiological functions during perinatal development.   Hormones such as glucocorticoids, catecholamines and glucagon can stimulate enzyme induction during development; on the other hand, insulin has been shown to antagonize these stimulatory effects.

Only the surface of the problem of hormonal regulation of enzyme differentiation during the perinatal period has been reached, especially as regards human development.   Each enzyme presents unique problems of chemical regulation; the functional consequences of these factors are not exactly the same in each tissue and perhaps not in each species.

The possibility of using inducing agents such as hormones, drugs and substrates to promote biochemical enzyme differentiation is a new and exciting aspect which needs to be explored further as a means of facilitating survival and ensuring optimal extrauterine development of the immaturely born human infant or the full-term infant with delayed enzymic development.   However, any intervention in the carefully programmed interplay of different hormones which regulate normal enzymic adaptation and development during the perinatal period should be undertaken only after careful consideration.   The possibilities of long-term harm must be weighed against short-term benefits.

For many decades scientists have collected descriptive information about morphological aspects of development, but the study of enzymic development and differentiation and, especially, its regulation is still only beginning.   Enzymic differentiation of any given tissue is the process whereby it acquires its characteristic quantitative enzyme pattern.   This process involves both positive changes, the appearance or increase in synthesis of enzymes *de novo*, and negative changes, the diminution in the amount of other enzymes.   The fundamental problem underlying this process is that of gene expression.

The carefully programmed normal formation of enzymes continues to a rather late stage in mammalian development, namely to the late fetal period and early postnatal life. It is only when enzymic differentiation has been completed that any organ or organism reaches full physiological maturity and function. The lack of complete enzymic development forms the biochemical basis for the concept of 'functional immaturity'. Many clinical problems associated with infants of low birth weight, dysmature infants and infants of diabetic mothers are those of functional immaturity or alterations in the normal course of enzymic development. Knowledge and understanding of the normal process of enzymic differentiation and its regulation, especially in the human fetus and neonate, are of the greatest importance in the care of the newborn infant with problems of functional immaturity.

The liver plays a central role in the process of metabolic adaptation necessary for maintaining homeostasis during the change from intrauterine to extrauterine life. The liver must take over metabolic duties which were performed by the placenta or the maternal tissues during fetal life. Thus, it is not surprising that the liver is the organ in which the largest number of enzymes have been studied as a developmental function, and the developmental patterns of several enzymes and groups of enzymes are well known.

COMPARISON OF ENZYME DEVELOPMENT IN HUMANS AND IN RATS

The rat is the experimental animal most commonly used in studies of enzyme development; only fragmentary and scattered reports exist for human development. If the results of experimental research on enzyme development and its regulation are to have any meaningful implications in clinical situations it will be important to collect all possible information about enzymogenesis in the human fetus and neonate. It is, however, possible to derive some general conclusions from data collected from experimental animals. Even though species differ with respect to length of gestation and maturity at birth, they have in common many important characteristics of intra- and extrauterine life. Greengard (1977) has recently collected data on the sequence in which different liver enzymes approach their adult concentrations in human and in rat liver. These studies suggest that the mechanisms responsible for the schedule of gene expression resemble each other fairly closely in the two species, with only a few exceptions. The fetal liver, like all rapidly growing tissues, is still rich in enzymes involved in the synthesis of nucleic acids, polyamines and pentoses. During neonatal development in both species these enzymes decrease towards the low adult values. The process of birth represents one similar event in both species, regardless of degree of maturation, and enzymes which are connected with functions necessary for extrauterine life would be expected to develop around the time of birth in both species.

Examples of such activities are gluconeogenesis (phospho*enol*pyruvate carboxykinase, EC 4.1.1.32; PEPCK) (Räihä & Lindros 1969), urea formation (argininosuccinate synthetase, EC 6.3.4.5; ASS) (Räihä & Suihkonen 1968a), and metabolism of some amino acids (tyrosine aminotransferase, EC 2.6.1.5; TAT) (Delvalle & Greengard 1977).

In rat liver the last step of biochemical maturation occurs around the weaning period, when the diet changes from the relatively low calorie, low protein milk to high protein solid food.

There is very little information about enzyme development during this period in man and we do not really know the exact postnatal age in man at which the hepatic enzymes, which are still lacking in the newborn, attain their adult levels. Some speculations have, however, been made on the basis of clinical feeding studies in premature infants (Räihä 1976).

Examples of enzymes which have different developmental behaviour in man and rat are cystathionase (cystathionine γ-lyase, EC 4.4.1.1) and ornithine aminotransferase. Cystathionase activity increases in the rat during the late fetal period (Heinonen 1975) and in the human sometimes after birth, probably after the second week of life (Gaull *et al.* 1977). Ornithine aminotransferase has a high activity in human fetal liver and does not rise in the rat until the weaning period (Kekomäki *et al.* 1969).

DEVELOPMENT OF TYROSINE AMINOTRANSFERASE, PHOSPHO*ENOL*PYRUVATE CARBOXYKINASE AND ARGININOSUCCINATE SYNTHETASE IN RAT LIVER

The best-studied enzymes, which all appear around birth in the rat, are those previously mentioned, TAT, PEPCK and ASS (Ghisalberti 1976; E. Edkins & N.C.R. Räihä, unpublished observations, 1977). The activity of these three enzymes is very low or undetectable in fetal liver up to the 20th day of gestation, but during the last two days of intrauterine life in the rat all three enzymes increase to about 30% of adult activity. After spontaneous delivery on day 22 the enzyme activities increase rapidly, within hours, to the adult level of activity. Premature delivery by Caesarean section on day 20 or 21 produces an increase in enzyme activities similar to the increase found in all three enzymes after spontaneous delivery. If, on the other hand, the pregnancy is prolonged beyond 22 days by maternal injection of progesterone, the activities increase to almost adult levels in the postmature fetal livers (Figs. 1 and 2). A direct effect of progesterone is unlikely since the hormone has no effect in the pre-term fetuses and does not increase the normal postnatal induction of the enzymes. These studies indicate that premature delivery of the rat fetuses produces a rapid appearance of these enzymes, similar to that found after spontaneous delivery at term; and, since the enzymes appear after prolongation of pregnancy at the normal time of birth, fetal age must also be a signal for enzyme induction.

STUDIES ON THE HORMONAL CONTROL OF ENZYME INDUCTION AROUND BIRTH

Effects of adrenalectomy and corticosteroids

The role of the adrenal cortex in the development of rat liver enzymes has been studied by experimental removal of the adrenal glands immediately after

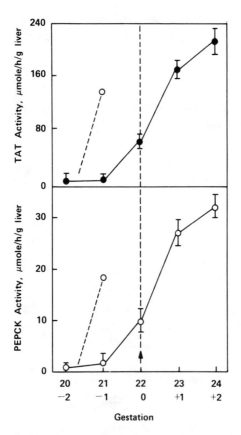

FIG. 1. Tyrosine aminotransferase (TAT) and phospho*enol*pyruvate carboxykinase (PEPCK) activities in rat liver after premature delivery by surgery, before term pregnancy and during prolonged gestation caused by maternal treatment with progesterone (Ghisalberti 1976).

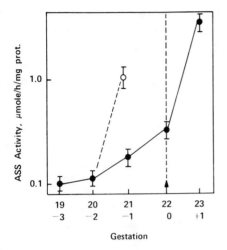

FIG. 2. Argininosuccinate synthetase (ASS) activity in rat liver after premature delivery by surgery and during prolonged gestation (Edkins & Räihä, unpublished observations, 1977).

birth.   Adrenalectomy almost completely inhibits the postnatal increase of ASS activity, but administration of the synthetic corticosteroid, triamcinolone, to adrenalectomized newborn animals prevents the effect of adrenalectomy, as seen in Fig. 3 (Räihä & Suihkonen 1968b).   Sereni *et al.* (1959), and Holt & Oliver (1969) have also shown that the postnatal increase of TAT activity can be repressed by adrenalectomy at delivery and that this enzyme activity can be restored by administration of corticosteroids.   These studies suggested that corticosteroids may be the natural triggers which induce enzyme activity at birth.   It was, however, soon shown that glucocorticoids injected into fetal animals *in utero,* could not induce either ASS (Schwartz 1972) or TAT (Ghisalberti 1976), although glucocorticoids were effective in increasing both ASS and TAT activity in postnatal animals after the normal increase in enzyme activity had occurred (Table 1).   In adult animals corticosteroids are also effective in increasing these enzyme activities.   It was further shown that injection of dibutyryl cyclic AMP, glucagon or catecholamines could replace TAT activity in adrenalectomized newborn rats (Holt & Oliver 1971; Ghisalberti 1976).   Since exogenous cyclic AMP replaced full enzyme activity in adrenalectomized animals and since corticosteroids cannot induce TAT or ASS activity when injected *in utero,* it is probable that corticosteroids are not the 'primary' inducers of enzyme activities at birth.   Measurements of plasma corticosteroids during development in the rat have shown that the concentration increases after the 17th day of gestation and is high until the 20th day,

after which it decreases; this low concentration is maintained during prolonged gestation, as seen in Fig. 4 (Ghisalberti 1976).   If the induction of enzyme
activities at birth depended only on the level of corticosteroids, enzyme
induction should occur *in utero*.   The rapid increase in enzyme activities
around the time of normal birth in the postmature fetuses in spite of low
corticosteroid levels also speaks against the theory that corticosteroids are the

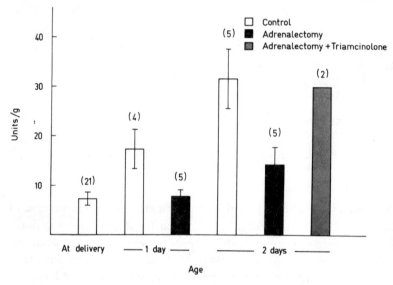

FIG. 3. Effect of adrenalectomy at birth and of triamcinolone on the development of the activity
of the arginine synthetase system in rat liver (Räihä & Suihkonen 1968*b*).

TABLE 1

Effect of triamcinolone on the activity of the arginine synthetase system during perinatal development of the rat (Schwartz 1972)

Age	Dose of triamcinolone	Arginine synthetase system activity: μmol urea formed/(30 min g liver)		
(days)	*(µg/animal)*	*Control*	*Experimental*	*P*
−2.5	190	7.2 ± 1.1 (5)	9.6 ± 2.4 (6)	n.s.
−1.5	19	5.1 ± 0.7 (4)	5.8 ± 1.9 (6)	n.s.
+1.0	19	37.9 ± 4.1 (3)	61.4 ± 9.6 (4)	<0.005
	190	29.6 ± 3.2 (3)	73.4 ± 3.3 (4)	<0.001
+5.0	190	40.3 ± 9.1 (4)	79.4 ± 14.0 (4)	<0.005

n.s. not significant
Mean ± S.D. (no. of experiments)

'primary' inducers.   It has been suggested that corticosteroids have a 'permissive' action and appear to 'sensitize' the system to other agents or to a second action of corticosteroid.

Effects of catecholamines, glucagon and insulin

It has been shown that catecholamines are able to induce both TAT and PEPCK activities when injected into the rat fetus *in utero* (Holt & Oliver 1968; Greengard 1969).   It is well known that an increase in catecholamine secretion immediately after birth occurs in both the rat (Ghisalberti 1976) and the human infant (Lagercrantz & Bistoletti 1973).   Catecholamines can increase hepatic cyclic AMP concentration by two mechanisms.   Both adrenaline (epinephrine) and noradrenaline (norepinephrine) stimulate liver adenylate cyclase (EC 4.6.1.1.) activity directly and in addition catecholamines modulate the insulin: glucagon ratio in the blood.   A decrease in this ratio increases hepatic cyclic AMP production.   During prolonged gestation in the rat, both plasma and liver catecholamines increase significantly, as shown by Ghisalberti (1976).   Simultaneously the concentration of hepatic cyclic AMP increases, as seen in Fig. 5.   The concentrations of catecholamine and cyclic AMP are already rising significantly between the 21st and 22nd days when the first sign of enzyme induction is seen in the liver.   There is much evidence that towards the end of gestation postmature mammals become hypoxic, due to the decrease in placental blood flow.   Ghisalberti (1976) has studied the effects of hypoxia on preterm induction of fetal enzymes.   Fig. 6 shows the response of both TAT and PEPCK activities in 19-day fetal rats exposed to hyp-

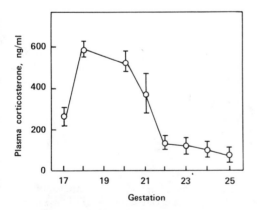

FIG. 4. Plasma corticosterone in the fetal rat before term and during prolonged gestation (Ghisalberti 1976).   The values are ng/ml (mean ± S.E.M).

oxia.   TAT activity can also be increased by injection into the fetuses of 2 μg
adrenaline/g body weight.   In preterm fetal rats it has been shown (Girard *et
al.* 1973*a*) that exogenous noradrenaline stimulates glucagon and inhibits
insulin release from the pancreas.   In experiments on prolonged gestation
(Ghisalberti 1976), an increase in plasma glucagon and a fall in serum insulin

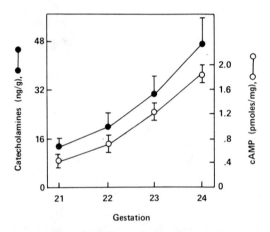

FIG. 5. Liver catecholamines and cyclic AMP before and during prolonged gestation.   Cyclic
AMP concentration (pmol/mg liver) is expressed as mean ± S.E.M.   Total liver catecholamines
(ng/g liver) also expressed as mean ± S.E.M. (Ghisalberti 1976).

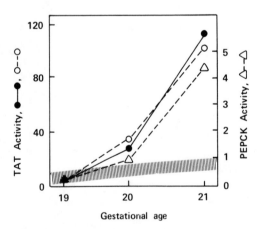

FIG. 6. Effects of hypoxia (o, Δ) and adrenaline injection (2 μg/g) into the rat fetus (●) on
tyrosine aminotransferase (TAT) and phospho*enol*pyruvate carboxykinase (PEPCK) activities.   The shaded area represents the enzyme activities during normal development.   The response of the enzymes increases with increasing gestational age (Ghisalberti 1976).

could be observed (Fig. 7). Between days 21 and 24 the plasma glucagon level increased 30-fold and the insulin concentration fell by 50%, with the largest decrease in insulin occurring between days 21 and 22. The insulin: glucagon ratio in blood fell from 19 on day 21 to 0.17 on day 24. Thus, the increased concentration of hepatic cyclic AMP observed during prolonged gestation probably results from increased catecholamine and glucagon release and decreased insulin secretion.

Enzyme induction after normal delivery in the rat has been thought to be a result of glucagon release triggered by postnatal hypoglycaemia (Greengard &

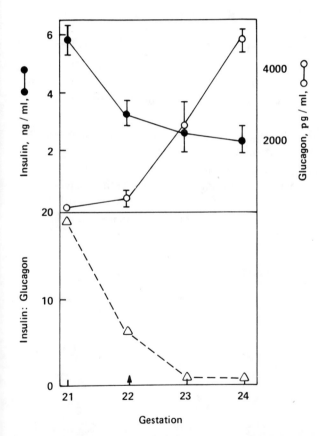

FIG. 7. Insulin and glucagon concentrations in fetal blood during gestation and during prolonged gestation. The concentrations of glucagon (pg/ml) in plasma is expressed as mean ± S.E.M. The concentration of insulin in serum (ng/ml) is expressed also as mean ± S.E.M. The insulin: glucagon molar ratio is calculated from the mean values of each parameter at each gestational age (Ghisalberti 1976).

Dewey 1967; Yeung & Oliver 1968). This hypothesis was strengthened when it was shown that massive doses of glucose at birth repressed the postnatal induction of TAT (Greengard & Dewey 1967; Holt & Oliver 1968) and of PEPCK (Yeung & Oliver 1968). It was thought that the glucose administration blocked the release of glucagon and thereby enzyme induction.

However, Girard *et al.* (1973*a*) demonstrated that, in contrast to expectations, the pancreatic cells of the perinatal rat did not respond to acute changes in blood glucose concentration by increased glucagon release. In addition it was shown that the postnatal increase in plasma glucagon occurred well before any significant change in blood glucose. These results seemed to rule out postnatal hypoglycaemia as the physiological stimulus for glucagon release in the newborn rat. It is now believed that postnatal increase in catecholamines, in addition to acting directly on adenylate cyclase in the liver, may induce enzyme activity by modulating the insulin : glucagon ratio in the plasma. Exogenous noradrenaline stimulates glucagon release and inhibits insulin release from the neonatal rat pancreas (Girard *et al.* 1973*a*). The repressive action of glucose administration on enzyme induction may be explained by insulin release.

During the fetal period in the rat, plasma insulin levels start to increase after the 17th day of gestation (Felix *et al.* 1968; Girard *et al.* 1973*b*), and are high until the 21st day, when a decrease occurs, as mentioned previously (Fig. 8). After normal birth on day 22 plasma glucagon increases and insulin decreases rapidly (Girard *et al.* 1973*b*). It has been proposed by Girard *et al.* (1973*b*) that the increased activity of the sympathetic nervous system induced by the stress of birth would trigger the release of noradrenaline at the pancrea-

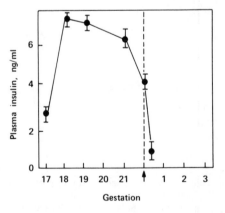

FIG. 8. Plasma insulin in the rat during late gestation and after birth. Values are expressed as mean ± S.E.M. (Felix *et al.* 1968; Girard *et al.* 1973*b*).

tic nerve endings, which in turn would stimulate the release of glucagon and inhibit the release of insulin.   The change in the insulin : glucagon ratio after birth, in combination with increased levels of hepatic catecholamines (Ghisalberti 1976), would further increase hepatic cyclic AMP and induce enzyme synthesis.

It is thus evident that glucocorticoids, catecholamines, glucagon and insulin participate in a complex interplay which determines the process of enzyme induction in the liver around the time of birth.

IN VITRO STUDIES OF FETAL LIVER IN ORGAN CULTURE

The organ culture system of fetal liver explants provides a technique for maintaining liver tissue in a chemically defined environment for a prolonged period of time, removed from the circulating factors present in utero.   This system allows for the study of enzyme induction and its regulation under controlled conditions, and also makes it possible to study regulation in human fetal tissues, which would not be possible in vivo.

Studies in fetal rat liver

Fetal rat liver in organ culture is competent to respond to hormonal stimulation by an increase in enzyme concentrations at a fairly early stage of gestation.   Our studies have shown that liver removed from 13-day-old rat fetuses responds to glucagon and cyclic AMP by increased TAT activity.   Corticosteroids also induce TAT activity in fetal rat liver in organ culture after the 14th to 15th day of gestation (Räihä et al. 1971).   The urea cycle enzymes (ASS) can be induced in fetal liver in culture by glucagon, cyclic AMP and by corticosteroid (triamcinolone or dexamethasone), as shown by Schwartz (1972) and Edkins & Räihä (1976).   The observations that a combination of optimal amounts of glucagon and cyclic AMP did not produce a greater effect than each agent alone but that a combination of cyclic AMP and corticosteroid produced an almost additive effect on ASS induction (Table 2) is compatible with the concept that cyclic AMP mediates the action of glucagon but that corticosteroids act through a different mechanism (Wicks 1969; Räihä & Schwartz 1973a).   The induction of TAT, ASS and PEPCK in fetal liver in organ culture by corticosteroids is in contrast to the effect of corticosteroids injected into fetal rats of the same age in utero.   Thus, Greengard et al. (1970) could not induce arginase (EC 3.5.3.1) activity in fetal rats in utero with cortisol, Schwartz (1972) could not induce ASS in utero with triamcinolone

TABLE 2

Effect of combinations of glucagon, dibutyryl cyclic AMP and triamcinolone on the arginine synthetase system in fetal rat liver explants in culture in the presence of theophylline (Schwartz 1972; Räihä & Schwartz 1973a)

	Concentration	Arginine synthetase system activity: μmol urea formed/(30 min g protein with theophylline)
Control	—	30.4 ± 2.6 (12)
Glucagon	67.0 μg/ml	69.9 ± 4.0 (8)
Dibutyryl cyclic AMP	0.1 mM	78.7 ± 6.2 (12)
Triamcinolone	20 μg/ml	94.0 ± 9.1 (6)
Dibutyryl cyclic AMP + triamcinolone	0.1 mM 20 μg/ml	129.1 ± 13.2 (6)

Mean ± s.e.m. (no. of duplicate determinations)

and Ghisalberti (1976) could not induce TAT *in utero* with dexamethasone. The lack of response *in utero* could be due to the presence of some inhibitor in the fetus which is not present *in vitro* in the organ culture system. One possibility is that the high plasma concentration of insulin in the fetus would antagonize the effect of corticosteroid during the late fetal period.

There is now evidence that this may be the case. Wicks *et al.* (1974) and Gunn *et al.* (1975) have shown that in rat hepatoma cells in culture insulin suppresses the increase in synthesis of PEPCK by either cyclic AMP or dexamethasone. Later we showed (Räihä & Edkins 1977) that insulin has an antagonistic effect on the increase in ASS activity induced with dexamethasone in cultured fetal rat liver (Table 3).

Since the concentrations of cyclic AMP, corticosteroids and insulin used in these experiments were close to the physiological range, it is probable that this antagonistic interaction between insulin and cyclic AMP and between insulin and corticosteroid also occurs *in vivo*. The results allow the important conclusion to be drawn that insulin does not always act simply by decreasing the cellular concentration of cyclic AMP, but that, through its suppression of corticosteroid action its effect can also be directed at specific enzyme synthesis. The cellular mechanism for the antagonistic effect of insulin on cyclic AMP or corticosteroid action is outside the scope of this review, but it has been suggested by Wicks *et al.* (1974) that insulin may act to prevent the release of enzyme at the polysomal level or by enhancing the rate of enzyme degradation.

TABLE 3

Effects of dexamethasone and insulin on argininosuccinate synthetase activity in fetal rat liver in organ culture (Räihä & Edkins 1977)

Additions	Argininosuccinate synthetase (units/mg protein)	
	24 h	48 h
None	0.10 ± 0.02 (4)	0.19 ± 0.02 (4)
Dexamethasone (4.6. x 10⁻⁶ M)	0.27 ± 0.06 (5)	0.62 ± 0.04 (5)
Insulin (1.8 x 10⁻⁶ M)	0.12 ± 0.01 (5)	0.28 ± 0.03 (5)
Dexamethasone + insulin	0.11 ± 0.02 (5)	0.42 ± 0.03 (5)

Mean ± s.e.m. (no. of experiments)

Studies in fetal human liver

Human fetal liver *in vitro* is 'competent' to respond to inducing hormones by increased enzyme production at a very early stage of development. Cystathionase activity can be increased in fetal human liver in organ culture after the 11th week of gestation by glucagon, dibutyryl cyclic AMP and dexamethasone (Heinonen & Räihä 1974). Glucose-6-phosphatase (EC 3.1.3.9) can be induced at the sixth week of gestation with dibutyryl cyclic AMP and this induction can be diminished by the addition of insulin (Schwartz *et al.* 1974). TAT can be induced in human fetal liver in organ culture by dibutyryl cyclic AMP in the presence of theophylline and after the 10th week of gestation also by the glucocorticoids, triamcinolone and dexamethasone (Räihä & Schwartz 1973*b*). Kirby & Hahn (1973) induced PEPCK activity in human fetal liver explants by adding dibutyryl cyclic AMP, and Schwartz & Rall (1975) stimulated the overall gluconeogenesis from labelled alanine to glucose in fetal human liver explants in culture by adding glucagon or dibutyryl cyclic AMP in the presence of theophylline. Schwartz & Rall (1975) also showed that triamcinolone stimulated glucose production from alanine by liver explants and that addition of insulin significantly decreased the stimulation obtained with dibutyryl cyclic AMP and glucagon.

These *in vitro* studies with human fetal liver suggest that enzyme induction during the perinatal period is regulated in the human by mechanisms very similar to those in the rat.

IN VIVO OBSERVATIONS IN THE HUMAN AND CLINICAL EXPERIENCES

Very little is known about the effects of hormone administration on the activities of liver enzymes in the human fetus or neonate. Corticosteroids are successfully used in the treatment of severe neonatal hypoglycaemia which cannot be overcome by glucose infusions alone, but the exact mechanism of action is not known. Kirby & Hahn (1973) have reported a 10-fold increase in the activity of liver PEPCK in a 12.5-week-old human fetus when the mother had received prednisone for eight weeks before abortion.

Menkes & Avery (1963) observed that administration of hydrocortisone (cortisol) to two infants who had high tyrosine concentrations in the blood during the first two weeks of life resulted in a prompt drop in tyrosine concentrations within 24 to 48 h after the injections. This finding suggests that tyrosine-oxidizing enzymes may have been induced in the liver of these infants.

Some conclusions concerning the effects of insulin on liver metabolism in the newborn infant can be drawn from studies of infants of insulin-dependent diabetic mothers. These infants have been shown to have hyperinsulinism due to fetal hyperglycaemia. In addition these infants fail to stimulate pancreatic glucagon release after birth and to increase urinary catecholamine excretion in response to postnatal hypoglycaemia (Bloom & Johnston 1972; Stern et al. 1968). The newborn infants of insulin-dependent diabetic mothers often develop severe hypoglycaemia in the neonatal period. Kalhan et al. (1977) have demonstrated that this is due to a lower rate of hepatic glucose production in these infants compared to normal infants. The decreased output of hepatic glucose may in part be due to hyperinsulinaemia causing perinatal induction of the enzymes of gluconeogenesis to fail.

Maturation-promoting effects of corticosteroids have been demonstrated in many other developing tissues in addition to the liver, such as intestine, lung, etc., but a detailed discussion of these effects is not possible in this paper. The studies by Liggins & Howie (1972) concerning the effects of corticosteroids on lung maturation are well known. These effects may well be mediated, partly or wholly, via corticosteroid stimulation or 'sensitization' of enzyme synthesis via transcriptional processes. Infants of diabetic mothers have an increased incidence of respiratory distress syndrome and this may be due to an antagonistic effect of insulin on the normal development of surfactant-synthesizing enzymes in the lung (Smith et al. 1975; Hallman & Kankare, unpublished work, 1977).

CONCLUSIONS

The liver enzymes PEPCK, TAT and ASS begin to increase in activity in fetal rat liver just before the end of gestation. This increase in specific enzyme synthesis is triggered by an increase in hepatic cyclic AMP produced by an increase in catecholamine and glucagon levels and a decrease in insulin levels. These hormonal changes may be due to relative hypoxia from decreased placental function towards the end of pregnancy. At birth a further release of adrenaline is induced by the stress of birth and by hypoglycaemia. This, together with the rapid fall in the insulin : glucagon ratio after birth, further increases hepatic cyclic AMP and induces enzyme production. Corticosteroids do not induce the synthesis of these enzymes *in utero,* perhaps due to an antagonistic effect of high insulin levels before birth in the rat. The corticosteroids, however, seem to 'sensitize' the system for the inducing action of cyclic AMP.

In vitro studies indicate that the hormonal control of induction of these enzymes in the human fetus and infant may be regulated by very similar mechanisms. Hyperinsulinaemia may interfere with the normal induction of important enzyme systems in infants of insulin-dependent diabetic mothers.

ACKNOWLEDGEMENTS

These studies have been supported in part by the Sigrid Jusélius Foundation.

References

BLOOM, S. R. & JOHNSTON, D. I. (1972) Failure of glucagon release in infants of diabetic mothers. *Br. Med. J. 4,* 453–454

EDKINS, E. & RÄIHÄ, N. C. R. (1976) Changes in the activities of the enzymes of urea synthesis caused by dexamethasone and dibutyryladenosine 3′ : 5′-cyclic monophosphate in foetal rat liver maintained in organ culture. *Biochem. J. 160,* 159–162

FELIX, J. M., JACQUOT, R. & SUTTER, B. Ch. J. (1968) Insulinémies maternelles et foetales chez le rat. *Horm. Metab. Res. 1,* 41-42

DELVALLE, J. A. & GREENGARD, O. (1977) Phenylalanine hydroxylase and tyrosine aminotransferase in human fetal and adult liver. *Pediatr. Res. 11,* 2–5

GAULL, G. E., RASSIN, D. K., RÄIHÄ, N. C. R. & HEINONEN, K. (1977) Milk protein quality and quantity in low-birth-weight infants III. Effects on sulfur amino acids in plasma and urine. *J. Pediatr. 90,* 348–355

GHISALBERTI, A. V. (1976) *Enzyme Induction in Perinatal Rat Liver.* Academic Dissertation, University of Western Australia

GIRARD, J., ASSAN, R. & JOST, A. (1973a) Glucagon in the rat foetus, in *Foetal and Neonatal Physiology (Proc. Sir Joseph Barcroft Centenary Symp),* pp. 456–461, Cambridge University Press, London

GIRARD, J. R., CUENDET, G. S., MARLISS, E. B., KERVARIN, A., RIEUTORT, M. & ASSAN, R. (1973b) Fuels, hormones, and liver metabolism at term and during the early postnatal period in the rat. *J. Clin. Invest.* 52, 3190–3200

GREENGARD, O. (1969) Enzyme differentiation in mammalian liver. *Science (Wash. D.C.)* 163, 891–895

GREENGARD, O. (1977) Enzymic differentiation of human liver: comparison with the rat model. *Pediatr. Res.* 11, 669–676

GREENGARD, O. & DEWEY, H. K. (1967) Initiation by glucagon of the premature development of tyrosine aminotransferase, serine dehydratase and glucose-6-phosphatase in fetal rat liver. *J. Biol. Chem.* 242, 2986–2991

GREENGARD, O., SAHIB, M. K. & KNOX, W. E. (1970) Developmental formation and distribution of arginase in rat tissues. *Arch. Biochem. Biophys.* 137, 447–482

GUNN, J. M., TILGHMAN, S. M., HANSON, R. W., RESHEF, L. & BALLARD, F. J. (1975) Effects of cyclic adenosine monophosphate, dexamethasone and insulin on phosphoenolpyruvate carboxykinase synthesis in Reuber H-35 hepatoma cells. *Biochemistry* 14, 2350–2357

HEINONEN, K. (1975) Induction of cystathionase in foetal rat liver explants. *Biochim. Biophys. Acta* 399, 113–123

HEINONEN, K. & RÄIHÄ, N. C. R. (1974) Induction of cystathionase in human foetal liver. *Biochem. J.* 144, 607–609

HOLT, P. G. & OLIVER, I. T. (1968) Plasma corticosterone concentrations in the perinatal rat. *Biochem. J.* 108, 339–341

HOLT, P. G. & OLIVER, I. T. (1969) Studies of the mechanism of induction of tyrosine aminotransferase in neonatal rat liver. *Biochemistry* 8, 1429–1437

HOLT, P. G. & OLIVER, I. T. (1971) Multiple forms of soluble rat liver tyrosine aminotransferase. *Int. J. Biochem.* 2, 212–220

KALHAN, S. C., SAVIN, S. M. & ADAM, P. A. J. (1977) Attenuated glucose production rate in newborn infants of insulin-dependent diabetic mothers. *N. Engl. J. Med.* 296, 375–376

KEKOMÄKI, M. P., RÄIHÄ, N. C. R. & BICKEL, H. (1969) Ornithine-ketoacid aminotransferase in human liver with reference to patients with hyperornithinaemia and familial protein intolerance. *Clin. Chim. Acta* 23, 203–208

KIRBY, L. & HAHN, P. (1973) Enzyme induction in human fetal liver. *Pediatr. Res.* 7, 75–81

LAGERCRANTZ, H. & BISTOLETTI, P. (1973) Catecholamine release in the newborn infant at birth. *Pediatr. Res.* 11, 889–893

LIGGINS, G. C. & HOWIE, R. N. (1972) A controlled trial of antepartum glucocorticoid treatment for prevention of respiratory distress syndrome in premature infants. *Pediatrics* 50, 515–525

MENKES, J. H. & AVERY, M. E. (1963) The metabolism of phenylalanine and tyrosine in the premature infant. *Bull. Johns Hopkins Hosp.* 113, 301–319

RÄIHÄ, N. C. R. (1976) Milk protein, quality and quantity, in the feeding of low birth weight infants. *Curr. Med. Res. Opin.* 4, Suppl. 1, 85–89

RÄIHÄ, N. C. R. & EDKINS, E. (1977) Insulin antagonism of dexamethasone-induced increase of argininosuccinate synthetase and argininosuccinate lyase activities in cultured fetal rat liver. *Biol. Neonate* 31, 266–270

RÄIHÄ, N. C. R. & LINDROS, K. O. (1969) Development of some enzymes involved in gluconeogenesis in human liver. *Ann. Med. Exp. Biol. Fenn.* 47, 146–150

RÄIHÄ, N. C. R. & SCHWARTZ, A. L. (1973a) Development of urea biosynthesis and factors influencing the activity of the arginine synthetase system in perinatal mammalian liver, in *Inborn Errors of Metabolism* (Hommes, F. A. & Van Den Berg, C. J., eds.), pp. 221–232, Academic Press, London

RÄIHÄ, N. C. R. & SCHWARTZ, A. L. (1973b) Enzyme induction in human fetal liver in organ culture. *Enzyme (Basel)* 15, 330–339

RÄIHÄ, N. C. R. & SUIHKONEN, J. (1968a) Development of urea-synthesizing enzymes in human liver. *Acta Paediatr. Scand.* 57, 121–124

RÄIHÄ, N. C. R. & SUIHKONEN, J. (1968b) Factors influencing the development of urea-synthesizing enzymes in rat liver. *Biochem. J. 107*, 793–797

RÄIHÄ, N. C. R., SCHWARTZ, A. L. & LINDROOS, C. M. (1971) Induction of tyrosine-α-ketoglutarate transaminase in fetal rat and fetal human liver in organ culture. *Pediatr. Res. 5*, 70–76

SERENI, F., KENNEY, F. T. & KRETCHMER, N. (1959) Factors influencing the development of tyrosine-α-ketoglutarate transaminase activity in rat liver. *J. Biol. Chem. 234*, 609–612

SCHWARTZ, A. L. (1972) Influence of glucagon, 6-N,2′-O-dibutyryladenosine 3′ : 5′-cyclic monophosphate and triamcinolone on the arginine synthetase system in perinatal rat liver. *Biochem. J. 126*, 89–98

SCHWARTZ, A. L. & RALL, T. W. (1975) Hormonal regulation of incorporation of alanine-U-14C into glucose in human fetal liver explants. *Diabetes 24*, 650–657

SCHWARTZ, A. L., RÄIHÄ, N. C. R. & RALL, T. W. (1974) Effect of dibutyryl cyclic AMP on glucose-6-phosphatase activity in human fetal liver explants. *Biochim. Biophys. Acta 343*, 500–509

SMITH, B. T. GIROUND, C. J. P., ROBERT, M. & AVERY, M. E. (1975) Insulin antagonism of cortisol action on lecithin synthesis by cultured fetal lung cells. *J. Pediatr. 87*, 953–955

STERN, L., RAMOS, A. & LEDUC, J. (1968) Urinary catecholamine excretion in infants of diabetic mothers. *Pediatrics 42*, 598–605

WICKS, W. D. (1969) Induction of hepatic enzymes by adenosine 3′ : 5′-monophosphate in organ culture. *J. Biol. Chem. 244*, 3941–3950

WICKS, W. D., BARNETT, C. A. & McKIBBIN, J. B. (1974) Interaction between hormones and cyclic AMP in regulating specific hepatic enzyme synthesis. *Fed. Proc. 33*, 1105–1111

YEUNG, D. & OLIVER, I. T. (1968) Factors affecting the premature induction of phosphopyruvate carboxylase in neonatal rat liver. *Biochem. J. 108*, 325–331

Discussion

Williamson: Someone remarked that when fetal insulin was increased by continuous injection there was an increase in liver size. This implies that insulin increases the activity of some processes and increases the concentration of some enzymes. You and others have shown, Dr Räihä, that insulin acts as a repressor of glucogenic enzymes. What enzymes do you think insulin increases in the liver? This is a very important question for the infant of the diabetic mother.

Räihä: I can't answer that. An increase in liver size may increase the total amount of enzymes.

Williamson: Does insulin change the morphology of the explants you studied?

Räihä: We have only looked at the morphology of the normally cultured liver explants to see whether they were viable. I am sure that insulin can stimulate the synthesis of some enzymes. I have been talking about changes in enzyme concentraion which would imply enzyme synthesis, protein synthesis.   We also have data from studies of glycogen metabolism in human fetal liver explants which show that incubation of liver explants with insulin produces an increase in glycogen synthetase (I-form) while the addition of cyclic AMP tended to decrease this enzyme activity.   These results suggest that glycogen levels in human fetal liver may be regulated by an antagonistic effect of cyclic AMP and insulin on the activity of glycogen synthetase (Schwartz *et al.* 1975).

Williamson: Is it worth looking into whether insulin actually increases the concentration of any of the enzymes of lipid synthesis?

Shafrir: My experience with pyruvate kinase and acetyl-CoA carboxylase activities indicates that fetal hyperinsulinaemia induces some increase in glycolysis and lipogenesis capacity in the liver.   I shall be talking about that in my paper.

Blázquez: Your studies on liver enzymic activation during the perinatal period might be related not only to the secretory dynamics of insulin and glucagon at this age but also to the number of receptors for both these hormones in liver.   In previous studies it has been reported that the circulating levels of insulin and glucagon change dramatically during development in the rat (Girard *et al.* 1972; Blázquez *et al.* 1972).   Insulin concentrations in fetal serum increase markedly during the last days of pregnancy, decrease immediately after birth, and remain low during the suckling period.   In contrast, a sharp rise in the concentrations of serum glucagon occurs as early as 15 minutes after birth and continues for the next 20 days.   These hormonal changes appear to control the prenatal accumulation of hepatic glycogen and its rapid breakdown and, thus, help to prevent hypoglycaemia in the immediate postnatal period of fasting.   In addition, these changes help to maintain a relatively high rate of gluconeogenesis throughout the suckling period, when a large percentage of the necessary glucose must derive from amino acids.

Although serum glucagon levels in the rat fetus are higher than in the adult animals, anabolic processes such as DNA and protein synthesis and deposition of hepatic glycogen occur at a high rate during fetal life.   To explain this paradox, we studied the response of adenylate cyclase to glucagon and the binding sites for insulin and glucagon on purified liver membranes during rat development (Blázquez *et al.* 1976).   The adenylate cyclase response to glucagon (10^{-9} M) was only 7% of the adult response on day 15 of fetal life and 20% on the 21st day.   Not until after the 30th day *post partum* did it reach maturity. However the adenylate cyclase response to stimulation by NaF was comparable to the adult response throughout fetal life.   The binding of ^{125}I-labelled glucagon by these membrane preparations was only 1% of the adult level on day 15 of fetal age and increased to 23% on the 21st day; like the adenylate cyclase response to glucagon, glucagon binding did not reach maturity until after the 30th day of postnatal life. In contrast, insulin binding on the 15th day of gestation was 11% of the adult level and on the 21st day 45%, reaching adult levels on the 30th postnatal day.

To exclude the possibility that these results might have been due to inclusion of membranes from haematopoietic elements, which become less abundant as gestation progresses, rather than to changes in the binding characteristics of the hepatocyte membrane, we conducted experiments with purified suspensions of hepatocytes from fetal, suckling and adult rats. These results revealed a pattern of insulin and glucagon binding similar to that observed with membranes obtained from mixed cell preparations, except that there was greater insulin binding by the hepatocytes of suckling rats, at the time when the circulating insulin levels were very low. In comparison the binding of insulin and glucagon by the other cell types found in the liver, such as haematopoietic elements, Küppffer cells and circulating erythrocytes, was negligible.

These results suggest that the secretory pattern of insulin and glucagon and the sequential development of receptors for these two pancreatic hormones could have an important role in controlling the metabolic activities of the liver during perinatal life.

Battaglia: Are you measuring binding per milligram of protein?

Blázquez: To determine whether fetal liver membranes can be purified as effectively as adult liver membranes, we determined 5-nucleotidase activities and glucagon and insulin binding at different steps of the liver membrane purification procedure. The results exclude the possibility that differences in the purity of isolated liver membrane preparations are responsible for the changes in the measurements already described. Hormone binding to liver membranes was expressed per milligram of protein.

Hoet: If glucagon is not present in blood do you find it in the fetal urine or in the amniotic fluid?

Blázquez: Glucagon is broadly distributed in the tissues and fluids of rat fetuses. In the amniotic fluid we have already reported (Blázquez *et al.* 1972) that glucagon concentrations on days 19, 20 and 21 of gestation are 240, 280 and 360 pg/ml respectively.

Räihä: Your findings do not contradict what I said. The fetus has insulin receptors present and this would speak in favour of insulin probably being very important during fetal life, perhaps blocking pre-partum enzyme development.

Girard: The fact that there are fewer receptors for glucagon and a lower adenylate cyclase activity in fetal liver does not mean that there is glucagon resistance. In adult rat liver only 10 to 20% occupation of glucagon receptors is required to obtain a maximal biological effect on the liver. Plas & Nunez (1975) have shown that cultured fetal hepatocytes were sensitive to physiological concentrations of glucagon (10^{-10} M). The absence of glycogen breakdown in the fetal liver in late gestation, despite relatively high levels of circulating glucagon, could be explained by the very high levels of plasma insulin rather than by glucagon resistance. It has been reported that glucagon injection into the rat fetus can induce liver glycogen degradation and the premature appearance of liver PEP-carboxykinase, the rate-limiting enzyme of gluconeogenesis (see Girard et al. 1977 for a recent review). However, the increase in activity of this enzyme that is induced by maximal doses of glucagon in the fetus in utero is not comparable to the spontaneous rise which occurs immediately after birth (Girard et al. 1973). An important difference between these two situations is that the level of plasma insulin decreases dramatically in the newborn, while it is increased to very high levels by injection of glucagon into the fetus. The injection of anti-insulin serum in the fetus to neutralize endogenous insulin markedly potentiates the effect of glucagon on liver PEPCK (Girard et al. 1977). This suggests that it is the insulin : glucagon ratio rather than the absolute level of glucagon which is important in the control of hepatic metabolism in neonatal rats.

Blázquez: It has already been reported in liver membranes of adult rats (Birnbaumer & Pohl 1973) that a maximal hormonal response can be obtained with 10–20% of the total glucagon receptor population. According to our results there is a close relationship between binding of ^{125}I-labelled glucagon and activation of adenylate cyclase by this hormone in the liver membranes of fetal, suckling and adult rats, despite the fact that the glucagon binding was 1% and 8% of the adult level in 15- and 17-day-old fetuses, and 38% and 50% in rats with 10 and 30 days of extrauterine life, respectively. Obviously one can obtain a hormonal effect at all ages, but there is a marked hyposensitivity to glucagon in younger rats which is potentiated by the earlier development of liver insulin receptors and the hypersecretion of this hormone during the last day of fetal life. After birth the low insulin : glucagon ratio and the progressive increase in the number of receptors for glucagon favours the biological action of this hormone.

Girard: I do not think that it is possible to conclude that there is glucagon resistance by studying only the binding of glucagon and the activation of adenylate cyclase in hepatic membranes. It will be necessary to look at a more distal response, e.g. activation of gluconeogenesis or glycogenolysis.

Blázquez: We can assume that a low number of liver receptors for glucagon indicates a relative resistance or hyposensitivity to this hormone when the adenylate cyclase response to glucagon fits well with the binding studies. This statement is reinforced because binding of glucagon to purified liver membranes or to isolated hepatocytes follows the same pattern during development in the rat.

Räihä: The trouble is that some people are studying hormone receptor sites, others are studying enzymes and others again are looking at substrate concentrations. We should get together and start to sort this out. The receptor site story fits in well with the insulin effects since receptors must be present before the hormone can have an effect. Dr Blázquez showed that, at least in the rat fetus, insulin receptors are present at a fairly early stage and should be present when the hormonal changes start to occur. Thus insulin receptors should be present when fetal insulin increases at the end of pregnancy.

Blázquez: Early development of insulin binding sites in fetal liver could explain the biological effects of this hormone during the last days of intra-uterine life. It has been reported that insulin stimulates glycogen synthesis in fetal rat liver (Manns & Brockman 1969) and also DNA and protein synthesis by fetal rat hepatocytes kept in culture (Leffert 1974). These insulin effects are relevant since growth hormone has no effect on the rat fetus (Jost 1966), and prolactin, a hormone with growth-hormone-like properties in rodents (Chen *et al.* 1972; Francis & Hill 1975; Richards 1975), possesses a small number of receptors on liver membranes during perinatal life (S. Duran *et al.* unpublished work).

Stowers: Dr Räihä, you mentioned that infants of diabetic mothers have a smaller rise in plasma glucagon after birth than do infants of normal mothers (Bloom & Johnston 1972). We repeated this, getting Dr L.G. Heding to do specific pancreatic glucagon measurements. She found that the infants of diabetic mothers have higher than normal plasma glucagon values, in parallel with the degree of diabetes of the mother (Stowers *et al.* 1979). It seems likely that the hypoglycaemia of the infants was stimulating glucagon secretion.

Räihä: Presumably it is a question of the insulin to glucagon ratio.

Stowers: In erythroblastosis fetalis due to Rh incompatibility there is a tendency for islet cell hyperplasia to occur, but usually without hypoglycaemia. We have looked at these too. They did not have hypoglycaemia and their pancreatic glucagon plasma level did not rise above normal 2 h after birth (Stowers *et al.* 1979).

Räihä: I thought that it had been shown (Raivio & Österlund 1969) that infants with erythroblastosis have a high incidence of hypoglycaemia?

Stowers: They don't have specific β cell hyperplasia at all (Van Assche & Gepts 1971).

Milner: My understanding of the erythroblastotic infant is that there is islet hyperplasia and the hyperplastic islet of the rhesus-affected infant differs from that of the infant of the diabetic mother. The endocrine cell types within the hyperplastic islets of the rhesus-affected infant remain in their normal proportions of β to α_1 to α_2 to the rest (Van Assche et al. 1970). The hyperplastic islet of the infant of a diabetic mother, however, is characterized by an absolute and relative β-cell hyperplasia. Most of the published evidence states that although hypoglycaemia in the erythroblastotic infant may not be so common as in the infant of the diabetic mother, it is commoner than in normal infants of the same gestational age (Barrett & Oliver 1968) and is associated with and probably due to hyperinsulinaemia (From et al. 1969). Dr Stowers' finding that these infants do not manifest hyperglucagonaemia is very interesting since from the β and α_2 cell hyperplasia in the erythroblastotic islet one might have anticipated hypersecretion of both insulin and glucagon.

Pedersen: We have studied insulin and glucagon concentrations in 30 infants of diabetic mothers from all of White's classes. The observations agree with what we have been told here about the concentrations. The infants of mothers in class A, who are near to the normal, have a more or less normal insulin: glucagon ratio, whereas infants of mothers in classes D and F have a very high insulin : glucagon ratio. Also the ratio diminishes at a slower rate than in classes A and B + C. The glucagon rises but it rises later in classes D + F than in A and B + C.

Kalkhoff: How long does that last?

Pedersen: The determinations were performed over the first 12 hours of life. At birth the plasma glucagon concentration was more or less equal in the three classes of infants investigated, although considerable differences between the plasma insulin and glucose concentrations of the different groups were noted. After birth an increment of just under threefold in plasma glucagon took place after two hours in the class A infants. In the class B + C infants a 3.5-fold increment in plasma glucagon was observed but maximal glucagon levels were first reached after 12 hours of life. Plasma glucagon of the class D + F infants rose 2.5 times after 12 hours, indicating that in these infants the increment in plasma glucagon was the smallest observed, even though the degree of hypoglycaemia was the greatest.

Girard: It is known that glucagon secretion cannot be decreased by glucose in normal newborn infants. The sluggish rise of glucagon in infants of diabetic mothers could result from the premature appearance of cell sensitivity to glucose or from the high insulin levels *in utero*. Is that a possible explanation?

Pedersen: It might be.

Battaglia: The published paediatric work is confusing on the issue of hypoglycaemia in erythroblastosis.

Milner: The incidence of spontaneous hypoglycaemia in erythroblastotic infants has been reported as 5 out of 16 (Barrett & Oliver 1968).

Battaglia: What percentage of babies is affected?

Milner: Three out of 10 of the erythroblastotic infants made hyperglycaemic by exchange transfusion with ACD blood became hypoglycaemic at some time within the first three hours after transfusion (Cser & Milner 1974). In most of them the hypoglycaemia was asymptomatic and self-correcting.

Battaglia: This is a bit like the discussions about patent ductus arteriosus (PDA) at high altitude. In Peruvian villages at 4300 metres there was said to be a 10–15-fold increase in the incidence of PDA. That sounds very impressive until one realizes that it is still only 1% or 2% of all births. The baby who doesn't get sick tells us more about biology than the one who does. In other words, most infants close the ductus arteriosus at very low oxygen tensions and that is more interesting than the occasional infant who keeps it open. Certainly most of the infants with erythroblastosis fetalis do not have problems with significant hypoglycaemia.

Räihä: Nobody argues that we have clinical problems with the newborn infants of insulin-dependent diabetic mothers. If these problems can be explained by the antagonistic effect of high insulin concentrations on normal enzymic development it clears up many points. In other words, all the organs in infants of diabetic mothers show signs of immature function, and the clinical problems are due to the functional immaturity.

Freinkel: Have you analysed your explants for lysosomal enzymes? In the adult liver, one of the major functions of glucagon may be to induce or integrate the development of lysosomes and there is some evidence that insulin may antagonize this action (Amherdt *et al.* 1974).

Räihä: We haven't studied that.

Girard: Lysosomes proliferate in the newborn rat liver within 4 or 6 h after birth and this could be related to the fall in plasma insulin and the rise in plasma glucagon (Girard *et al.* 1973).

References

AMHERDT, M., HARRIS, V., RENOLD, A. E., ORCI, L. & UNGER, R. H. (1974) Hepatic autophagy in uncontrolled experimental diabetes and its relationships to insulin and glucagon. *J. Clin. Invest. 54*, 188–193

BARRETT, C. T. & OLIVER, T. K. JR. (1968) Hypoglycemia and hyperinsulinism in infants with erythroblastosis foetalis. *N. Engl. J. Med. 278*, 1260–1263

BIRNBAUMER, L. & POHL, S. L. (1973) Relation of glucagon-specific binding sites to glucagon-dependent stimulation of adenylyl cyclase activity in plasma membranes of rat liver. *J. Biol. Chem. 248*, 2056–2061

BLÁZQUEZ, E., SUGASE, T., BLÁZQUEZ, M. & FOÀ, P. P. (1972) The ontogeny of metabolic regulation in the rat, with special reference to the development of insular function. *Acta Diabetol. Lat. 9*, 13–35

BLÁZQUEZ, E., RUBALCAVA, B., MONTESANO, R., ORCI, L. & UNGER, R. (1976) Developmc... insulin and glucagon binding and the adenylate cyclase response in liver membranes of the prenatal, postnatal and adult rat: evidence of glucagon 'resistance'. *Endocrinology 98*, 1014–1023.

BLOOM, S. R. & JOHNSTON, D. J. (1972) Failure of glucagon release in infants of diabetic mothers. *Br. Med. J. 4*, 453–454

CHEN, H. W., HAMER, D. H., HEINIGER, H. J. & MEIER, H. (1972) Stimulation of hepatic RNA synthesis in dwarf mice by ovine prolactin. *Biochim. Biophys. Acta 287*, 90–97

CSER, A. & MILNER, R. D. G. (1974) Metabolic and hormonal changes during and after exchange transfusion with heparinized or ACD blood. *Arch. Dis. Child. 49*, 940–945

FRANCIS, M. J. O. & HILL, D. J. (1975) Prolactin-stimulated production of somatomedin by rat liver. *Nature (Lond.) 255*, 167–168

FROM, G. L. A., DRISCOLL, S. G. & STEINKE, J. (1969) Serum insulin in newborn infants with erythroblastosis foetalis. *Pediatrics 44*, 549–553

GIRARD, J., BALL, D. & ASSAN, R. (1972) Glucagon secretion during the early postnatal period in the rat. *Horm. Metab. Res. 4*, 168–170

GIRARD, J. R., CUENDET, G. S., MARLISS, E. B., KERVRAN, A., RIEUTORT, M. & ASSAN, R. (1973) Fuels, hormones and liver metabolism at term and during the early postnatal period in the rat. *J. Clin. Invest. 52*, 3190–3200

GIRARD, J. R., FERRE, P., KERVRAN, A., PEGORIER, J. P. & ASSAN, R. (1977) Influence of insulin-glucagon ratio in the change of hepatic metabolism during development of the rat, in *Glucagon: its Role in Physiology and Clinical Medicine* (Foa, P.P. *et al.*, eds.), pp. 563–581, Excerpta Medica, Amsterdam

JOST, A. (1966) In *The Pituitary Gland*, vol. 2 (Harris, G. W. & Donovan, B.T., eds.), p. 299, University of California Press, Berkeley

LEFFERT, H. L. (1974) Growth control of differentiated fetal rat hepatocytes in primary mono-layer culture. VII. Hormonal control of DNA synthesis and its possible significance to the problem of liver regeneration. *J. Cell Biol. 62*, 792–801

MANNS, J. G. & BROCKMAN, R. P. (1969) The role of insulin in the synthesis of fetal gluco-gen. *Can. J. Physiol. Pharmacol. 47*, 917–921

PLAS, C. & NUNEZ, J. (1975) Glycogenolytic response to glucagon of cultured fetal hepatocy-tes. Refractoriness following prior exposure to glucagon. *J. Biol. Chem. 250*, 5304–5311

RAIVIO, K.O. & ÖSTERLUND, K. (1969) Hypoglycemia and hyperinsulinemia associated with erythroblastosis fetalis. *Pediatrics 43*, 217–225

RICHARDS, J. F. (1975) Ornithine decarboxylase activity in tissues of prolactin-treated rats. *Biochem. Biophys. Res. Commun. 63*, 292–299

SCHWARTZ, A. L., RÄIHÄ, N. C. R. & RALL, T. W. (1975) Hormonal regulation of glucogen metabolism in human fetal liver. *Diabetes 24*, 1101–1112

STOWERS, J. M., HEDING, L. G., FISHER, P. M., TREHARNE, I. A. L., ROSS, I. S., SUTHERLAND, H. W., BEWSHER, P. D., RUSSELL, G. & PRICE, H. V. (1979) The relationship between gluca-gon and hypocalcaemia in infants of diabetic mothers in *Carbohydrate Metabolism in Preg-nancy and the Newborn* (Sutherland, H. W. & Stowers, J. M., eds.), Springer-Verlag, Berlin

VAN ASSCHE, F. A. & GEPTS, W. (1971) The cytological composition of the fetal endocrine pancreas. *Diabetologia 7*, 434–444

VAN ASSCHE, F. A., GEPTS, W., DE GASPARO, M. & RENAER, M. (1970) The endocrine pancreas in erythroblastosis fetalis. *Biol. Neonate 15*, 176–185

Regulation of placental enzymes of the carbohydrate and lipid metabolic pathways

ELEAZAR SHAFRIR and YORAM Z. DIAMANT

Departments of Biochemistry, and Gynecology and Obstetrics, Hadassah University Hospital and Hebrew University-Hadassah Medical School, Jerusalem, Israel

Abstract   The activity of enzymes with a regulatory function in the pathways of glycolysis, gluconeogenesis, NADPH generation and fatty acid synthesis was measured in the placenta and liver of rats.   Compared with the liver, a high activity of pyruvate kinase was found in the placenta, indicating a high glycolytic potential; a small capacity for gluconeogenesis was also present and a moderate to low activity of enzymes associated with lipogenesis.

The activity of all placental enzymes fell from day 15 to 20 of gestation irrespective of the pathway they represented.   The pattern of decline continued when the gestation was prolonged up to day 26 by the administration of chorionic gonadotropin.   The rates of activity disappearance over 11 days of gestation differed for each enzyme, with half-lives ranging from 2.7 days for NADP-malate dehydrogenase to 7 days for glucose-6-phosphate dehydrogenase.   In contrast, the activity of hepatic enzymes either remained unchanged or showed individual adaptation to the advancing pregnancy.

The regression in placental metabolic capacity after day 15 of gestation was also evident by the decrease in glucose uptake and its channelling to lactate, CO_2, glycerol and fatty acids.   In addition, placental ageing was associated with triglyceride accumulation, mainly due to the decrease in free fatty acid oxidation.

Treatment of pregnant rats with several hormones, while markedly affecting the hepatic enzyme activities, failed to induce appreciable changes in the corresponding placental enzymes.   This was illustrated in the case of triiodothyronine treatment.   Similarly, insulin deficiency induced by streptozotocin failed to elicit adaptive changes in placental enzyme activities typical of diabetes like those occurring in the maternal liver; some converse responses in the placenta were attributed to hyperglycaemia.   On the other hand, responses in some fetal liver enzymes were suggestive of fetal hyperinsulinaemia.

These observations indicate that placental enzymes are not susceptible to endocrine regulation and imply that placental metabolism is largely independent of the physiopathological alterations affecting the maternal organism.   The gradual activity decreases with gestation suggest that the enzyme complement of the placenta, once developed, is designed to last through its limited lifespan without continuous replenishment.   Within this context, no mechanism seems to operate to induce the adaptive synthesis of individual enzymes, and the age of the placenta appears to be the primary factor determining its enzyme activity and metabolic performance.

161

The placenta is known today to be much more than a selective two-way barrier for metabolite transport between mother and fetus. It performs complex metabolic functions for which it is endowed with a multitude of enzymic activities on its own.

Although the lifespan of the placenta is relatively limited, the endocrine responses and patterns of metabolism of the feto-maternal system change at different stages of fetal development. Therefore it was of interest to study whether the enzymic activities of the placenta adapt to these changes. In addition it seemed important to establish the pattern of responses of placental enzymes to various endocrine challenges and to diabetes.

Pregnant albino rats of the Hebrew University strain were used in our studies. They weighed about 200 g and were fed a regular pelleted chow *ad libitum*. Experimental procedures and methods for liver and placental homogenate preparation and enzyme assays were outlined in our previous publications (Y.Z. Diamant & Shafrir 1972; Beyth *et al.* 1977). Enzyme activities were measured at 37 °C and expressed as nanomoles of substrate metabolized per minute per milligram of cytoplasmic protein.

PLACENTAL ENZYME ACTIVITIES COMPARED TO MATERNAL LIVER

Table 1 shows the effect of gestation on several enzymes of regulatory importance within the pathways of glycolysis, gluconeogenesis and transamination, NADPH generation and fatty acid synthesis. Table 2 lists the activity of these enzymes in the liver of pregnant rats.

A comparison of the corresponding enzymes in the placenta and the liver on day 15 of gestation (see column 1 in Tables 1 and 2) shows that pyruvate kinase (EC 2.7.1.40) exhibited a very high activity in the placenta, about fourfold that in the liver. This demonstrates the presence of a very potent glycolytic pathway and suggests that glucose is the main metabolic fuel in the placenta. Similarly, high activity of pyruvate kinase relative to liver was found in sheep (Dhand *et al.* 1970) and human (Y.Z. Diamant *et al.* 1975a) placenta.

A distinct activity of phospho*enol*pyruvate carboxylase (PEP carboxylase, EC 4.1.1.32) was also found in the placenta, indicating its ability to channel 3-carbon precursors into glucose, glycerol or glycogen formation. However the activity of this enzyme, as well as of aspartate and alanine aminotransferases (EC 2.6.1.1 and EC 2.6.1.2) associated with the pathway of gluconeogenesis, was quite low in the placenta as compared to the liver.

The activity of enzymes directly participating in lipogenesis, ATP citrate

TABLE 1

Effect of pregnancy on placental enzyme activity

Enzyme	Normal gestation			Postmaturity	
	Day 15	Day 18	Day 20	Day 23	Day 26
	$n\ mol\ min^{-1}\ mg^{-1}$				
Pyruvate kinase	2490 ± 104	1640 ± 173*	615 ± 68*	402 ± 64*	221 ± 26*
PEP carboxylase	23 ± 1	15 ± 1*	11 ± 1*	8.6 ± 0.9	3.9 ± 0.6*
Aspartate amino- transferase	21 ± 2	13 ± 2*	10 ± 1	8.2 ± 0.9	5.4 ± 0.4**
Alanine amino- transferase	6.8 ± 0.9	3.3 ± 0.7*	1.7 ± 0.3*	1.1 ± 0	0.6 ± 0.1*
G6P dehydrogenase	42 ± 4	34 ± 4	28 ± 3*	22 ± 3*	14 ± 2*
6PG dehydrogenase	50 ± 4	37 ± 4*	30 ± 2	25 ± 3*	18 ± 1*
NADP-malate dehydrogenase	33 ± 6	16 ± 1*	11 ± 1*	4.9 ± 0.3*	2.2 ± 0.1*
ATP-citrate lyase	11 ± 1	9.5 ± 1.0	5.2 ± 1.5*	2.8 ± 0.3*	1.8 ± 0.2*
Acetyl-CoA carboxylase	2.3 ± 0.4	1.4 ± 0.3*	0.7 ± 0.2*	0.3 ± 0.1*	0.15 ± 0.08

Values are means ± S.E. for groups of 8 to 14 rats.
Postmaturity was induced by a single i.v. injection of 500 units/rat of HCG on day 18 of
pregnancy. The values are derived in part from our previous work (Y.Z. Diamant & Shafrir
1972; Beyth et al. 1977), and in part have been redetermined with improved procedures. Asterisk denotes a statistically significant difference from the preceding value at $P < 0.05$ at least.

(pro-3S)-lyase (citrate cleavage enzyme, EC 4.1.3.8) and acetyl-CoA carboxylase (EC 6.4.1.2), was also present in the placenta, indicating the capacity for
de novo fatty acid synthesis. These activities in the placenta amounted to half
and one-sixth of those in the liver respectively.

The activity of enzymes supporting lipogenesis by NADPH production, that
is glucose-6-phosphate and 6-phosphogluconate dehydrogenases (EC
1.1.1.49 and EC 1.1.1.43) and malate dehydrogenase (oxaloacetate-
decarboxylating) (NADP$^+$) ('malate enzyme', EC 1.1.1.40), in the placenta
was one-third to one-sixth of their activities in the liver. This suggests an
ample capacity for NADPH generation, taking into the account that the
NADPH requirement in the placenta is not extensive in view of the limited
direct lipogenesis in this tissue.

EFFECT OF GESTATIONAL AGE ON PLACENTAL AND LIVER ENZYMES

Whereas the placental enzyme content was shown to represent a wide
spectrum of metabolic capacity, the activities of all enzymes fell with gesta-

TABLE 2

Effect of pregnancy on liver enzyme activity

Enzyme	Normal gestation			Postmaturity	
	Day 15	Day 18	Day 20	Day 23	Day 26
	$nmol\ min^{-1}\ mg^{-1}$				
Pyruvate kinase	628 ± 32	563 ± 20	602 ± 30	545 ± 42	416 ± 33*
PEP carboxylase	165 ± 25	189 ± 20	226 ± 19	425 ± 62*	620 ± 58*
Aspartate amino- transferase	289 ± 21	241 ± 22	392 ± 24*	485 ± 62*	695 ± 67*
Alanine amino- transferase	167 ± 22	130 ± 13	112 ± 16	179 ± 22*	228 ± 48*
G6P dehydrogenase	184 ± 23	175 ± 10	152 ± 17	168 ± 20	182 ± 14
6PG dehydrogenase	350 ± 10	302 ± 17	292 ± 8	320 ± 42	335 ± 36
NADP-malate dehydrogenase	96 ± 7	50 ± 6*	51 ± 3*	25 ± 3*	16 ± 2*
ATP-citrate lyase	24 ± 4	12 ± 2*	7.2 ± 1.2*	8.8 ± 1.5	5.4 ± 1.0*
Acetyl-CoA carboxylase	12 ± 1	9.5 ± 1.0	8.4 ± 0.9*	6.0 ± 0.4*	4.1 ± 0.5*

Values are means ± S.E. for groups of 8 to 14 rats. Postmaturity was induced by a single i.v. injection of 500 units/rat of HCG on day 18 of pregnancy. The values are derived in part from our previous work (Y.Z. Diamant & Shafrir 1972; Beyth et al. 1977), and in part have been redetermined with improved procedures. Asterisk denotes a statistically significant difference from the preceding value at $P < 0.05$ at least.

tion. Although the enzymes of various metabolic pathways usually respond in different directions to changing physiopathological conditions in deference to alterations in substrate and/or hormone availability, placental senescence was associated with a consistent decrease in enzyme activities, irrespective of the particular pathway they represent.

Table 1 shows the pattern of the decrease during the last five days of normal gestation in the rat. Since this was relatively a short time span and it is difficult to measure placental enzyme activities in very young placentas, the pregnancy was prolonged by five days by giving human chorionic gonadotropin (HCG) to the rat, and enzyme activities were followed up to the 26th day of gestation. The results demonstrate a continuing decrease and indicate that the factor(s) determining the activity of placental enzymes continue(s) to operate beyond term.

In contrast to the changes in the placenta, the maternal liver enzymes (Table 2) did not show a unidirectional pattern of changes, but rather adaptation to advancing pregnancy.   The glycolytic capacity, as inferred from the activity of pyruvate kinase, remained without change except late in postmaturity when it decreased.   The hepatic capacity for lipogenesis decreased more markedly, even earlier in gestation, as seen from the decreased activity of the three enzymes concerned with this pathway.   The activity of enzymes related to gluconeogenesis increased, particularly in postmaturity.   These changes reflect the metabolic responses to the prolonged gestation which accentuates the trend of maternal starvation, already discernible at the end of normal gestation, into a diabetes-like situation.

It should be noted that the decrease in placental enzyme activities during the course of normal and delayed gestation was apparent despite the continuing growth of the placenta and the fetus (Table 3).   The placenta did not histologically show any signs of deterioration.

Since the enzyme activities were expressed per milligram of cytoplasmic protein (the concentration of which did not appreciably change during the gestation) the decrease in specific enzyme activities might have been somewhat compensated by the increase in placental size.   However, such compensation was relatively small, as exemplified by pyruvate kinase: from days 15 through 26 of pregnancy the activity of this enzyme decreased nearly 11-fold whereas the placental weight increased only about threefold.   This fact speaks against the possibility that the placental enzymes were located in a particular tissue compartment which remained constant during gestation, while other non-functional cells continued to grow.

The kinetic aspects of the decrease in placental enzyme activities are depicted in Fig. 1.   It can be seen that the rate of disappearance of the individual

TABLE 3

Placental and fetal weight during normal and prolonged gestation

Day of gestation	Placental weight (g)	Fetal weight (g)
15	0.21 ± 0.01	1.1 ± 0.1
18	0.38 ± 0.01	1.9 ± 0.1
20	0.46 ± 0.01	3.2 ± 0.1
23	0.53 ± 0.01	5.1 ± 0.1
26	0.59 ± 0.02	7.1 ± 0.2

Pregnancy was extended by a single i.v. administration of HCG, 500 units/rat on day 18.   Values are means ± S.E. for groups of 8 to 20 rats, in each case representing an average of 5 placentas and fetuses.

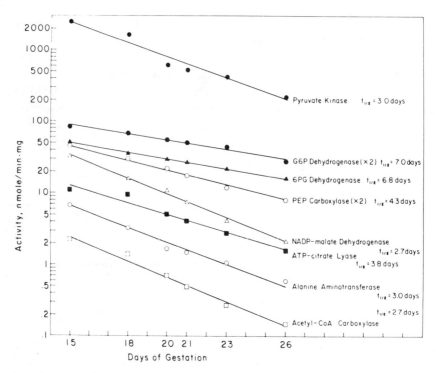

FIG. 1.   Rates of disappearance of the activity of placental enzymes during normal and prolonged gestation.

enzymes was not uniform, ranging from half-lives of 2.7 days for NADP-
malate dehydrogenase and acetyl-CoA carboxylase to 6.8 to 7 days for G6P
and 6PG dehydrogenases.   These kinetics do not describe enzyme turnover
since the synthesis and degradation rates were not measured and it is not
known whether the decrease in activity results from retarded synthesis or
accelerated breakdown.   The different half-lives do demonstrate, though, an
individual fate of each enzyme within its own cellular metabolism rather than a
uniform decay pattern of placental cells.

EFFECT OF GESTATIONAL AGE ON GLUCOSE AND FATTY ACID METABOLISM

The activities of placental enzymes shown in Table 1 actually represent maximal enzyme capacities measured under optimal assay conditions.   To support
the conclusions reached on the basis of decrease in enzyme activity, we studied
the utilization of glucose by placental slices *in vitro*.   The results shown in
Table 4 confirm the conclusion that placental glycolysis and lipogenesis dimi-

TABLE 4

Placental glucose utilization during normal and prolonged gestation

Day of gestation	Glucose conversion to:			
	Lactate $\mu mol\ 2\ h^{-1}\ (g\ tissue)^{-1}$	CO_2	Lipid glycerol	Fatty acids
15	15.2	1.42	2.24	0.36
18	11.5	1.06	2.06	0.28
20	9.5	0.85	2.40	0.24
23	7.7	0.56	1.62	0.10
26	5.8	0.51	1.16	0.04

Results of representative experiment (mean of 2 rats for each day). Placental slices weighing about 300 mg were incubated for 2 h in 5 ml of [U-^{14}C]glucose solution in 2% bovine albumin. CO_2 was trapped to measure its radioactivity, lactate production was measured in the medium; the tissue was extracted and the extract hydrolysed for the determination of radioactivity in total lipid components. Pregnancy beyond day 21 was extended by a single i.v. injection of HCG, 500 units/rat, on day 18 of gestation.

nished with advancing gestation. Between days 15 and 26 of gestation, lactate and CO_2 production from glucose was reduced by about 60%, and fatty acid synthesis by as much as 89%. Lipid glycerol synthesis was least affected (reduced by 48%), probably because in late pregnancy the placenta is exposed to increasing levels of circulating free fatty acids, to the esterification of which a larger share of glucose carbons is shifted. Of interest is the large proportion of glucose carbons converted into lactate relative to those metabolized to CO_2. This points out a limited capacity of full glucose oxidation in the placenta and repeatedly indicates that glycolysis is the principal energy source of this tissue.

Table 5 shows, indeed, the presence of an increased triglyceride content in the aged placenta together with a reduction in fatty acid metabolism. With albumin-bound oleate as the substrate, placental slices exhibited a significantly increased esterification of the free fatty acid to tri- and diglycerides but, at the same time, oxidation to CO_2 remained virtually unchanged. The decrease in fatty acid utilization seems thus to be linked to the general decrease in metabolic capacity of the placenta and to contribute to the accumulation of triglycerides in this tissue in late pregnancy.

Whereas the extent of transfer of free fatty acids through the placenta seems to be species-dependent (Robertson & Sprecher 1968), Szabo & Szabo (1974) and Hull & Elphick (1979, this volume) postulated that the excessively high

TABLE 5

Placental triglyceride (TG) synthesis and turnover

Day of gestation	TG content (mg/ml DNA)	[1–^{14}C]oleate incorporation ($\mu mol/mg$ DNA)			Specific activity (dpm/mg TG × 10^3)
		TG	DG	CO_2	
15	0.68 ± 0.02	2.5 ± 0.2	0.03 ± 0.01	3.0 ± 0.5	41.1 ± 3.1
20	2.13 ± 0.15*	3.9 ± 0.2*	0.08 ± 0.01*	3.4 ± 0.4	15.1 ± 1.5*

Unpublished data of Y.Z. Diamant and N. Freinkel.
Fresh placental slices from rats fed *ad libitum* and weighing 150 to 180 g were incubated for 1 h with 2 ml albumin solution containing 0.75 μmol [1-^{14}C]oleate.
Values are means ± S.E. of 8 experiments.   Asterisk denotes a significant difference at $P < 0.05$ at least.

concentrations of maternal free fatty acids in diabetic pregnancy may become available to the fetus and be in part responsible for its increased weight.   In the rat a direct passage of preformed fatty acids has not been observed (Koren & Shafrir 1964) but an increased removal to the fetal side, of the triglycerides that accumulate in the placenta, by a lipolytic process remains a possibility to be investigated.

Our results on the reduction of metabolic activity of the ageing placenta are in general accord with those of Sakurai *et al.* (1969), who found a decrease in the incorporation and oxidation of [U-^{14}C]glucose in human placentas at term, with those of Walker *et al.* (1967), who reported a decrease in the activity of hexose monophosphate shunt enzymes towards term, and with those of Villee (1953), who noted a decrease in oxygen consumption and pyruvate and lactate production and utilization in human placentas at term.

RESPONSE OF PLACENTAL ENZYMES TO ENDOCRINE CHALLENGES

To explore whether the pattern of placental enzyme changes is influenced by hormonal alterations during the course of gestation and whether the enzymes are susceptible to adaptive responses to hormones, we treated pregnant rats with several hormones known to affect the metabolism of liver and several reproductive tissues.   In view of the gradual decreases with age of the placenta, special care was taken to measure the enzyme activity on a particular day of gestation.   In general the hormones were given for three days to rats weighing about 200 g, starting on day 15 of gestation.   Conjugated oestrogen (0.1

mg/day), HCG (50 units/day), progesterone (5 mg/day), and triamcinolone (5 mg/day) failed to induce changes in most placental enzyme activities, as reported elsewhere (Y.Z. Diamant et al. 1975b), although they affected the activity of glycolysis, lipogenesis and gluconeogenesis enzymes in the liver. In particular the glucocorticoid triamcinolone, which promoted hepatic gluconeogenesis and was found in male rats to induce lipogenesis enzymes in the liver while suppressing the activity of the same enzymes in adipose tissue (S. Diamant & Shafrir 1975), did not affect lipogenesis enzymes in the placenta (Y.Z. Diamant et al. 1975b).

The different effects of a hormone on liver and placenta are illustrated in Table 6 for the case of triiodothyronine (T_3). This hormone was previously reported to induce the activity of several hepatic and adipose tissue enzymes associated with lipogenesis in male rats (S. Diamant et al. 1972). As shown in Table 6, the activity of enzymes taking part in NADPH generation and fatty acid synthesis was pronouncedly increased in the liver of pregnant rats treated for five days with T_3; the gluconeogenesis capacity was also increased whereas that of glycolysis was lowered. None of these changes were seen in the respective placental enzymes.

TABLE 6

Effect of T_3 treatment on maternal hepatic and placental enzymes (E. Shafrir & R. Kiselevitch, unpublished work)

	Pyruvate kinase	PEP carboxyl-ase	G6P dehydro-genase	6PG dehydro-genase	NADP-malate dehydro-genase	Acetyl-CoA carboxylase
			$nmol\ min^{-1}\ mg^{-1}$			
Liver						
Control	623 ± 62	239 ± 31	154 ± 12	219 ± 19	46 ± 5	9.1 ± 1.0
T_3-treated	304 ± 19*	445 ± 32*	211 ± 15*	317 ± 17*	89 ± 9*	21.1 ± 1.6*
Placenta						
Control	646 ± 90	9.1 ± 1.9	32.6 ± 3.4	25.7 ± 3.3	18 ± 3	2.0 ± 0.3
T_3-treated	673 ± 35	7.4 ± 1.8	28.9 ± 4.1	27.4 ± 2.3	20 ± 4	1.7 ± 0.2

Values are means ± s.e. for groups of 14 to 16 rats. T_3, 100 μg/kg, was injected s.c. daily from day 15 to day 20 of pregnancy. Asterisk denotes a significant difference from the control value at $P < 0.05$ at least.

EFFECT OF DIABETES ON PLACENTAL ENZYME ACTIVITIES IN RELATION TO
MATERNAL AND FETAL LIVER

Although hormonal treatments did not affect the placental enzymes it
should be borne in mind that these treatments were given for three to five days
late in gestation.   To further explore whether the placental enzymes may
become affected by a drastic and long-standing metabolic change on the
maternal side, due to lack rather than to excess of a hormone, we have studied
the effect of streptozotocin-induced diabetes.   On day 20 of pregnancy, after
eight days of diabetes, the rats were markedly insulin-deficient as shown by the
hyperglycaemia of 440 mg/dl, serum insulin < 10% of the control value and
pancreatic immunoassayable insulin ~ 5% of that in the non-diabetic pregnant
rats.

Table 7 records the enzyme activities in the placenta, maternal and fetal
liver.   On the maternal side the hepatic glycolytic capacity, as represented by

TABLE 7

Effect of diabetes on enzyme activities in the placenta and in the maternal and fetal liver of the rat
(results derived from work by Y.Z. Diamant & E. Shafrir 1978)

	Placenta		Maternal liver		Fetal liver	
	Control	Diabetes	Control $nmol\ min^{-1}$	Diabetes mg^{-1}	Control	Diabetes
Pyruvate kinase	886 ± 62	1401 ± 110*	592 ± 54	304 ± 49*	294 ± 15	411 ± 35 *
PEP carboxylase	24 ± 3	13 ± 2*	229 ± 22	936 ± 108*	32 ± 4	28 ± 2
Aspartate amino-transferase	34 ± 3	47 ± 5	494 ± 54	1989 ± 218*	206 ± 24	168 ± 22
Alanine amino-transferase	53 ± 10	7.6 ± 2.8	176 ± 22	360 ± 37*	31 ± 2	28 ± 4
G6P dehydro-genase	28 ± 3	35 ± 3	139 ± 11	66 ± 7*	54 ± 4	68 ± 6
NADP-malate dehydrogenase	17 ± 2	17 ± 2	52 ± 5	25 ± 3*	12 ± 1	18 ± 1*
ATP-citrate lyase	5.1 ± 0.9	6.5 ± 0.8	24 ± 2	11 ± 2*	8 ± 1	12 ± 1*
Acetyl-CoA carboxylase	0.8 ± 0.1	0.7 ± 0.1	11 ± 2	5 ± 1*	1.4 ± 0.2	2.3 ± 0.3*

Values are means ± S.E. for groups of 10 to 12 rats.   Streptozotocin, 65 mg/kg, was injected i.v.
on day 12 of pregnancy and enzyme activities were determined on day 20 of pregnancy.
Asterisks denote a statistically significant change at $P < 0.05$ at least.

pyruvate kinase activity, was reduced; the gluconeogenesis capacity, as represented by the rate-limiting enzyme, PEP carboxylase, and by alanine and aspartate aminotransferases, was markedly increased.   The activity of NADPH-generating enzymes, as well as that of ATP citrate lyase and acetyl CoA carboxylase, which are directly involved in lipogenesis, fell considerably.   This enzyme pattern shown here in the liver of pregnant rats is known to be characteristic of insulin deficiency (Chang & Schneider 1971; Dolkart *et al.* 1964; Migliorini 1971).

In contrast to maternal liver, the fetal liver did not exhibit a diabetic enzyme pattern.   There was no increase in enzymes associated with gluconeogenesis.   Conversely, a small though significant increase was seen in the activity of pyruvate kinase and of the lipogenic enzymes NADP malate dehydrogenase, ATP citrate lyase and acetyl CoA carboxylase, suggesting a state of fetal hyperinsulinaemia.   This contention was supported by the finding of an increase in the glycogen content of the fetal liver and is discussed elsewhere (Y.Z. Diamant & Shafrir 1978).

In the placenta, diabetes did not induce changes in the activity of most of the investigated enzymes, such as those related to transamination, NADPH generation and lipogenesis, in agreement with our observations in other hormonal deviations.   There was no evidence of premature ageing and deterioration of placental enzyme activities like that seen in placentas from toxaemic patients (Y.Z. Diamant *et al.* 1976).   However, there was a small but surprising rise in the activity of pyruvate kinase, whereas that of PEP carboxylase fell somewhat.   The response of these two enzymes in the placenta was the inverse of their response in the liver, although not as extensive, and this response was considered to be incompatible with the circumstances of enhanced gluconeogenesis.   The fact that the activity of these two enzymes was not altered in the placenta of starving pregnant rats (Y.Z. Diamant & Shafrir 1978) indicated that these changes may be related to the direct effect of glycaemia rather than to adaptation to insulin deficiency.

In our previous experiments with pregnant triamcinolone-treated rats (Y.Z. Diamant *et al.* 1975*b*) we also observed similar reciprocal changes in the activity of pyruvate kinase and PEP carboxylase in the liver and placenta.

A common feature of the diabetic and triamcinolone-treated rats is hyperglycaemia.   High glucose concentrations are known to suppress PEP carboxylase activity (Dodek *et al.* 1975; Shrago *et al.* 1967) and to promote at the same time pyruvate kinase activity by the feed-forward activation effect of phosphorylated hexoses, particularly FDP (Llorente *et al.* 1970; Van Berkel & Koster 1973).   A further feature of the placenta is its increased glycogen content in diabetes (Gabbe *et al.* 1972; Hagerman 1962; Sybulski & Maughan

1972).   Coupled with glycogen loss in the liver this is another instance of reciprocal behaviour, most probably to be attributed to different responses of the placental and hepatic glycogen synthetase-phosphorylase system.

These observations indicate that the means of enzyme control differ in the placenta and the liver.   The adaptive enzymes in the latter tissue are sensitive to suppression or induction by insulin deficiency or to the information transmitted by hormones in general, whereas some of the placental enzymes may show a limited response to changing substrate availability, such as hyperglycaemia.   It is pertinent that a reciprocal fashion of responses of pyruvate kinase and PEP carboxylase in relation to the liver in diabetes has been also reported in other tissues with non-adaptive enzymes, such as the duodenum (Anderson & Zakim 1970) and kidney (Anderson & Stowring 1973).

CONCLUDING COMMENTS

Our results showing the lack of changes in placental enzyme activities in insulin-deficient diabetes, together with the findings showing that the enzymes do not respond to an excess of glucocorticoids, T_3, oestrogen, progesterone or chorionic gonadotropin, give rise to the concept that placental enzymes are not susceptible to hormonal regulation, at least not in the later stages of gestation.   This concepts fits well with the physiological purpose of the placenta, which is to support fetal growth irrespective of the metabolic vicissitudes afflicting the maternal organism.   The overriding requirement to protect the fetus carries with it a lack of capacity for enzyme adaptation and thus dissociation from factors regulating the maternal metabolism.   This metabolic independence and stability applies mainly to long-range adjustments usually linked to de novo enzyme synthesis and does not include moment-to-moment control of enzyme activity through substrate flow and fluctuations in the concentration of intracellular effectors.

The only consistent changes we found in enzyme activities were the gradual but individual decreases related to the age of the placenta during normal and prolonged gestation.   On the basis of these findings we suggest that the age of the placenta is the primary factor determining its enzyme activity and metabolic performance.   It may be surmised that the placenta during its early rapid biogenesis towards full functional maturity receives a fixed endowment of enzymes to last through its limited lifespan.   While the initial production of these enzymes is regulated by central programming the subsequent regression of their activity is probably due to the cessation or reduction of their synthesis at some point of the advancing gestation.   Within this context no mechanism appears to be available for metabolic or hormonal stimuli to specifically induce the synthesis of individual enzymes.

The clinical relevance of our observations cannot be fully assessed at present. We have found a general trend for enzyme activities to decrease in human placentas between 6 to 10 weeks of gestation and term (Y.Z. Diamant *et al.* 1975*a*). In a preliminary study, clues were obtained suggesting an accelerated fall in enzyme activities in term placentas from pregnancies complicated by pre-eclamptic toxaemia; in placentas from non-toxaemic pregnancies with small-for-date babies the enzyme activities were higher than in normal term placentas, as if the ageing of the placenta became slowed down (Y.Z. Diamant *et al.* 1976). However, more metabolic and enzyme studies will have to be performed on human placentas to validate the suggestion that the fall in enzyme activities responsible for the supply of metabolic energy from glycolysis contributes to the functional insufficiency of toxaemic, senescent or postmature placentas, whereas a rise in activity signifies an arrested development.

ACKNOWLEDGEMENTS

The investigations reviewed here were supported in part by grants from the Hebrew University-Hadassah Joint Research Fund. E.S. is an Established Investigator of the Chief Scientist's Bureau, Ministry of Health.

The experimental assistance of Shulamit Neuman and Nina Mayorek is gratefully acknowledged.

References

ANDERSON, J. W. & STOWRING, L. (1973) Glycolytic and gluconeogenic enzyme activities in renal cortex of diabetic rats. *Am. J. Physiol. 224*, 930–936

ANDERSON, J. W. & ZAKIM, D. (1970) The influence of alloxan diabetes and fasting on glycolytic and gluconeogenic enzyme activities of rat intestinal mucosa and liver. *Biochim. Biophys. Acta 201*, 236–241

BEYTH, Y., NEUMAN, S., GUTMAN, A. & SHAFRIR, E. (1977) Effect of prolonged gestation on placental and maternal liver enzyme activities in the rat. *Diabète Métab. 3*, 91–96

CHANG, A. Y. & SCHNEIDER, D.I. (1971) Hepatic enzyme activities in streptozotocin diabetic rats before and after insulin treatment. *Diabetes 20*, 71–77

DHAND, U. K., JEACOCK, M. K., SHEPHERD, D. A. L., SMITH, E. M. & VARNAM, G. C. E. (1970) Activities of enzymes concerned with pyruvate, oxaloacetate, citrate, acetate and acetoacetate metabolism in placental cotyledons of sheep. *Biochim. Biophys. Acta 222*, 216–218

DIAMANT, S. & SHAFRIR, E. (1975) Modulation of the activity of insulin-dependent enzymes of lipogenesis by glucocorticoids. *Eur. J. Biochem. 53*, 541–546

DIAMANT, S., GORIN, E. & SHAFRIR, E. (1972) Enzyme activities related to fatty acids synthesis in liver and adipose tissue of rats treated with triiodothyronine. *Eur. J. Biochem. 27*, 553–559

DIAMANT, Y. Z. & SHAFRIR, E. (1972) Enzymes of carbohydrate and lipid metabolism in the placenta and liver of pregnant rats. *Biochim. Biophys. Acta 279*, 424–430

DIAMANT, Y. Z. & SHAFRIR, E. (1978) Placental enzymes of glycolysis, gluconeogenesis and lipogenesis in the rat in diabetes and starvation. *Diabetologia 15*, 1–5

DIAMANT, Y. Z., MAYOREK, N., NEUMAN, S. & SHAFRIR, E. (1975a) Enzymes of glucose and fatty acid metabolism in early and term human placenta. *Am. J. Obstet. Gynecol. 121*, 58–61

DIAMANT, Y. Z., NEUMAN, S. & SHAFRIR, E. (1975b) Effect of chorionic gonadotropin, triamcinolone, progesterone and estrogen on enzymes of placenta and liver in rats. *Biochim. Biophys. Acta 385*, 257–267

DIAMANT, Y. Z., BEYTH, Y., NEUMAN, S. & SHAFRIR, E. (1976) Activity of placental enzymes of carbohydrate and lipid metabolism in normal, toxemic and small for date pregnancies. *Isr. J. Med. Sci. 12*, 243–247

DODEK, P., KIRBY, L., FROHLICH, Y., HAHN, P. & HO-YUEN, B. (1975) High glucose concentration and phosphoenolpyruvate carboxykinase activity in human and rat fetal liver cultures. *Proc. Soc. Exp. Biol. Med. 150*, 7–10

DOLKART, R. E., TOROK, E. E. & WRIGHT, P. H. (1964) Hepatic enzyme activities in rats made diabetic with alloxan and with guinea pig anti-insulin serum. *Diabetes 13*, 78–82

GABBE, S. G., DEMERS, L. M., GREEP, R. O. & VILLEE, C. A. (1972) Placental glycogen metabolism in diabetes mellitus. *Diabetes 21, 1185–1191*

HAGERMAN, D. D. (1962) Metabolism of tissues from pregnant diabetic rats in vitro. *Endocrinology 70*, 88–89

HULL, D. & ELPHICK, M. C. (1979) Evidence for fatty acid transfer across the human placenta, in this volume, pp. 75–86

KOREN, Z. & SHAFRIR, E. (1964) Placental transfer of free fatty acids in the pregnant rat. *Proc. Soc. Exp. Biol. Med. 116*, 411–414

LLORENTE, P., MARCO, R. & SOLS, A. (1970) Regulation of liver pyruvate kinase and the phosphoenolpyruvate crossroads. *Eur. J. Biochem. 13*, 45–54

MIGLIORINI, R. H. (1971) Early changes in the levels of glycolytic enzymes after total pancreatectomy in the rat. *Biochim. Biophys. Acta 244*, 125–128

ROBERTSON, A. F. & SPRECHER, H. (1968) A review of placental lipid metabolism and transport. *Acta Paediatr. Scand. Suppl. 183*, 3–18

SAKURAI, T., TAKAGI, H. & HOSOYA, N. (1969) Metabolic pathways of glucose in human placenta. Changes with gestation and with added 17β-estradiol. *Am. J. Obstet. Gynecol. 105*, 1044–1054

SHRAGO, E., YOUNG, J. W. & LARDY, H. A. (1967) Carbohydrate supply as a regulator of rat liver phosphoenolpyruvate carboxykinase activity. *Science (Wash. D.C.) 158*, 1572–1573

SYBULSKI, S. & MAUGHAN, G. (1972) Use of streptozotocin as diabetic agent in pregnant rats. *Endocrinology 89*, 1537–1540

SZABO, A. J. & SZABO, O. (1974) Placental free-fatty-acid transfer and fetal adipose tissue development: an explanation of fetal adiposity in infants of diabetic mothers. *Lancet 2*, 498–499

VAN BERKEL, Y. Y. C. & KOSTER, J. F. (1973) M-type pyruvate kinase of leukocytes: an allosteric enzyme. *Biochim. Biophys. Acta 273*, 134–139

VILLEE, C. A. (1953) The metabolism of human placenta in vitro. *J. Biol. Chem. 205*, 113–123

WALKER, O. G., LEA, M. A., ROSSITER, G. & ADDISON, M. E. B. (1967) Glucose metabolism in the placenta. *Arch. Biochem. Biophys. 120*, 646–653

Discussion

Chez: In your consideration of what regulates placental enzymes did you find that placental lactogen, prolactin or any of the oestrogens have any influence on placental enzymes?

Shafrir: We have not studied prolactin, but we injected the rat with progesterone and oestrogen for the last 3 to 5 days of gestation and did not find any change in activity.

Chez: And placental lactogen and somatomammotropin?

Shafrir: We have not injected them.

I don't know the cause of growth retardation in the small-for-dates babies, associated with the high placental enzyme activity, as there was no morphological follow-up. The babies were born after apparently normal pregnancies, at 38–40 weeks of gestation (Diamant *et al.* 1976). The only common denominator was the higher enzyme activity than in the matched placentas from babies of normal weight supplied on more or less the same day. However, when the pregnancy was complicated by toxaemia, the placental enzyme activities were lower than normal.

Pedersen: Were the gestation times the same?

Shafrir: Yes. I should add that the increases in enzyme values were based on calculations per unit of tissue weight or per milligram of cytoplasmic protein. Since the 'small for dates' placenta is also smaller in size, the enzyme activities when expressed per total placenta might show less conspicuous differences. It remains, therefore, open to question whether we are dealing with a selective lack of placental cells less rich in enzyme activities or with an arrested course of placental ageing.

Räihä: It is a little disturbing that the enzymes in the placenta were not affected when you administered various hormones, including corticosteroids. How do you administer the hormones? Does the hormone actually get to the placenta? In all tissues PEP-carboxykinase, for example, should be stimulated by corticosteroids. I don't understand why the placental cells, which structurally should be like any other cells, would not respond to this when most other cells in the body do.

Shafrir: The glucocorticoid triamcinolone was injected intramuscularly for 3 days in a rather high dose of 25 mg/kg. We have good evidence that it was absorbed and was active because it produced typical and remarkable changes in the liver and in many serum constituents. With regard to PEP-carboxykinase I would like to say that it may not necessarily respond in the same way in all tissues; although it is markedly stimulated in the liver, it is suppressed in adipose tissue (Gorin *et al.* 1969). The absence of response in placental enzyme activities when hormonal treatment started on day 15 of gestation may be because the enzyme synthetic apparatus is no longer active in the placenta. Therefore no stimulation could reactivate protein synthesis.

Räihä: Then the cells must be dead.

Shafrir: Not necessarily. The cell and its enzymes are intact but may have lost the capacity for additional adaptive enzyme synthesis. The enzymes in the cell are now decaying slowly, while other functions proceed unchanged.

Räihä: It would be interesting to see whether placental cells react to hormonal stimulation *in vitro*. Degradation of the injected hormone in the placenta may be so rapid that it doesn't reach the inside of the cells. If the placental cells were in an organ culture system or cell culture system there might be an effect.

Shafrir: We haven't got the proper system for separating and growing placental cells as yet.

Williamson: Most of the energy obtained by the placenta is presumably supplied by glycolysis. Does the lactate which accumulates eventually reach the fetus? Secondly, pyruvate kinase is a very important regulatory enzyme for glycolysis in other tissues. In liver we now know that this enzyme exists in a phosphorylated and a dephosphorylated form. It can also be controlled by alanine, which is an inhibitor of the enzyme. If there were regulatory effects on pyruvate kinase this could affect the whole energy supply to the fetus and therefore perhaps affect fetal growth. Have you investigated this?

Shafrir: I presume that the lactate elaborated in the placenta is available to both the maternal side and the fetal side. There is quite a significant concentration of lactate in the amniotic fluid, for instance. In preliminary studies we find that pyruvate kinase in the placenta is of the so-called non-adaptive M type. But this variant of pyruvate kinase could be regulated by the intracellular changes in metabolites such as FDP and PEP and by the ADP/ATP ratio. It appears to be sensitive to inhibition by alanine.

Beard: The regular fall in activity of placental enzymes as gestation proceeds suggests that the maturing fetus is starting to supply itself with the nutrients and metabolites. Have you measured enzyme activities in the fetal liver in parallel?

Shafrir: We started to do this in fetal liver but only in diabetic animals. From our preliminary experience and from the evidence in the literature it appears that the activities of most of these enzymes are present quite early but in low activity. There is no gradual increase in the activity of these enzymes but a rather rapid rise just before or after birth.

Beard: In the growth-retarded fetus, can premature induction of enzyme activity be regarded as an attempt by the feto-placental unit to overcome some of the nutritional deficiencies caused by a small placenta?

Räihä: We know very little about enzyme development in the growth-retarded fetus.

Kalkhoff: Although you showed no changes in many placental enzymes in animals with severe diabetes, there was a tremendous accumulation of glycogen, Professor Shafrir. This might relate to what Dr Chez might say about glycogen synthetase.

Secondly you showed that the fall in enzyme activities in the placenta began on day 15. When does activity reach its maximum before the fall starts? This is relevant to diabetes and the infants of diabetic mothers.

Shafrir: Placental glycogenesis is a well-known phenomenon in diabetic pregnancy but does not occur in starvation. This goes together with the observation that placental pyruvate kinase activity was increased in hyperglycaemia but not in starvation. Therefore, it should be attributed to the effect of hyperglycaemia.

With respect to your second question it is very difficult to determine when the initial endowment of enzymes was received. I would assume that enzyme protein synthesis occurs very early during placental biogenesis. We cannot look earlier than day 12, when the placenta is extremely small and very difficult to separate. Some of our unpublished results indicate that on day 12 the enzyme activity per milligram of cytoplasmic protein is still higher than on day 15. But if the activity is expressed per total placenta, which increases very much in size during this time period, it appears not appreciably different from that on day 15. We assume, tentatively, that the peak of enzyme biogenesis takes place between day 10 and day 15.

Freinkel: The placenta is fascinating in this regard. In the rat placenta, DNA synthesis and hence new cell formation ceases on the 17th day whereas total organ weight, protein and RNA all continue to rise until the 19th day (Winick & Noble 1966). Thus, in its 21–22-day lifetime, the rat placenta appears capable of hyperplastic or replicative growth only up to about day 17. It would be important to relate your enzyme measurements to DNA or some other estimate of actual cell number, especially since proliferative growth is so finite. Your data have the fascinating implication that adaptive changes, perhaps hormonally mediated, may occur only while placental cells retain some replicative capacity. Perhaps the most rewarding period in which to examine the placenta in this regard would be during day 12–17.

Battaglia: I question whether changes in an organ with age should be called ageing or senescence. Measurements of organ function in the placenta *in vivo* show a tremendous increase in function of the organ up to the end of term. You seem to be saying that if the enzyme activity goes up you'll call it maturation and if it goes down you'll call it ageing. That bothers me very much. I also question whether you should express the enzyme activity per milligram of cytoplasmic protein if you are not isolating just trophoblastic cells in an organ with cell types that are changing markedly with development. How would you separate something you would call maturation from something you would call ageing?   Such terms imply a value judgement about the changes.

Shafrir: I am glad to hear you say this.   The words senescence and ageing were not something I invented, and they should not be construed to mean a regression of placenta after its maturation.   The gradual decrease in enzyme activities might represent a selective cessation of synthesis of certain proteins and may mean some change in placental function or be confined only to a particular cell type.   We are now approaching the question of different cellular moieties of the placenta by trying to isolate and separate placental cells and to repeat the enzyme determinations in isolated cell types.

Naismith: You expressed your enzyme values in relation to protein.   This could be misleading.   The total amount of protein and the size of the placenta increase continuously.   Have you expressed these values as total enzyme activities?

Shafrir: The cytoplasmic protein content does not change.   I have indicated that while placental weight between days 15 and 25 may double, the enzyme activities fall to one-twelfth of the initial activity.   They would still fall quite considerably if the values were expressed per total placental weight.

Naismith: Are the very high enzyme activities that you find up to day 15 perhaps a reflection of energy production for cell multiplication of the placenta itself, which ceases shortly thereafter?

Shafrir: All the enzyme activities are of the energy production and energy storage type.   Energy for any anabolic process would be dependent on the activity of these enzymes.

Naismith: But cell division, which would have a higher energy cost, ceases at about day 17.   One would expect a big reduction in energy requirement at that time.

Shafrir: Yes.   But enzyme activities were found to decrease gradually over the whole lifespan of the placenta.

Hoet: I have been struck by the marked increase in the glycogen content of the placenta from your diabetic rats.   Do you have any explanation for this?

Shafrir: This is indeed a very interesting phenomenon which has been described to occur in diabetes in animal and human placentas.   It does not, however, occur in the insulin deficiency of fasting so it must be related to the prevalent hyperglycaemia.   As you well know, the enzyme system responsible for glycogen synthesis and breakdown is very sensitive to insulin, the absence of which results in glycogen depletion, as is the case in the liver.   We have investigated the activity of glycogen synthetase and of phosphorylase, as well as of their phosphorylation– dephosphorylation enzymes in the placenta, and we did not find any marked deviations from normal.   It is unlikely, then, that there is an excessive stimulation of glycogen synthesis or an inhibition of glycogen breakdown. It is probable that glucose remains available to the placenta in diabetes and becomes phosphorylated to glucose-6-phosphate, but that its further metabolism along the glycolytic pathway is obstructed. This is likely to occur at the phosphofructokinase, pyruvate kinase or other steps which become inhibited by some diabetes-specific metabolites. The resulting back-pressure would tend to push the glucose-6-phosphate towards glycogen formation. Although this course of events has not been directly shown for the placenta, I am drawing an analogy to muscle, in which a cross-over between fructose-6-phosphate and fructose diphosphate has been shown in diabetes, in association with glycogen accumulation. There is also an analogy to adipose tissue in starved/re-fed animals in which the renewed availability of glucose in the face of still obstructed glycolysis results in a pronounced glycogen deposition.

References

DIAMANT, Y. Z., BEYTH, Y., NEUMAN, S. & SHAFRIR, E. (1976) Activity of placental enzymes of carbohydrate and lipid metabolism in normal, toxemic and small for date pregnancies. *Isr. J. Med. Sci. 12*, 243–247

GORIN, E., TAL-OR, Z. & SHAFRIR, E. (1969) Glyceroneogenesis in adipose tissue of fasted, diabetic and triamcinolone treated rats. *Eur. J. Biochem. 8*, 370–375

WINICK, M. & NOBLE, A. (1966) Quantitative changes in ribonucleic acids and protein during normal growth of rat placenta. *Nature (Lond.) 212*, 34–35

Culture *in vitro* as a means of analysing the effect of maternal diabetes on embryonic development in rats

ELIZABETH M. DEUCHAR

Department of Biological Sciences, University of Exeter

Abstract Rodents have been used by many investigators for studies of the effects that maternal diabetes during pregnancy may have on developing fetuses. In Wistar rats, the induction of mild chronic diabetes at the onset of pregnancy by alloxan or streptozotocin results in abnormalities of the nervous system and the heart, recognized in embryos at 11–13 days' gestation. Thus, early organogenesis is evidently affected in these embryos. With a method which enables rat embryos to be cultured *in vitro* in serum for the period of their early organogenesis, the growth and differentiation of embryos from normal and from diabetic rats can be observed in some detail. It is also possible to compare the effects of normal and of diabetic maternal serum on their development. The results reported here show that embryos from diabetic animals are more likely to be retarded or abnormal than those from non-diabetic animals when cultured in identical serum. The development of both types of embryo is more successful in diabetic than in non-diabetic serum, however, possibly because of the higher glucose content of diabetic serum. Cultures of fetal organs may also be used as test systems for the effects of diabetic maternal serum. Sacral vertebrae, some of which fail to ossify in fetuses from diabetic rats, are now being grown in media containing diabetic serum. It is planned to test the effects of insulin on these cultures..

In animals as well as in man there is now ample evidence that maternal diabetes mellitus can cause abnormalities or death in fetuses. For example, Mintz *et al.* (1972) found that if pregnant female macaque monkeys were made diabetic with the drug streptozotocin, deaths of fetuses and neonates occurred. Watanabe & Ingalls (1963) and Horii *et al.* (1966) found a wide range of malformations in mouse fetuses when the mothers were made diabetic with alloxan. The incidence of most malformations, and of deaths, was highest when the mice had been given alloxan on the 9th, 10th or 11th day of pregnancy: a period when the main organ systems of the embryo are forming (New 1966*a*). If the mice were given insulin to relieve their diabetic condition, hardly any malformations occurred.

181

In the rat, which is the animal chosen for the culture work to be reported here, previous studies have shown that as a result of maternal diabetes fetal deaths occur, as well as a retardation of fetal growth. Davis *et al.* (1947), Sinden & Longwell (1949) and Ferret *et al.* (1950) found that diabetes induced by alloxan in the pregnant rat caused deaths of fetuses mid-way through gestation: this could be prevented by treatment of the rats with insulin.   Small size in rat fetuses of diabetic mothers has been reported by Lazarow *et al.* (1960), Golob *et al.* (1970) and Van Assche (1975).   Birth weight, on the other hand, is higher than normal, because gestation is prolonged by several hours in diabetic animals.   These effects can also be prevented by insulin treatment.   Since the discovery that the antibiotic streptozotocin can be used to induce stable chronic diabetes in rats and has fewer undesirable side-effects than alloxan (Rudas 1969; Rerup 1970), the rat and its organs have become used increasingly for experimental studies on diabetes.   Hitherto the work on fetuses of diabetic animals has referred to their development *in vivo*, observed at a few arbitrarily chosen stages.   It is the purpose of the present paper, however, to introduce some possibilities of investigating the effects of maternal diabetes on embryos and their organs grown *in vitro*, where some of the conditions can be more carefully controlled than *in vivo*.

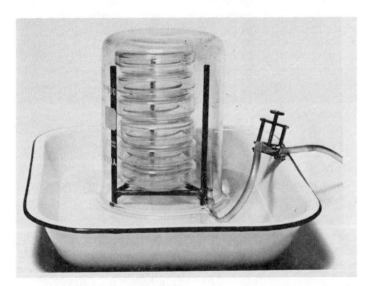

FIG. 1.   Simplest form of watch-glass culture apparatus for early rat embryos (cf. New 1966*b*), × 0.35. Embryos are placed in serum in the watch-glasses in moist Petri dishes which are then stacked under a beaker in a tray of liquid paraffin.   The gas mixture (95 % O_2 : 5 % CO_2) is led in via plastic tubing for 10 min, then the tubing is clamped and the apparatus placed in the incubator.

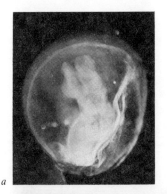

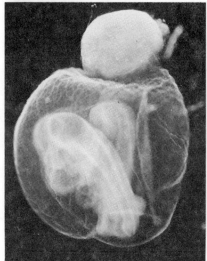

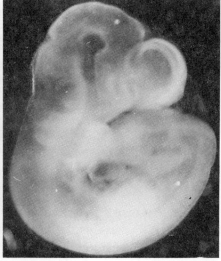

a

b

c

FIG. 2.   Cleared specimens of cultured rat embryos.
(*a*) $10^1/_2$-day embryo in its membranes.   Head and anterior trunk are seen in ventral view.   Head neural folds are not yet closed.   Heart rudiment is seen ventral to head.   × 30
(*b*) $11^1/_2$-day embryo in its membranes, after 24 h in watchglass culture.   The head (dorsal side) is towards the camera.   The embryo has rotated so that it is convex dorsally.   The tail is seen to the right of the head.   Heart, and forelimb buds, can also be seen.   The trophoblast mass lies at the top of the picture, while the transparent yolk sac envelops the embryo.   × 24
(*c*) $12^1/_2$-day embryo, removed from its membranes after culture in a roller tube.   Note advanced development of brain and somites.   × 24

New (1966*b*) described a simple and effective method for growing early rat embryos during their initial phases of organ formation, from 9–11 days' gestation.   The embryos are placed in watch glasses containing rat serum and are gassed with 95 % O_2 : 5 % CO_2, then incubated at 37 °C.   Fig. 1 shows the apparatus in its simplest form.   Embryos grow well, up to the $11^1/_2$-day stage,

TABLE 1

Abnormalities in early rat embryos from alloxan-diabetic mothers

	No. of rats used	Deaths/ resorptions	Total live embryos	CNS abnormal	Heart abnormal
Experimental	17	34	120	7	2
Control	15	10	136	3	0

TABLE 2

Abnormalities in early rat embryos from streptozotocin-diabetic mothers

	No. of rats used	Deaths/ resorptions	Total live embryos	CNS abnormal	Heart abnormal
Experimental	20	38	190	19	10
Control	16	8	176	5	3

in this limited volume of serum.   More recently, New *et al.* (1973) and New & Coppola (1977), have used roller bottles to support development up to the 13½-day stage, when the embryo is about equivalent to a 7-week human embryo, with all its organ systems established, fore- and hindlimbs present, and a fully developed chorioallantoic circulation.   The external appearance of rat embryos cultured during these stages of organogenesis is shown in Fig. 2.   The embryos provide a useful test system for agents that might affect these early but crucial steps in development, and the culture method mirrors conditions *in vivo*, in that the embryonic membranes are maintained intact and are in direct contact with maternal serum (review: New 1978).

In Wistar rats, recent evidence (Deuchar 1977) shows that maternal diabetes causes an increased incidence of abnormalities of the brain and heart in early embryos.   These are found at 11–13-day stages: Tables 1 and 2 give the data, obtained from rats made diabetic with alloxan and streptozotocin.   As a follow-up to these findings, it was decided to study the immediately preceding stages of development in more detail *in vitro*.   The stage from 10½ to 11½ days' gestation was chosen, as it includes the most crucial steps in formation of the brain and heart.   The development of embryos from diabetic rats over this period has been compared with that of embryos from normal rats.   In addition, the effects of using diabetic serum as the culture medium have been investigated.

MATERIAL AND METHODS

On the day after mating, female Wistar rats were injected intravenously with 45 mg streptozotocin (Upjohn Ltd)/kg body weight; the streptozotocin was dissolved immediately before use in ice-cold 0.01M-citrate buffer, pH 4.7.   Control animals were injected with buffer alone.   Four days later, tests with Dextrostix (Ames Ltd.) showed a blood glucose level of 175–250 mg/100 ml, which could be confirmed by hexokinase assays, in the diabetic animals.   Controls showed values of 90–130 mg/100 ml.

On Day 10 of pregnancy, one control and one experimental rat were bled by heart puncture to provide serum for the culture media; they were then killed and the embryos were removed from the uteri as described by New (1966 a,b).   Each embryo was placed in a watch-glass containing 0.3 ml serum.   Four types of culture were set up: embryos from the control rat, in either control serum or diabetic serum, and embryos from the diabetic rat, in either control serum or diabetic serum.   Cultures were examined after 24 hours, then fixed in Bouin's fixative, dehydrated in alcohols and cleared in methyl benzoate.   Paraffin sections 8 μm thick were stained in Ehrlich's haematoxylin and eosin.

RESULTS

In the 24 hours from $10^{1}/_{2}$–$11^{1}/_{2}$ days' gestation, the embryos developed *in vitro* from a late neurula with 10–15 pairs of somites (cf. Fig. 2a) to a fully rotated, larger embryo with a well developed brain, forelimb buds, beating heart and active circulation of red blood cells in the embryo and yolk sac (cf. Fig. 2b).   Embryos which attained all these features externally are classed as good in Table 3.   Development which had not reached quite this stage (for instance, rotation not being complete: Deuchar 1971) was classed as fair, and embryos which were stunted or otherwise abnormal-looking were classed as poor.   The final category in Table 3 is dead embryos, in which blood circulation had ceased and the embryonic body was white and opaque.

Table 3 gives the frequencies of these different categories of development in each type of culture.   It can be seen that the embryos from normal rats do better than those from diabetic rats, in both types of serum.   In both normal and diabetic serum, the numbers of good control embryos are significantly higher than those of embryos from diabetic rats (χ^2 = 9.06 for the difference between embryos of controls and those of diabetic rats, in control serum, and χ^2 = 6.95 for this difference in diabetic serum: $P<0.01$). Conversely, the numbers of only 'fair' embryos among those from diabetic rats are significantly higher than among the controls (χ^2 = 10.44 for the difference in control serum and 4.04 for the difference in diabetic serum: $P<0.01, P<0.05$, respectively). It can also be seen from Table 3 that the diabetic serum has no apparent deleterious effects on development.

Besides these preliminary observations on the external appearance of the embryos, the final size they attained was measured. Table 4 shows the data for the diameter of the membranes, the crown-rump length and the tail length. There were considerable variations, as the standard errors indicate. It was apparent, however, that in the control embryos all the dimensions measured were significantly larger after culture in diabetic serum than after culture in normal serum (t = 2.39, $P<0.02$; t = 2.60, $P<0.02$; t = 2.03, $P<0.05$, for the differences in membrane diameter, crown-rump length and tail length respectively). In the embryos from diabetic animals, there appear-

TABLE 3

External appearance of cultured 11½-day embryos

	Total	% 'Good'	% 'Fair'	% 'Poor'	% Dead
Diabetic					
diabetic serum	52	ᐃ58	■25	11	6
normal serum	60	☆55	●28	8	8
Controls					
diabetic serum	30	ᐃ83	■ 7	7	3
normal serum	59	☆76	● 5	7	12

ᐃᐃ
☆☆ } pairs of data that show significant differences
■■
●●

TABLE 4

Dimensions of cultured $11^{1}/_{2}$-day embryos (mm ± S.E.)

	Diameter of membranes	Length of trunk	Length of tail
Diabetic			
diabetic serum	3.18 ± 0.07	2.26 ± 0.09	2.07 ± 0.07
normal serum	3.00 ± 0.08	2.08 ± 0.06	1.91 ± 0.05
Controls			
diabetic serum	△3.30 ± 0.08	•2.45 ± 0.09	☆2.15 ± 0.07
normal serum	△3.01 ± 0.07	•2.18 ± 0.06	☆1.94 ± 0.06

△△
•• } pairs of data showing significant differences
☆☆

ed to be size differences in the same sense, but these are not significant on the data obtained so far.

Histologically, the development of several organs (e.g. brain, spinal cord, sense organs, heart, gut, somites and limb buds) in the embryos could be compared. Only a very few abnormalities were observed, exclusively in the brain and the heart, and in some embryos the organ systems as a whole were slightly retarded in development. For simplicity all the abnormalities are grouped together in Table 5. It can be seen that a significantly higher proportion of the control embryos were normal than were embryos of diabetic animals, both when cultured in normal serum and when cultured in diabetic serum ($\chi^2 = 24.9$, $P<0.001$; $\chi^2 = 5.41$, $P<0.02$, for the differences in normal serum and in diabetic serum respectively). On the other hand, more of the embryos from diabetic rats were retarded in their development than among the controls, in both sera ($\chi^2 = 4.01$, $P<0.02$ for this difference). A further interesting finding was that embryos from both control and diabetic rats had fewer cases of cell death within their organs when cultured in diabetic serum than when in normal serum ($\chi^2 = 10.72$, $P<0.01$; $\chi^2 = 4.74$, $P<0.02$,

TABLE 5

Histology of cultured 11$\frac{1}{2}$-day embryos

	Total embryos	% with normal organs	% with abnormal organs	% with retarded development	% with cell death
Diabetic					
diabetic serum	44	+50	9	29	$^{\triangledown}$18
normal serum	52	$^{\triangle}$40	8	$^{\bullet}$19	$^{\triangledown}$38
Controls					
diabetic serum	27	+78	11	18	* 4
normal serum	50	$^{\triangle}$56	4	$^{\bullet}$6	*38

++
ΔΔ
●● } pairs of data showing significant differences
∇∇
☆☆

for the difference between diabetic and normal serum, in control and diabetic embryos respectively).   This finding, together with the observations on size mentioned above, indicate that the diabetic serum had some beneficial effects in the maintenance of the embryos *in vitro*.

DISCUSSION AND CONCLUSIONS FROM EMBRYO CULTURE WORK

Three main points emerge from what is, admittedly, a small body of data so far.   The first is that over this brief but crucial period of organogenesis, embryos from diabetic rats are slightly less viable and slightly more prone to abnormality or retardation in development than are the embryos of normal rats, when tested under identical conditions *in vitro*.   The lower viability of the diabetic embryos must be due to influences that reach them from the diabetic mother *in vivo*, before the 10$\frac{1}{2}$-day stage, since they show the lower viability whether cultured in normal or in diabetic serum subsequently.   Evidently, in Wistar rats at least, maternal diabetes can have harmful effects on embryos either during the period before or during that immediately after their implantation in the uterus (which occurs at 7 days after mating). Other experiments (Deuchar 1979) have shown that preimplantation embryos flushed from the uteri of diabetic Wistar rats are perfectly normal in appearance: so it looks as if the diabetic mother rat's ill-effects on embryos are not exerted until after implantation.

The finding that growth is enhanced and cell death less frequent when diabetic serum is used instead of normal serum for embryo cultures is probably explained by its higher glucose content. Cockroft & Coppola (1977) estimated that each cultured rat embryo uses about 0.4 mg glucose in 24 h, which is near the maximum glucose content of 0.3 ml normal serum. So, in the present cultures, some of the embryos in normal serum may have gradually run short of glucose while those in diabetic serum would not have done so. In their work Cockroft & Coppola (1977) showed also that excess glucose can cause abnormalities in cultured embryos, but only at high concentrations of 12–15 mg/ml serum, which is a great deal higher than in any of our mildly diabetic rats.

The final point to emerge from the present study is that diabetic serum has no apparent ill-effects on early organogenesis in rat embryos. There are evidently no deleterious factors permanently present in the maternal serum. This suggests that it is either factors from the blood cells, or longer-term physiological influences due to the diabetic mother's deranged metabolism, that act deleteriously on the newly implanted rat embryo.

Unfortunately present techniques do not yet allow very long-term studies on rat embryos in culture to be made to test the effects of changes in the environment such as might occur in a diabetic mother: fluctuations in glucose content, for instance, or increases in free fatty acids. Cockroft (1973, 1976) has managed to keep rat embryos alive in culture up to 14 days, but only by deflecting their membranes, so that exchanges between the embryo and the maternal serum are no longer equivalent to those *in vivo*. If one is to study fetal development *in vitro* under controlled conditions, one is limited to organ cultures. It is still possible, however, to obtain specific information from these studies that is relevant to the effects of maternal diabetes. Recently I have been exploring the possibility of culturing sacral vertebrae of fetal rats, from 17–20 days' gestational age. The reason for special interest in these is that 20-day rat fetuses from diabetic mothers frequently have some of their sacral vertebrae unossified (Deuchar 1977), and it is well known that ossification can be deranged by abnormally high levels of insulin. This has been shown with limb bones cultured *in vitro* (Chen 1954; Hay 1958; review: Reynolds 1972). It has also been found that high doses of insulin induce abnormalities of the vertebrae in chick and mouse embryos (Landauer 1945;

Duraiswami 1950; Smithberg & Runner 1963). Moreover, there is evidence that rat fetuses of diabetic mothers secrete more insulin than normal during the last few days of gestation, in response to the mother's hyperglycaemia (Kim *et al*. 1960; Van Assche 1975). So cultures of sacral vertebrae *in vitro* could be used to test whether sacral ossification is deranged by high levels of insulin, and also whether sacral vertebrae of fetuses from diabetic rats have any intrinsic inability to ossify.

It is too soon to report results from the very few cultures of sacral vertebrae carried out so far. The sacral vertebrae have been isolated from 17-day fetuses of both normal and diabetic rats, and they appear to grow successfully *in vitro* up to the 20th day, in media that contain either normal or diabetic serum. The degrees of ossification achieved, and the effects of adding insulin at levels comparable to those in the fetal blood, have yet to be studied.

It would not be fair to end this report without voicing the main question and criticism that must be levelled at all results obtained from cultures of mammalian embryos or their organs *in vitro*. Do they really reflect conditions *in vivo*, and could not equivalent or better experiments be carried out with the embryos or fetuses retained in the mother? With the rat, which is in other ways one of the most convenient mammals for embryological work, such *in vivo* experiments have seldom been successful. Any surgical, injection or sampling procedure applied to the rat embryo *in utero* is likely to cause it to be reabsorbed, so that only a necrotic mass of cells is left. So it is certainly better to have short-term results in carefully controlled conditions *in vitro*, where the dosage of substances to the embryo can also be known accurately, than to risk this high failure rate *in vivo*. With short-term *in vitro* cultures, the effects on embryonic development of hormones or other metabolites that may be found in abnormal concentrations in the blood of diabetics can easily be tested; and this should increase our understanding of the mechanisms whereby the diabetic mother sometimes produces abnormal offspring.

ACKNOWLEDGEMENTS

This work was supported by the British Diabetic Association. Thanks are due to Mrs C. Jeynes for skilled technical assistance and to Mr M. Alexander for photography: also to the Department of Biological Sciences, The University of Exeter for their laboratory facilities.

References

CHEN, J. M. (1954) The effect of insulin on embryonic limb-bones cultivated *in vitro*. *J. Physiol. (Lond.) 125*, 148–162

COCKROFT, D. L. (1973) Development in culture of rat foetuses explanted at 12.5 and 13.5 days of gestation. *J. Embryol. Exp. Morphol. 29*, 473–483

COCKROFT, D. L. (1976) Comparison of *in vitro* and *in vivo* development of rat foetuses. *Dev. Biol. 48*, 163–172

COCKROFT, D. L. & COPPOLA, P. T. (1977) Teratogenic effects of excess glucose on head-fold rat embryos in culture. *Teratology 16*, 141–146

DAVIS, M. E., FUGO, N. V. & LAWRENCE, K. G. (1947) Effect of alloxan diabetes on reproduction in the rat. *Proc. Soc. Exp. Biol. Med. 66*, 638–641

DEUCHAR, E. M. (1971) The mechanism of axial rotation in the rat embryo: an experimental study in vitro. *J. Embryol. Exp. Morphol. 25*, 189–201

DEUCHAR, E. M. (1977) Embryonic malformations in rats, resulting from maternal diabetes: a preliminary study. *J. Embryol. Exp. Morphol. 41*, 93–99

DEUCHAR, E. M. (1979) Experimental evidence relating fetal anomalies to diabetes. *Carbohydrate Metabolism in Pregnancy and the Newborn* (Sutherland, H. W & Stowers, J. M., eds.) (2nd Aberdeen Int. Colloq.), Springer, Berlin

DURAISWAMI, P. K. (1950) Insulin-induced skeletal abnormalities in developing chickens. *Br. Med. J. 2*, 384–390

FERRET, P., LINDEN, O. & MORGANS, M. E. (1950) Pregnancy in insulin-treated alloxan diabetic rats. *J. Endocrinol. 7*, 100–102

GOLOB, E. K., RISHI S., BECKER, K. L. & MOORE, C. (1970) Streptozotocin diabetes in pregnant and non-pregnant rats. *Metabolism 19*, 1014–1019

HAY, M. F. (1958) The effect of growth hormone and insulin on limb-bone rudiments of the embryonic chick cultivated *in vitro. J. Physiol. (Lond.) 144*, 490–504

HORII, K., WATANABE, G. & INGALLS, T.H. (1966) Experimental diabetes in pregnant mice. Prevention of congenital malformations in offspring by insulin. *Diabetes 15*, 194–204

KIM, J. N., RUNGE, W., WELLS, L. & LAZAROW, A. (1960) Pancreatic islets and blood sugars in prenatal and postnatal offspring from diabetic rats: beta granulation and glycogen infiltration. *Anat. Rec. 138*, 239–249

LANDAUER, W. (1945) Rumplessness of chicken embryos produced by the injection of insulin and other chemicals. *J. Exp. Zool. 98*, 65–73

LAZAROW, A., KIM, J. N. & WELLS, L. J. (1960) Birth weight and fetal mortality in pregnant subdiabetic rats. *Diabetes 9*, 114–117

MINTZ, D. H., CHEZ, R. A. & HUTCHINSON, D. L. (1972) Subhuman primate pregnancy complicated by streptozotocin-induced diabetes mellitus. *J. Clin. Invest. 51*, 837–843

NEW, D. A. T. (1966*a*) *The Culture of Vertebrate Embryos*, Logos/Academic Press, London

NEW, D. A. T. (1966*b*) Development of rat embryos cultured in blood sera. *J. Reprod. Fertil. 12*, 509–524

NEW, D. A. T. (1978) Whole embryo culture and the study of mammal embryos during organogenesis. *Biol. Rev. 53*, 8

NEW, D. A. T. & COPPOLA, P. T. (1977) Development of a placental blood circulation in rat embryos in vitro. *J. Embryol. Exp. Morphol. 37*, 227–235

NEW, D. A. T., COPPOLA, P. & TERRY, S. (1973) Culture of explanted rat embryos in rotating tubes. *J. Reprod. Fertil. 35*, 135–138

RERUP, C. C. (1970) Drugs inducing diabetes through damage of the insulin-secreting cells. *Pharmacol. Rev. 22*, 485–520

REYNOLDS, J. J. (1972) Skeletal tissue in culture, in *The Biochemistry and Physiology of Bone*, 2nd edn. (Bourne, G. H., ed.), pp. 69–126, Academic Press, New York

RUDAS, B. (1969) Über das Verhalten von Ratten mit chronischem Streptozotocin-Diabetes. *Klin. Wochenschr. 47*, 1120–1121

SINDEN, J. A. & LONGWELL, B. B. (1949) Effect of alloxan on fertility and gestation in the rat. *Proc. Soc. Exp. Biol. Med. 70*, 607–610

SMITHBERG, M. & RUNNER, M. N. (1963) Teratogenic effects of hypoglycemic treatments in inbred strains of mice. *Am. J. Anat. 113*, 479–489

VAN ASSCHE, F. A. (1975) The fetal endocrine pancreas, in *Carbohydrate Metabolism in Pregnancy and the Newborn* (Sutherland, H. & Stowers, J., eds.), pp. 68–85, Churchill Livingstone, Edinburgh

WATANABE, G. & INGALLS, T. H. (1963) Congenital malformations in the offspring of alloxan-diabetic mice. *Diabetes 12*, 66–72

Discussion

Milner: The dose of 45 mg/kg which you gave the rats is in the middle of the diabetogenic dose range for streptozotocin. I have the impression that the animals were hyperglycaemic but not in need of .exogenous insulin therapy. Did you treat the diabetic mothers with exogenous insulin in your experiments?

Deuchar: Not in these cases, no.

Milner: It seems likely then that the diabetic mothers still had endogenous insulin in their circulation but an inadequate amount to maintain normoglycaemia. In interpreting the quasi-protective effect of diabetic serum on the control and the diabetic embryos, we have to think not only of the potential benefit conferred by the high glucose concentration of the diabetic serum but also of a possible effect of endogenous insulin. Have you measured the diabetic maternal serum for its insulin content?

Deuchar: No, we have not the means to do insulin assays in our laboratory at present. Are you suggesting that the insulin has a protective effect on the embryo?

Milner: I am intrigued to know whether diabetic serum confers its beneficial effect on the control embryo by virtue of its hyperglycaemia alone or by virtue of hyperglycaemia in the presence of some insulin which is biologically active. To test that I would spike diabetic serum with anti-insulin antibody to remove any insulin present in the diabetic serum. The question that intrigues me goes back to Dr Blázquez's point earlier (p. 154). In those early embryos, is glucose entry into the cell independent of insulin? In later life one would expect glucose entry to be insulin-dependent.

Deuchar: I do not know if insulin can get across to the embryo *in vitro*. The embryo certainly does not produce any insulin itself until much later in development.

Milner: It is generally accepted that in later pregnancy, in the species we have been discussing, the placenta is impermeable to insulin. You said that the period from 4 to 9 days of gestational age is the time when there is some inimical effect on the diabetic fetuses. I am still preoccupied with the possibility that streptozotocin given after mating could have had some effect. You may know more about the kinetics of streptozotocin clearance from the mated mother, but could something happen at the time of fertilization which would not be morphologically manifest at day 5 but which could become manifest at day 10?

Deuchar: I think that is possible.

Milner: In that case should not streptozotocin be given before mating, despite all the consequent difficulties of mating diabetic female rats, before we can be sure that it wasn't the streptozotocin which was making those animals more vulnerable?

Deuchar: In earlier experiments where I gave streptozotocin before mating we got the same malformations in fetuses when streptozotocin was given at any time from 5 to 10 days before pregnancy. The oestrous cycle is often upset and it is difficult to mate these animals. I agree that the possibility that streptozotocin has an effect on early embryos has not been completely ruled out. So far I have looked only at the morphology of the early embryos.

Williamson: It is well established that in the short term streptozotocin decreases the NAD concentration in various tissues and this effect lasts for about 48 h (Schein *et al.* 1971). Have you increased the glucose concentration of the control sera to see whether this has the same effect as in the diabetic sera?

Deuchar: I haven't done that, but David Cockroft and Pat Coppola have, and there seemed to be an enhanced growth of embryos. Later they used abnormally high concentrations of glucose, equivalent to about 800 mg/100 ml (44.4 mmol/l) of whole blood, and these caused malformations. At 800 mg/100 ml there would be very severe diabetes: more severe than is found in our streptozocin-treated rats.

Hoet: Did the serum contain any ketone bodies? This may already be a sign of insulin insufficiency.

Deuchar: We haven't measured that.

Pedersen: I was interested to hear that you found that these fetuses were less viable and were retarded.

Deuchar: The retardation and lowered viability were seen in early embryos only, not in fetuses. There was a high frequency of sacral ossification defects in fetuses, however, which may represent retardation of a special kind.

Pedersen: To our surprise, in 70 cases from all of White's classes, we found, by ultrasound, that between weeks 7 and 14 the diabetic fetuses were on average 5 days delayed compared with normal fetuses. This intrigued us. One has to be very cautious about this because it is crucial to know the day of gestation. In at least 10% of those cases we had the basal temperature measurements etc., so we are quite sure that the diabetic fetuses were delayed (J. Fog-Pedersen, unpublished work, 1977).

Shafrir: Have you any information on malformations if diabetes is induced by streptozotocin administration on day 8, 10 or 12 of pregnancy rather than before mating or on day 2? Professor Chez and collaborators gave streptozotocin late in pregnancy to primates and found very little disturbance in metabolic measurements of the fetus. The fetal pancreas seemed to be either immune to streptozotocin or streptozotocin was rapidly degraded so that pancreatotoxic levels on the fetal side were not reached.

Deuchar: Golob *et al.* (1970) administered streptozotocin as late as 5 days but I think never as late as 12 days. The main effect was a reduction in size of the fetuses. These workers did not give any biochemical data on the fetuses. They reported some fetal deaths, but no abnormalities.

Chez: Over the years we have examined about 70 pregnancies in non-human primates in which streptozotocin was given to the mother at the end of the first trimester. We have looked at an equal number of pregnancies in which the mother received streptozotocin before conception. We have also looked at the placental transfer of radioactively labelled streptozotocin (Reynolds *et al.* 1974). In the primate it crosses the placenta and is degraded in the fetus at the same rate as in the adult. There is a relative limitation to its transfer to the fetus in the sense that maximum fetal concentrations are only about a third of the simultaneous maternal concentrations. This occurs at the time that the maternal concentration levels off. Using light microscopy we cannot demonstrate morphological differences in the fetal pancreas near term in mothers who received streptozotocin before conception and those who received it when they were already pregnant. In the 140 pregnancies we saw no gross physical congenital anomalies that we could identify. Ann Reynolds (unpublished work, 1978), who also has a colony of streptozotocin-treated monkeys, found only one congenital anomaly, a forked tongue.

The next question in my mind is whether, as well as species differences in terms of susceptibility to congenital anomalies, there is a possibility that we see no anomalies because anything that does develop in the monkey is a lethal anomaly and results in spontaneous abortion. We have an abortion rate of about 25–30% in these animals, which is not very different from the rate in controls. We would not be able to recognize subtle differences in anomalies but isn't it a possibility, in any one species, that spontaneous abortions would cover the differences in incidences of anomalies and therefore they would not be apparent?

In the non-human primate in about 400 normal pregnancies I have not found congenital anomalies at birth. We have seen various anatomical variations in the placentas that in the human at least we would also describe as variations in the normal placental configuration. The monkey may not be a good animal to think about in terms of the relationship between glucose intolerance and congenital anomalies.

We have always been concerned about using the term diabetes mellitus to describe streptozotocin-induced glucose intolerance. Perhaps we should all be rigorous about this. There may be political expediencies in using the term diabetes fom the point of view of funding. Our belief is that diabetes mellitus is a multi-organ disease of which glucose intolerance is one element. I would question whether we should be using the term diabetes for streptozotocin glucose intolerance. Streptozotocin, we think, is a specific β-cell cytotoxic agent. In the monkey, for instance, the basal plasma insulin concentrations are the same in the streptozotocin-treated mothers as in the controls. The difference is only the failure to increase circulating insulin when challenged by glucose, with resultant glucose intolerance.

Deuchar: Whatever you like to call the condition, if you give these animals insulin you don't get any fetal malformations. There is a disease that is remediable by exogenous insulin.

Battaglia: You presented data on embryos *in vitro* and on embryos removed from the uterus after they had developed *in vivo*. Which were you referring to in that comment?

Deuchar: The insulin correction was achieved in experiments in which I was recording fetal anomalies at a later stage (20 days). It doesn't apply to the work on embryos *in vitro*.

Williamson: In rats the diabetic effect depends on the dose of streptozotocin. With graded doses we and others have shown that the animals get the whole spectrum of diabetes, from no increase in basal glucose to 1000 mg/100 ml (50 mmol/l), plus or minus dramatic ketoacidosis (Schein *et al.* 1971). It is very important to decide whether the rats are ketoacidotic and what the insulin levels are. Unfortunately in the first 24 hours after streptozotocin is given, as with alloxan, there are effects on the liver including a decrease in NAD and ATP concentrations. These are over within 48 hours and it doesn't have the renal effects that alloxan has.

Chez: At the same injected dosage in the monkey we get the spectrum of chemical diabetes all the way to a glucose intolerance that is associated with ketoacidosis.

Deuchar: Even in different strains of rats one gets variable responses to streptozotocin. I have just started with a new strain and this needs 50 mg streptozotocin to induce mild diabetes, per kilogram of body weight, whereas Wistar rats need only 45 mg.

Milner: In streptozotocin-induced diabetes one sees nephropathy (Slater *et al.* 1978). I would accept streptozotocin as an appropiate model for diabetes mellitus in the rat.

Williamson: It would be important to carry out all the measurements which are required to define diabetes.

Hoet: Your work confirms what Horii *et al.* (1966) reported, Dr Deuchar. Diabetes had to be controlled fairly strictly in order to prevent the appearance of congenital malformations. They had to administer insulin twice daily to get the glucose levels exactly right. The presence of skeletal malformation was related to blood sugar control.

Beard: Is it possible to remove the conceptus before the critical time of organogenesis and growth?

Deuchar: I assume that you refer to times after implantation. One can remove and culture it at 9 days quite easily. At 8 days, the primitive streak stage, it is also possible to remove it, but not to culture it successfully.

Beard: So you can't get at the conceptus before the critical time of 4–9 days?

Deuchar: So far people haven't been able to get these early stages of the rat to grow *in vitro*. Preimplantation stages, up to 5 days, can be washed out of the uterine tubes but do not develop normally *in vitro*. With mice, there are better possibilities of this.

Beard: If you were able to get them out and then test out the two sera it would be very interesting, don't you think?

Räihä: Is streptozotocin completely specific for the pancreatic cells or does it affect the metabolism of other cells?

Deuchar: I can't answer that question.

Freinkel: This is an extraordinarily exciting preparation, Dr Deuchar. It may well be the ideal arena in which to test the implications of alternative fuels for differentiating cell structures. In this regard, it is important to recognize some of the unique features of fuel metabolism in these experimental forms of diabetes. With streptozotocin- as with alloxan-induced diabetes, fat mobilization and ketogenesis are greatest in the early stages as islets are being destroyed. After diabetes has become established, fat depots have become depleted, hyperglycaemia persists but full-blown ketoacidosis is no longer seen although there is still some ketonaemia. Therefore, when you culture rat embryos with serum from day 10, the likelihood of obtaining the full spectrum of potential substrate actions may be restricted because maximal ketonaemia is no longer operative. I hope that you will add ketones to the suspending medium in some of your future experiments. It is conceivable that a given degree of hyperglycaemia plus or minus the added contributions of a given amount of ketones may exert considerably different actions at this stage of cell proliferation and differentiation.

Deuchar: One can correct for the osmotic effects. It is perfectly feasible to add up to 1/2 volume of Tyrode saline or other diluents to the medium. Another variant would be to use the serum from rats over the 4–9-day period of pregnancy rather than at 10 days and see whether that serum had any deleterious effects on cultured embryos.

Freinkel: This may be an effective approach for testing the whole gamut of potential substrate mixtures.

Gillmer: Once you have set the experiment up, do you have to leave it for 24 hours or could you change the substrate environment?

Deuchar: There is no reason why we shouldn't change it. Cockroft uses a much better system, a continuous circulating medium with a point of entry where substances can be added.

Gillmer: So you could test the effects of rapid changes in substrate concentrations?

Deuchar: I haven't got this set-up myself, but that seems possible with Cockroft's apparatus.

Hoet: Could you grow a fertilized egg from a diabetic animal in a normal animal?

Deuchar: I think egg transfer could easily be done. Anne McLaren and her associates have been doing this.

Hoet: All this makes me wonder whether insulin is really a growth-promoting hormone or whether at certain concentrations it inhibits rather than promotes growth or specific functions of fetal tissues. The sensitivity of certain cell functions to different insulin concentrations should be taken into account in our discussion.

References

GOLOB, E. K., RISHI, S., BECKER, K.L. & MOORE, C. (1970) Streptozotocin diabetes in pregnant and non-pregnant rats. *Metabolism 19,* 1014–1019

HORII, K., WATANABE, G. & INGALLS, T. H. (1966) Experimental diabetes in pregnant mice. Prevention of congenital malformations in offspring by insulin. *Diabetes 15,* 194–204

REYNOLDS, W. A., CHEZ, R. A., BHUYAN, B. K. & NEIL, G. L. (1974) Placental transfer of streptozotocin in the rhesus monkey. *Diabetes 23,* 777–782

SCHEIN, P. S., ALBERTI, K. G. M. M. & WILLIAMSON, D. H. (1971) Effects of streptozotocin on carbohydrate and lipid metabolism in the rat. *Endocrinology 89,* 827–834

SLATER, D. N., MANGNALL, Y., SMYTHE, A., MILFORD WARD, A. & FOX, M. (1978) Neonatal islet cell transplantation in the diabetic rat: effect on the renal complications. *J. Pathol. 124,* 117–124

General discussion II

Young: As I have indicated previously, we have been investigating the influence of insulin on tissue protein turnover rates in the fetus. We were interested in this because so little is known about any hormonal regulation of fetal growth and because of the current view that insulin may cause the macrosomia of the large infant of the diabetic mother, a matter dear to all your hearts – and to my own! Most of the evidence for insulin being a possible growth hormone depends on observations in a variety of isolated fetal and adult tissues which, when examined closely, are very conflicting. The *in vivo* observations are also conflicting; those of Picon (1967) cited by Jean Girard earlier suggest a nitrogen-retaining action of insulin in the rat fetus, whilst those of Pain & Garlick (1974) showed that insulin had little effect on muscle protein synthetic rate in the adult rat.

Our observations were made in the fetal lamb *in utero* during the third trimester, using the continuous infusion of a labelled amino acid. Steady-state whole-body synthetic rate was calculated from the plasma clearance or flux of the [^{14}C]lysine used; the half-life of the mixed protein in the individual organs was calculated from the rate constant for the fractional synthetic rate obtained from the ratio of the specific activities of the lysine taken up by the protein and that of the intracellular precursor pool. In the control animals, the half-life of the mixed protein was about one day in the brain, liver and cardiac muscle and seven days in skeletal muscle (Fig. 1). These values are much shorter than in the adult, with less differentiation between the tissues, as might be anticipated in a growing animal.

A six to tenfold increase in steady state plasma insulin levels apparently reduced the fractional organ protein synthetic rates, but this was significant only in cardiac muscle (Fig. 2). These changes were difficult to interpret because of the fall in the tissue free amino acids which suggested decreased protein breakdown, and the extensive metabolism of the labelled lysine, both of which were most marked in skeletal muscle (Chrystie *et al.* 1977).

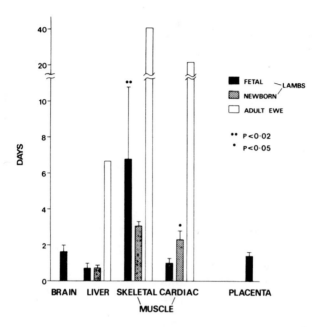

FIG. 1 (Young). Effect of age on mixed protein half-life (days^{-1}, mean ± S.E.).

Insulin may have different effects on protein synthesis rate in the normal fetus and that of a diabetic mother for, although Pain & Garlick (1974) observed little effect of insulin on the protein synthetic rate in skeletal muscle of normal rats, the hormone stimulated the depressed protein synthetic rate of muscle in streptozotocin diabetic rats.

Kalkhoff: How low did the blood sugar concentrations go in the fetus?

Young: Blood glucose was reduced by insulin from a mean value of 16 mg/100 ml (0.9 mmol/l) to levels which were not measurable.

Kalkhoff: How long is gestation in sheep?

Battaglia: It lasts about 145 days.

Kalkhoff: In these animals near the end of pregnancy, with the fetuses having that low blood sugar level, could the fetus be mobilizing a substantial amount of catabolic hormones?

Young: We have done further experiments maintaining normal plasma glucose and free amino acid levels by constant infusion, but found that protein synthetic rate was not influenced by such manoeuvres.

Räihä: When you speak about the half-life of mixed protein, can you distinguish between synthesis and degradation? In other words, when there is an increased half-life is there decreased degradation?

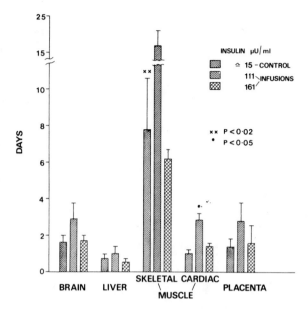

FIG. 2 (Young). The effect of insulin on mixed protein half-life in the organs of fetal lambs (days[-1], mean ± S.E.). In control fetuses the half-lives were 0.67 for liver, 1.0 for cardiac muscle, 1.4 for placenta and 1.62 for brain; the half-life of 7.81 for skeletal muscle was significantly longer. Insulin prolonged the half-life slightly; this was only significant for cardiac muscle at a plasma level of $111 \, \mu U/ml$.

Young: No, unfortunately we cannot distinguish clearly between synthesis and degradation. The method used measured protein synthetic rate. In the steady state, this is equivalent to turnover rate, with degradation equalling synthesis. In the fetus, both protein accumulation and turnover rates are faster than in the adult, and the latter is accompanied by high free amino acid concentrations in the tissues. The low concentration of tissue free amino acids which we found during insulin infusions (Fig. 3) suggests that there was a decrease in degradation; the metabolic clearance rate of labelled amino acids was also decreased, so insulin appears to decrease protein anabolism as well as catabolism. Norbert Freinkel suggested to me that insulin might act as a growth hormone by altering the balance between anabolism and catabolism; growth might occur at any protein synthetic rate so long as the balance was in favour of anabolism.

Räihä: Wicks *et al.* (1974), who worked with PEP-carboxykinase, suggested that insulin may decrease the enzyme by enhancing the enzyme degradation. The effect of insulin on a specific enzyme protein may be completely different from the effect on general tissue protein.

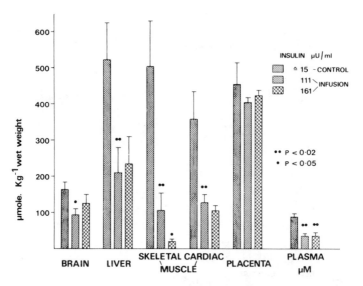

FIG. 3 (Young). The effect of insulin on free lysine pools in fetal lambs (mean ± s.e.).   In control
fetuses the concentrations of free amino acids in the tissues are all high in comparison with those in
the adult; that for brain is significantly lower than for the other fetal organs ($P < 0.05$).
    Insulin significantly reduced the concentration of free amino acids in the plasma and all the
organs; this effect was most marked in skeletal muscle and, because this tissue forms 30–40% of
the body mass and will contribute most to the interorgan traffic of amino acids, the fall in the other
tissues may be secondary to the reduction in muscle.

Young: We studied mixed protein synthetic rate in organs because we were
interested in growth generally.

Naeye: In human diabetic gestations it is not always easy to differentiate the
effects of insulin from other influences.   One setting in which fetal hyperinsulinaemia appears to exist without ketosis or other complications of diabetes is transposition of the great vessels.   The resultant abnormal haemody-
namic pattern directs blood with a relatively high level of glucose to the
abdominal organs, including the pancreas.   Under these circumstances the
fetus develops some of the characteristics of the infant of the diabetic mother,
i.e. pancreatic islet cell hyperplasia and a hypertrophy of cells in most of the
visceral organs (Naeye 1966).

Hoet: This type of malformation is a special situation too, presumably
characterized by a greater activity of the gastrointestinal tract because of the
blood turnover rate.   At this meeting we haven't taken into account the
activity of the gastrointestinal tract and its absorption of glucose.   In sheep at
126–136 days of gestation, there is very little absorption of glucose (Wright &
Nixon 1961).   One of the building stones might be in the gastrointestinal

tract, for instance glucose or amino acid in gastrointestinal juice. We have data that indicate that glucose may be absorbed preferentially in relation to the time of gestation.

Battaglia: I don't understand that. If I don't eat, then even with all the gastrointestinal juices in the world I won't grow. Something has to be put into the gastrointestinal tract. You are really talking about amniotic fluid nutrients. When people refer to amniotic fluid as a source of nutrition they are mixing up unidirectional flux with net change. There are minor changes in amniotic fluid concentrations of solutes but for the most part the concentrations of amino acids and glucose are fairly constant and volumes are not changing markedly. Thus, it is not easy for me to hypothesize a net utilization of solute sufficient to sustain metabolism for a long period of time. If solute is taken out it is obviously being put in from somewhere else. That is the trouble I have in thinking of amniotic fluid as a major source of nutrients over the whole of gestation. It might be used for an hour or two but for 40 weeks it doesn't make sense.

Hoet: The function of the gastrointestinal tract changes in the course of fetal development. If the rat is fasted at 19.5 days or 21.5 days, the glucose content of the gastric juice will behave in a completely different fashion. At 19.5 days the rat will not be able to call upon that reservoir and the glucose content remains unchanged. At 21.5 days glucose will have disappeared completely from the gastrointestinal juice during fasting. Similarly, if glucose is given to the rat mother for five days up to 19.5 days, the glucose will be increased in the amniotic fluid and in the gastric juice. There seems not to be an easy increased absorption at that gestational age. When the same amount of glucose is given to the mothers up to 21.5 days, the glucose will have disappeared from the gastric juice, showing presumably that it has been absorbed through the tract. In relation with fetal hyperinsulinaemia, which is apparent after a glucose load up to 21.5 days and not at 19.5 days, we have to take into account the effect of the maturation of the gastrointestinal tract (Reusens *et al.* 1979).

Chez: I have a different thought about why transposition may result in pancreatic cell hyperplasia, as Dr Naeye mentioned. It has to do with how much challenge the fetal β cell requires before it can be prematurely induced to elaborate insulin. When the great vessels are transposed, the possibility is that blood with slightly more glucose than normal after body metabolic extraction (3–4 mg/100 ml; 0.17–0.22 mmol/l) reaches the pancreas than if the vessels were normal. The suggestion therefore is that this slightly richer blood, which is still within the normal range, is enough to induce the β cell prematurely.

Naeye: During fetal life the heart and the brain are the major users of glucose. In transposition of the great vessels, the brain and heart do not take up glucose before it reaches the fetal pancreas.

Chez: If the brain and the heart are not taking up glucose before the fetal pancreas sees this blood, because of the transposition, then that uptake difference will be increased by the extra amount of glucose presented.

Milner: The theme running through Dr Chez's comments is the classical Pedersen hypothesis. In considering what will make the β cell divide, he immediately thinks of glucose. Dr Freinkel earlier gave appropriate credit to the original hypothesis but now talks about an extended hypothesis in which we have to consider other metabolites or substances in addition to glucose.

We have demonstrated that if fetal rat pancreas explanted on day 14 is grown in organ culture in glucose-enriched medium for 6 days there is no effect on the number of β cells. But if the pancreatic explants are grown in an amino acid-enriched medium, twice as many β cells are produced in the organ culture as would have developed *in utero,* despite poorer overall growth of the organ *in vitro* (de Gasparo *et al.* 1978). Is it possible that glucose is the marker which is characteristic of diabetes mellitus but that some other metabolic perturbation, as Freinkel suggested, which occurs early in pregnancy is the actual trigger, or which coupled with glucose is a combined trigger, for increased β cell mitosis? When one considers amino acid fluctuations in the mother it is interesting that gestational diabetics, albeit at 33–39 weeks of gestation, showed higher peak plasma concentrations of isoleucine and serine postprandially. Studies in adult male diabetics given a protein meal have shown higher postprandial concentrations of arterial amino acid than in normal controls. Splanchnic efflux was similar in the two groups but the diabetics had poorer peripheral uptake of amino acids as measured in the leg. This affected in particular the branch chain amino acids: leucine, isoleucine and valine, which accounted for 50% of the excess in plasma concentration (Wahren *et al.* 1976). Professor Young has demonstrated that branch chain amino acids traverse the placenta in proportion to the plasma concentration (Young & Prenton 1969). These are all pointers which may permit us to make a more specific extension of the Pedersen hypothesis: namely that amino acids as well as glucose play a part in the endocrine pancreatic dysmorphogenesis that occurs in the fetus of the diabetic mother (Milner *et al.* 1979).

Williamson: Our work on newborn rats shows that the transaminases responsible for branched-chain amino acid metabolism are very low in skeletal muscle (P. Ferré & D.H. Williamson, unpublished results). There may therefore be increased delivery to the fetal pancreas and continual stimulation of the β cell.

Stowers: Only small changes in maternal plasma glucose are required to effect the changes in the fetus. We have correlated the birth weights of babies with the blood sugar concentrations in fasting mothers in the last few weeks of pregnancy. There is a positive correlation within the normal range of fasting blood sugar.

Beard: We found an inverse relationship between the glucose tolerance test and the degree of relative hypoglycaemia in the newborn at all stages, even well within the normal range. The concept of a sharp cut-off between normality and diabetes is quite erroneous as far as the effect on the glucose concentration of the newborn that we observed is concerned. We found that the relationship held good even for women whom clinically one would regard as having normal glucose tolerance.

References

CHRYSTIE, S., HORN, J., SLOAN, I., STERN, M., NOAKES, D. & YOUNG, M. (1977) Effect of insulin on protein turnover in fetal lambs. *Proc. Nutr. Soc. 36,* 118A

DE GASPARO, M., MILNER, G. R., NORRIS, P. D. & MILNER, R. D. G.(1978) Effect of glucose and amino acids on foetal rat pancreatic growth and insulin secretion *in vitro. J. Endocrinol., 77,* 241–248

MILNER, R. D. G., DE GASPARO, M., MILNER, G. R. & WIRDNAM, P. K. (1979) Amino acids and development of the beta cell, in *Carbohydrate Metabolism in Pregnancy and the Newborn,* (Sutherland, H. W. & Stowers, J. M., eds.), Springer Verlag, Berlin

NAEYE, R. L. (1966) Transposition of the great arteries and prenatal growth. *Arch. Pathol. 82,* 412–418

PAIN, V. M. & GARLICK, P.J. (1974) Effect of streptozotocin diabetes and insulin treatment on protein synthesis in tissues of the rat *in vivo. J. Biol. Chem. 249,* 4510–4514

PICON, L. (1967) Effect of insulin on growth and biochemical composition of the rat fetus. *Endocrinology 81,* 1419–1421

REUSENS, B., DE GASPARO, M., KUHN & HOET, J. J. (1979) Controlling factors of fetal nutrition, in *Carbohydrate Metabolism in Pregnancy and the Newborn* (Sutherland, H. W. & Stowers, J. M., eds.) Springer Verlag, Berlin

WAHREN, J., FELIG, P. & HAGENFELDT, L. (1976) Effect of protein ingestion on splanchnic and leg metabolism in normal man and in patients with diabetes mellitus. *J. Clin. Invest. 57,* 987–999

WICKS, W. D., BARNETT, C. A. & MCKIBBIN, J. B. (1974) Interaction between hormones and cyclic AMP in regulating specific hepatic enzyme synthesis. *Fed. Proc. 33,* 1105–1111

WRIGHT, G. H. & NIXON, D. A. (1961) Absorption of amniotic fluid in gut of fetal sheep. *Nature (Lond.) 190,* 816

YOUNG, M. & PRENTON, M. A. (1969) Maternal and fetal plasma amino acid concentration during gestation and in retarded fetal growth. *J. Obstet. Gynaecol. Br. Commonw. 76,* 333

Congenital anomalies and the diabetic and prediabetic pregnancy

PETER H. BENNETT, CARYLL WEBNER and MAX MILLER

National Institute of Arthritis, Metabolism, and Digestive Diseases, Epidemiology and Field Studies Branch, Phoenix, Arizona

Abstract   Congenital anomalies are two to four times more frequent in the offspring of diabetic mothers than in those of non-diabetic mothers, and represent an increasingly important cause of perinatal mortality.   These anomalies involve multiple organ systems more often than those found in the children of non-diabetic mothers.   The excess of anomalies associated with maternal diabetes occurs in many organ systems.

Anomalies are no more frequent in the offspring of diabetic fathers and pre-diabetic mothers than among those of non-diabetics, suggesting that non-genetic factors are the important determinants.

Anomalies are most frequent in the offspring of mothers who have developed diabetes at an early age, many of whom have diabetes of long duration, are insulin-treated, and may have vascular complications.   The relative importance of each of these factors in the pathogenesis of anomalies is unknown, but present evidence is consistent with a hypothesis that anomalies are the result of metabolic disturbances in the intrauterine environment during the first trimester of pregnancy.   Whether or not their incidence can be reduced by optimum metabolic control of maternal diabetes during this period is unknown.

Congenital anomalies are now recognized to be more frequent in the offspring of diabetic women than among those of non-diabetic women.   The infants of diabetic mothers also tend to be heavier and suffer increased rates of stillbirth and neonatal death.   In recent years, however, a decline in perinatal death rate among such infants has been observed, yet congenital malformations continue to contribute to perinatal deaths and, as other causes diminish in frequency, appear to represent an increasingly important cause of death as well as contributing considerably to the morbidity of those who survive.   It has been estimated that about 25% of the perinatal deaths associated with diabetic pregnancies are now the direct consequence of congenital anomalies (Soler *et al.* 1976).

The excessive frequency of malformations in the infants of diabetic mothers has now been clearly established by many investigators.   However, difficulties in the definition of anomalies and indeed in classifying various types of diabetic pregnancies, led for many years to discussion of the truth of the association, and continue to impede the investigation of the nature of the association.   Definitional problems usually preclude direct comparisons of reports of the frequency of anomalies between different centres, and multicentre studies require elaborate definitions, and hence prospective, rather than retrospective, data collection.   In most populations the diabetic pregnancy occurs in only one of 200–400 pregnancies.   Yet centres specializing in the care and management of the diabetic pregnancy may draw a select group of pregnancies and this bias may severely limit the conclusions that may be reached from investigations in such centres.   Furthermore, as the perinatal mortality rate for infants of diabetic mothers is high, especially when anomalies are present, the infant of a diabetic mother is more likely to be examined in detail, e.g. at autopsy, and because of the many potential problems of these infants, those who survive are almost certain to receive greater scrutiny than those of non-diabetic mothers.   Hence, there is the potential bias that the degree of ascertainment of anomalies in the children of diabetics will be greater than that in non-diabetics.

Important questions remain concerning the pathogenesis of the excessive frequency of malformations in the infants of diabetic mothers.   The magnitude of the increased risk of malformation is not well established, nor are the issues of whether the determinants are primarily genetic or environmental; whether or not the effect of diabetes is system-specific; whether the effect is related primarily to insulin therapy or to the severity, duration or age of onset of diabetes, or to the presence of vascular or metabolic abnormalities.

The purpose of this review is to present recent findings relating to these questions.   Data from the Pima Indian pregnancy study will be considered in conjunction with findings reported from the Collaborative Perinatal Project (Berendes & Weiss 1970).   These studies each collected data systematically on diabetic and non-diabetic pregnancies in a standardized manner.

Briefly, the Pima Indian results represent the pooled data from two subgroups; (a) data concerning 1207 offspring of 237 women, aged 25–44 years, each of whom had had at least one pregnancy before 1966 and received a glucose tolerance test in the period 1965–67 (Comess et al. 1969), and (b) data from 1441 children born between 1966 and 1977 of Pima/Papago mothers who resided on the Gila River Indian Reservation in Arizona, USA, and who were eligible to participate in a prospective study of the natural history of diabetes mellitus and its complications.   During this period data were collected systematically on all pregnant women and their offspring and, whenever possible, glucose tolerance testing was carried out in the third trimester and 24–72 hours *post partum,* as well as at two-yearly intervals on all persons resident on the reservation.   Thus, in this group the age of onset of diabetes, and hence the diabetic status of each pregnancy, can be ascertained with unusual precision.   The characteristics of diabetes in the Pima Indians, which are similar to those found in other races, and the diagnostic criteria for diabetes and anomalies, have been detailed previously (Bennett *et al.* 1976; Comess *et al.* 1969).

CONGENITAL ANOMALIES AND MATERNAL DIABETES

Diabetic pregnancies accounted for 4.3% or 1 in 23 of all pregnancies in the Pima Indian women, compared to rates of 1 in 200–400 pregnancies in other centres thought to be representative of the general US population (Chung & Myrianthopoulos 1975; Miller 1965).   This rate is in accord with the 10–15-fold greater prevalence of diabetes in the Pima Indian population.

Congenital anomalies were encountered more frequently in the diabetic than in the non-diabetic and prediabetic pregnancies.   Anomalies in the Pima were found in 11% of the children of diabetic pregnancies, a rate four times greater than that in the non-diabetic pregnancies (Table 1).   However, among prediabetic pregnancies – pregnancies occurring in women before the onset of diabetes–the rates were no different than in the non-diabetic pregnancies. These rates can be compared to data from the Collaborative Perinatal Project (Chung & Myrianthopoulos 1975) (Table 2), which showed higher anomaly rates in both White and Negro diabetic pregnancies, with 2.1- and 1.6-fold increases, respectively.   Although the reported rates of major mal-

TABLE 1

Congenital anomalies and maternal diabetes status in Pima Indians

Maternal diabetes status	No. of children	With anomalies	
		No.	%
Normal	2013	51	2.53
Prediabetic	511	18	3.52
Diabetic	114	13	11.40
Total	2638	82	3.11
		$\chi^2_2 = 28.54; P < 0.001$	

TABLE 2

Collaborative Perinatal Project:major malformations in children according to mother's diabetes status in Whites and Negroes (from Chung & Myrianthopoulos 1975)

Diabetes status of mother	Whites			Negroes		
	Pregnancies No.	Major malformations No.	%	Pregnancies No.	Major malformations No.	%
Non-diabetic	23000	1919	8.3	24408	2063	8.5
Gestational	189	22	11.6	183	11	6.0
Overt diabetes	457	82	17.9^a	110	15	13.6^b

^{a} $P < 0.001$ ^{b} $P < 0.1$

formation in this study are higher than in the Pima, differences in the definition of anomalies may be responsible. Nevertheless, a relative increase in the frequency of anomalies in diabetics of each racial group was found.

NATURE OF MALFORMATIONS

Malformations in the offspring of the diabetic pregnancy are more numerous, but are also more often multiple. Multiple anomalies were considered to be structural abnormalities occurring in two or more organ systems. Table 3 shows that 4% of the diabetic pregnancies in the Pima were associated with multiple anomalies compared to 0.3% ($P < 0.005$) of other pregnancies. Furthermore, the proportion of anomalous offspring with multiple

TABLE 3

Incidence of multiple malformations in Pima Indian children by maternal diabetes status

	Non-diabetic ($n = 2013$)	Prediabetic ($n = 511$)	Diabetic ($n = 114$)
With anomalies	51	18	13
With multiple anomalies	5(0.3%)	3(0.6%)	5(4.4%) $P < 0.005$
Percent of anomalous with multiple anomalies	9.8	16.7	38.5
		11.6%	
			$P < 0.05$

TABLE 4

Frequency of major malformations in children of non-diabetic and diabetic pregnancies (from Chung & Myrianthopoulos 1975)

System	Non-diabetic (n = 47 408)		Diabetic (n = 567)		Ratio diabetic/ non-diabetic
	No.	%	No.	%	
CNS	322	0.68	13	2.29	3.4
Musculoskeletal	1666	3.51	30	5.29	1.5
Sensory	114	0.24	2	0.35	1.5
Cardiovascular	209	0.44	14	2.47	5.6
Respiratory	337	0.71	11	1.94	2.7
Genitourinary	440	0.93	19	3.35	3.6
Alimentary	906	1.91	20	3.53	1.8
Total	3982		97		

malformations was significantly greater in the diabetic (39%) than among the other pregnancies (12%: $P < 0.05$).   Similar conclusions were drawn in the Collaborative Perinatal Project.

The types of anomalies found in relation to the diabetic pregnancy, for the most part, do not appear to be specific.   In the Collaborative Perinatal Project significant excesses were noted in major malformations in all systems listed in Table 4, except for sensory abnormalities, but the excesses were particularly notable in the CNS, cardiovascular and genitourinary systems.   In the Pima study also, the increases appeared to be excessive in all systems, although the diabetics showed a disproportionate number of musculoskeletal abnormalities compared to those in the non-diabetics.   The only abnormality which appears to be relatively specific for the diabetic pregnancy is the caudal regression syndrome, also known as sacral dys- or agenesis, or phocomelic diabetic embryopathy.   This syndrome is rare, and was identified in only two anomalous children in the Collaborative Perinatal Project and one of the Pima Indians – each the products of diabetic pregnancies.

MATERNAL FACTORS

As the average age of the mother was greater in the Pima diabetic than the

TABLE 5

Congenital anomalies and maternal age at delivery in Pima Indians

Maternal age at dlivery	Non-diabetic and prediabetic			Diabetic		
	Total	With anomalies		Total	With anomalies	
		No.	%		No.	%
<15	10	–	–	1	–	–
15-24	1411	36	2.6	23	3	13.0
25-34	923	23	2.5	60	9	15.0
35-44	180	10	5.6	30	1	3.3
Total	2524	69	2.7	114	13	11.4

other pregnancies, the frequency of anomalies in relation to age at delivery was examined (Table 5). In the non-diabetic and prediabetic pregnancies the frequency of anomalies tended to increase with age, whereas the converse was found in the diabetic group. Consequently, the frequency of anomalies in diabetic pregnancies according to the mother's age at the onset of diabetes was examined (Table 6). Women with an onset of diabetes before 25 years of age were shown to have an unusually high risk of having anomalous children (Comess et al. 1969). Similar results have been presented by Koller (1953), and Soler et al. (1976), who found that 11% of pregnancies in women with an onset before 20 years of age led to an anomalous child compared to 6% in

TABLE 6

Age of onset of maternal diabetes and congenital anomalies in Pima Indians

Age of onset of diabetes in mother (yrs) %	No. of pregnancies	Anomalies	
		No.	%
≤ 24	42	9	21.4
25-34	56	4	7.1
35-44	16	0	0.0
Total	114	13	11.4

$P < 0.05; \chi^2 = 7.24$

those with a later age of onset.   These workers, however, failed to find any relationship to duration of maternal diabetes at the time of pregnancy and the occurrence of anomalies, as was the case in the Pima Indian Study.

Another study of the outcome of pregnancy in diabetics, reported by Neave (1967), also failed to find evidence of an association with the duration of maternal diabetes, but a contrary conclusion was reached in the Collaborative Perinatal Project (Table 7); however, the effect of the age of onset of diabetes in the mother was not reported in this investigation.   Since an earlier age of onset of diabetes is related to a longer average duration at the time of pregnancy, additional data relating to simultaneous influences of age of onset and duration would be informative.

Among the Pima diabetic pregnancies an excess of malformed children was found in the subgroup treated with insulin (Table 8).   This finding is in accord with the reports of Day & Insley (1976), but no significant differences were found in the Collaborative Perinatal Project, or in the series reported by Soler *et al.* (1976).   No evidence of an excessive occurrence of anomalies has been described in diabetic pregnancies treated with oral hypoglycaemic agents compared to those treated by other means in any of these studies.   The possible effects of exogenous insulin as a teratogenic agent must be entertained, but it is important to consider that the earlier the age of onset of diabetes and the longer its duration, the greater the likelihood that the diabetic patient will receive insulin treatment.

TABLE 7

Incidence of malformations by duration of diabetes in mothers receiving insulin therapy

Diabetes duration	No. of pregnancies	Major malformations		Significance
		No.	%	
Collaborative Perinatal Project				
< 5 years	188	21	11.2	
≥ 5 years	368	74	20.1	$P < 0.01$
Joslin Clinic[a]				
≤ 5 years	543	71	18.08	
> 5 years	1401	204	14.56	

[a] From Neave (1967)

TABLE 8

Congenital anomalies and hypoglycaemic medication used by Pima Indian diabetic mothers during pregnancy

Hypoglycaemic medication	Children	Anomalies No.	%	Significance
Insulin	46	10	21.7	
				$P < 0.005$
Oral agents	9	0	0.0 ⎫	
			⎬ 4.4	
None	59	3	5.1 ⎭	
Total	114	13	11.4	

The Pima data tend to suggest that age of onset of diabetes may be the more important variable, as anomalies resulted in five (38.5%) of 13 pregnancies in women with an age of onset of less than 25 years, where insulin was used in the first trimester, compared to three (37.5%) of eight where insulin was not used (Comess *et al.* 1969).

Nevertheless, the available data do not unequivocally exclude the possibility that the administration of insulin during pregnancy may be implicated in the genesis of malformations. Such an action of insulin has been reported in (non-diabetic) chickens, rats, rabbits and mice, yet in mice with alloxan-induced diabetes, the administration of insulin early in pregnancy has been claimed to reduce the frequency of such malformations (Horii *et al.* 1966).

PATERNAL FACTORS

Since there is evidence of genetic predisposition to many types of congenital anomalies, the possibility that the excessive rate of anomalies found in diabetic pregnancies has a genetic basis must be considered. As the predisposition to diabetes is believed to be determined by autosomal genes the possibility exists that linked genes might be responsible for the excessive occurrence of anomalies in infants of diabetic mothers. If so, the offspring of diabetic fathers should also demonstrate an increased frequency of anomalous children. Both the Collaborative Perinatal Project and the Pima Study have examined this possibility, but, as shown in Table 9, no evidence was found that either diabetic or prediabetic fathers sire children with a greater frequency of anomalies than do non-diabetic fathers. This evidence, taken together with the earlier evidence that prediabetic mothers do not bear an excessive number

TABLE 9

Incidence of malformations and paternal diabetes

Father's status	No. of pregnancies[a]	Malformations		Significance
		No.	%	
Collaborative Perinatal Project				
Non-diabetic	51 803	4289	8.28	NS
Diabetic	253	23	9.09	
Pima Indians				
Non-diabetic	395	13	3.3	NS
Prediabetic	197	7	3.6 ⎫ 3.7	
Diabetic	44	2	4.5 ⎭	

[a] Pregnancies in which mother had diabetes are excluded. NS: $P > 0.05$

of anomalous offspring, eliminates the possibility that the excess of congenital anomalies found in the offspring of diabetic mothers is simply a consequence of genetic determinants which are linked to diabetes-related genes.

DISCUSSION

There is now a consensus that congenital anomalies are more frequent in the offspring of diabetic mothers. Anomalies appear to be more frequent in the offspring of diabetic mothers of all races, with an incidence two to four times that of the non-diabetic. Besides their greater incidence, anomalies in the offspring of diabetic women more commonly affect multiple organ systems, and are now responsible for a considerable and increasing proportion of the perinatal deaths associated with diabetic pregnancies.

Genetic factors do not appear to be the predominant determinants of the anomalies associated with diabetic pregnancies. Firstly, the offspring of diabetic fathers do not have any increased incidence, and secondly, no significant increase has been found in pregnancies that clearly preceded the onset of diabetes in the mother. Furthermore, it is unlikely that increases in such a heterogeneous group of malformations could be attributed to genetic determinants linked to the gene or genes responsible for diabetes. It seems more likely that such a spectrum of malformations would result from factors operating in the fetal environment at the time of organogenesis during the first trimester.

The diabetic women most prone to bear children with malformations are those with a relatively early age of onset of diabetes.   The onset of diabetes often precedes the first pregnancy and is usually severe enough to require insulin therapy.   Many of these women exhibit the vascular complications of diabetes before their child-bearing years are over.   Because of the multitude of factors which occur in such women the determinants of anomalies in their offspring are difficult to ascertain.   Several authors, e.g. Pedersen *et al.* (1964) and Soler *et al.* (1976), have shown a relationship of anomalies in children to the White classification of diabetes in the mother (White 1974).   This classification depends on the concurrent consideration of age of onset, duration of diabetes and the presence of vascular complications.   As a result the classification has prognostic significance, but its use does little to enhance understanding of the possible aetiology of congenital anomalies.

There is no convincing evidence that the presence of gestational diabetes – that is abnormal glucose tolerance during but not after the termination of pregnancy – is associated with any excess of anomalies in the offspring.   Conversely, women with evidence of vascular complications at the time of pregnancy appear to have an unusually high risk of bearing malformed children (Pedersen *et al.* 1964; Neave 1967), but these women are also those with diabetes of long duration and an early age of onset, and are almost invariably insulin-treated.   As early-onset diabetes without clinical evidence of vascular disease is also associated with an excessive risk of anomalies it seems more likely that the severity of the metabolic derangement during the first trimester may be a more important determinant than the presence of vascular disease or insulin treatment.   Nevertheless, the interrelationships between age at onset of maternal diabetes, insulin treatment in the first trimester, and severity and duration of diabetes require further exploration.

The association of anomalies with early-onset diabetes suggests that perhaps only a subset of diabetic women may be prone to develop anomalies. Since juvenile-onset insulin-requiring diabetes is also associated with the HLA types B8 and B15 in Caucasians, the question of whether congenital anomalies might show similar associations can be raised.   We believe that while these histocompatibility antigens are characteristically found in those diabetics prone to have offspring with congenital anomalies, these antigens will not explain the observed associations with age of onset.   In the Pima Indians, where such antigens are extremely rare, the association of anomalies with early-onset diabetes is also found, yet the vast majority of the diabetics are of the 'maturity-onset type', even though some develop the disease at an early age. Consequently, it seems likely that the severity of metabolic derangement in early pregnancy offers the most reasonable explanation for the pathogenesis of these diabetes-related congenital malformations.

The major unanswered question is whether congenital malformations, which are responsible for an increasing proportion of perinatal mortality related to diabetes, are preventable. Although insulin itself has been shown to be teratogenic in some animals, the reported prevention of anomalies in alloxan-diabetic mice by the administration of insulin suggests that congenital anomalies in human diabetes may also be preventable. This hypothesis could be tested in a controlled clinical trial in which insulin was used to maintain meticulous diabetic control during the critical period for organogenesis.

ACKNOWLEDGEMENTS

We would like to express our thanks to the members of the Gila River Indian Community, who participated in this investigation, the staff of the Indian Health Service, whose help made the study possible, and the staff of the Southwestern Field Studies Section for the coding and analysis of data and help in preparing the manuscript.

References

BENNETT, P. B., RUSHFORTH, N. B., MILLER, M. & LECOMPTE, P. M. (1976) Epidemiologic studies of diabetes in the Pima Indians. *Recent Prog. Horm. Res. 32,* 333–376

BERENDES, H. W. & WEISS, W. (1970) The NIH Collaborative Study. A progress report, in *Congenital Malformations* (Clarke-Fraser, F. & McKusick, V. A., eds.), (I.C.S. No. 204), pp. 293–298, Excerpta Medica, Amsterdam

CHUNG, C. S. & MYRIANTHOPOULOS, W.C. (1975) Factors affecting risks of congenital malformations. Report from the Collaborative Perinatal Project, in *Birth Defects Orig. Article Series* (Bergsma, D., ed.), vol. 11, No. 10, pp. 23–38, The National Foundation-March of Dimes Symposia Specialists, Miami

COMESS, L. J., BENNETT, P. H., BURCH, T. A. & MILLER, M. (1969) Congenital anomalies and diabetes in the Pima Indians of Arizona. *Diabetes 18,* 471–477

DAY, R. E. & INSLEY, J. (1976) Maternal diabetes mellitus and congenital malformation. Survey of 205 cases. *Arch. Dis. Child. 51,* 935–938

HORII, K., WATANABE, G. & INGALLS, T. H. (1966) Experimental diabetes in pregnant mice: prevention of congenital malformation in offspring by insulin. *Diabetes 15,* 194–204

KOLLER, O. (1953) Diabetes and pregnancy. *Acta Obstet. Gynecol. Scand. 32,* 80–103

MILLER, M. (1965) Diabetic pregnancy and foetal survival in a large metropolitan area, in *On the Nature and Treatment of Diabetes* (Leibel, B.S. & Wrenshall, G. E., eds.), (I.C.S. No. 84), pp. 714–717, Excerpta Medica, Amsterdam

NEAVE, C. (1967) Congenital malformations in offspring of diabetics, D. P. H. Thesis, Harvard University, Boston

PEDERSEN, L. M., TYGSTRUP, I. & PEDERSEN, J. (1964) Congenital malformations in newborn infants of diabetic women. *Lancet 1,* 1124–1126

SOLER, N. G., WALSH, C. H. & MALINS, J. M. (1976) Congenital malformations in infants of
    diabetic mothers. *Q.J. Med. 45,* 303–313
WHITE, P. (1974) Diabetes mellitus in pregnancy. *Clin. Perinatol. 1,* 331

Discussion

Pedersen: This study is very important on at least two points.   You have
shown that infants of true prediabetic women do not have more congenital
malformations than infants of normal mothers.   Therefore, you have spared
us an investigation of the children of non-diabetic sisters of diabetic women
which would provide the best scientific evidence on the role of the diabetic
state.   You have also shown that there is no increase in malformations in the
progeny of diabetic fathers.   Since there does not seem to be any increase in
chromosomal failures in these infants we can be sure that malformations must
have something to do with the diabetic state.

There are difficulties in establishing the exact rate of congenital malformations but you found just about the same rate in the Pima Indians as others have
found.   In Copenhagen we have shown that the frequency is three times
higher than in the offspring of non-diabetic mothers.   Kučera (1971) collected everything he could find about congenital malformations in the world
literature, and the figure was again three times higher.

As regards the caudal regression syndrome it seems that the Pima Indians
have the same frequency (3 cases out of about 700) as we have in Denmark (1
in 200).   Which minimum malformations did you see?

Bennett: We considered anything that looked like an obvious morphological
condition, such as heart disease, but also including things like syndactyly.

Pedersen: Did you include warts?

Bennett: No.   If we could agree to look at a select list of well-defined and
reasonably obvious malformations, it would be very easy to compare rates
between various places.   But when people include minor aberrations – things
like minor haemangiomas – the non-diabetic group gets filled up with more
and more trivia and one can't see the difference between diabetic and non-
diabetic.   The most clear-cut ratios come from considering major malformations.   Collaborative studies could be done on this subject but it is a matter of
agreeing on definitions.

Another problematic area concerning definitions is the White classification,
where one has to consider at least three things simultaneously.   I would like
to see a study where each of those items – age of onset, duration, and presence
of vascular complications – are separately characterized.   One could then
examine the rates of malformations among the offspring of the rare individuals

who have diabetes of long duration without vascular complications.

Pedersen: Whether one uses the age of onset, the duration or the White classification one gets more or less the same groups of women. Thousands of diabetic pregnancies are needed to pick up those with onset between 5 and 15 years and divide them into those with and those without vascular complications. I don't think that could be done.

Bennett: In the Pima very few diabetics have an onset below age 15, and the pregnancies in the diabetics occur mostly among those who have diabetes of about 5 years' duration. They haven't yet had time to develop vascular complications, yet the frequency of anomalies at that age is just as high as you see in pregnant women with diabetes of longer duration where the vascular complications may have developed. My tentative interpretation of the Pima data is that the clinical evidence of vascular complications is not necessary for the very high frequencies of anomalies in women with an early age of onset.

Pedersen: Later I hope to show you that in some cases the strong positive correlation between malformations and the White groups can be overcome.

Beard: It seems to me that the usefulness of the White classification in looking at the congenital anomalies will soon end. All that the White classification can do is tell us the severity of the diabetic state. What we now need is some index of the severity of the metabolic disturbance within the first three months when organogenesis is occurring. In this way we are most likely to find the link between metabolic disturbance in the mother and fetal congenital anomaly.

Chez: I am trying to separate the effect of age of onset of disease from the effect of age for the particular pregnancy in which the infant has an anomaly. Also, have you been able to dissect out any additional variable of gravidity or parity?

Bennett: We have looked for such a variable and we can't find one, but the series is very small for that sort of analysis.

Chez: Is there any evidence that the same women will bear subsequent infants with anomalies?

Bennett: We can't prove that some women are more predisposed to bear children with anomalies but there are several women who have had two or more such infants.

Chez: When a woman who has diabetes mellitus has a baby with anomalies can we say something to her about the anticipated outcome in subsequent pregnancies? Can we say that the frequency will be the same as in her non-diabetic sister who has not had a baby with anomalies?

Bennett: This is where we really need a good controlled clinical trial. Women who have had one anomalous child are very motivated to come through pregnancy and follow instructions carefully in the first trimester or before conception. This is the only way we will ever get a final answer to the question of whether the risk of a child with anomalies can be controlled early in pregnancy.

Chez: Is the spontaneous abortion rate in the diabetic women any different from that in the controls?

Bennett: The stillbirth rate in the diabetic women is greater but we haven't been able to get data on spontaneous abortions.

Chez: You specified what you meant by malformations. The Iowa study of Stehbens *et al.* (1977) suggests that after five years other anomalies become apparent, perhaps not as blatant as physical anomalies but more in the realm of behavioural, social and intellectual effects, with a 25% incidence.

Battaglia: Are you saying, Dr Bennett, that we still don't know whether an increased anomaly rate is associated with diabetes where insulin was not used as therapy?

Bennett: It hasn't been sorted out in human pregnancies.

Hoet: It is not quite so confusing in animals. When Duraiswami (1950) used insulin in the chicken, the exogenous insulin reached the eggs and there were skeletal abnormalities. In *in vitro* experiments, high insulin concentrations will stimulate bone resorptions (Puche *et al.* 1973). The experiments of Horii *et al.* (1966) in experimentally diabetic mice are also very convincing. They regulated diabetes carefully, giving insulin twice a day, and they were able to prevent the appearance of congenital abnormalities.

Deuchar: In most of the experimental work in which malformations were caused by insulin, I think very much higher doses were used than are used for therapy, because people wanted to investigate the effects of insulin shock, which was believed to cause deaths and malformations in human fetuses.

Brudenell: There was an incidence of 8.3% for major malformations in the non-diabetic population in the Collaborative Perinatal Project. That is surprisingly high. It perhaps underlines the fact that congenital anomaly is multifactorial in origin, which is what makes it difficult to explain. Have you any information about congenital abnormalities which contribute to perinatal mortality? A fatal congenital abnormality is a more definite feature than a non-fatal malformation. I am trying to get at why there was such a high incidence of major malformations in the larger series.

Bennett: Those are not my data. The series has been fully reported, with details of the malformations (Chung & Myrianthopoulos 1975). Among the Pima a major malformation was present in about 40% of the cases of perinatal deaths, though we don't know whether the malformation was the cause of death.

Pedersen: What was the perinatal death rate in the Pima?

Bennett: In our series between 1960 and 1965 the perinatal death rate was 25% in the diabetic pregnancies. Between 1970 and 1975 it was 7%.

Pedersen: And 40% of those had a malformation. Then you conclude that the fatal malformation rate is now about 2–3%, which is just what we have found.

Bennett: All we can say is that 40% of the perinatal deaths had a malformation present. We can't say that it was the cause of death.

Kalkhoff: You mentioned that the Pima Indian is characterized mostly by a maturity-onset type of diabetes as opposed to a ketosis-prone type of diabetes. What percentage are on insulin before they become pregnant?

Bennett: The vast majority were not on insulin before pregnancy but many received insulin during pregnancy. Roughly half of White class B and beyond are on insulin at some time during pregnancy. All the relationships one would expect are there – the longer the duration, the higher the likelihood of anomalies; the earlier the age of onset, the higher the likelihood. I don't think one can dissect out of these observational data the sort of information on the possible effects of insulin treatment which you want.

Kalkhoff: Will you eventually have data that will provide controls as well as make it clear how many are receiving insulin? Will the computer be able to show whether control plays a role?

Bennett: Only a controlled trial of the effects of insulin will yield this sort of information. We have not embarked on such a trial at this time.

Kalkhoff: Do many of these women become ketotic easily when they are pregnant if they have maturity-onset diabetes?

Bennett: There is ketonuria but diabetic ketosis in the sense of having a high level of blood ketones is a rare event.

O'Sullivan: Could you break down the figure for anomalies among the fetal deaths according to whether the woman had diabetes or not?

Bennett: Again, about 40% of deaths among offspring of diabetic mothers were associated with anomaly. The rate in non-diabetics is uncertain.

O'Sullivan: You mentioned that the frequency of perinatal mortality dropped from 25% to 7%. Was the number of anomalies associated with perinatal deaths in the earlier period any higher than in the later period?

Bennett: There was a slight fall in the later period but it is not statistically significant.

O'Sullivan: An interesting point that has nothing to do with the anomalies is that there are cyclical changes in disease frequency. A good example is the association between streptococcal infection and rheumatic fever. There is some evidence that suggests that the frequency was falling before penicillin was introduced.   While we don't deny that penicillin made a dramatic change, the incidence was actually falling before it was introduced.   We may be seeing the same phenomenon with perinatal mortality in the diabetic.   We ascribe all the beneficial results today to improved methodology – fetal monitoring, assessment of placental function and so on – but I am not completely convinced, and part of the improvement may be due to a cyclical change.   The Pima Indians probably don't have this kind of sophisticated treatment in pregnancy, yet the perinatal mortality has dramatically improved.

Bennett: There has certainly been no real attempt to introduce sophisticated diabetic pregnancy care, yet we have seen a fall in perinatal mortality of the same order of magnitude as in the best university centre.   The only thing we have consciously done is to test the women in the third trimester and *post partum.*

O'Sullivan: But insulin treatment is not responsible for the dramatic change that we have seen in the past decade.   The improved salvage is associated with individual timing of delivery, using sophisticated techniques, and thus avoiding the exposure of all maternal diabetics to the hazards of very early delivery in an attempt to avoid the unexplained stillbirth.   We have no evidence that insulin *per se* produced the significant difference.

Pedersen: We have pointed out that we cannot in a scientific way show what is the trigger for the decrease in perinatal mortality (Pedersen *et al.* 1974).

Beard: How many of the gestational diabetics returned to a normal carbohydrate tolerance after delivery?

Bennett: All of them, because our definition of gestational diabetes included normal post-partum glucose tolerance.

Chez: Anomalies may provide a clue that mothers were going to become diabetics.   How many normal mothers who had infants with anomalies went on to develop diabetes subsequently?

Bennett: None of those classified as non-diabetic in Table 1 (p. 209) and those who subsequently developed diabetes were classified as prediabetic, in retrospect.

Gillmer: The incidence of genitourinary anomalies in the Collaborative Perinatal Project (Table 4, p.211) is very high.   Stilboestrol has effects on the urogenital tracts of both male and female fetuses.   Would some of these patients have been treated with stilboestrol?

Bennett: Possibly, but I do not have any information.

Gillmer: Does this high incidence also occur in areas where stilboestrol was not used widely?

Bennett: I don't know.

Hull: Some of the conditions seen are known to be polygenic and have a known frequency. Did you follow that up along the father's line where there isn't diabetes? Or is this an extra that diabetes introduces into the risk?

Bennett: The Pima data are relatively limited in number. We attempted to look at that question but one is severely limited by the number of generations one can go back. We couldn't find anything, but a negative answer doesn't mean much in the size of series we have available.

Hull: Are you suggesting it is the diabetes that increases the risk?

Bennett: There may well be a genetic predisposition to an anomaly in both the non-diabetic and the diabetic, but for some reason it becomes manifest only in the diabetic.

Milner: Dr Deuchar spoke earlier about culturing runts. When one reviews the published work, it looks as though the sacrum is a vulnerable area in the chicken, in the same way as the palate is in rodent fetuses (Tuchman-Duplessis 1970). There are strains of chicken in which rumplessness is an inherited feature. I found to my srprise that Landauer (1945) had reported that in one strain even shaking the eggs would produce this defect. There seems to be a wide spectrum of insults that will produce sacral agenesis in the right species. Have you any comments on this?

Bennett: I have only seen one case. The specificity depends on the strict definition of sacral agenesis. If one extends the definition it is clearly not specific. Other anomalies may be diabetes-associated but we may recognize only sacral agenesis as being specific to diabetes because it is such a rare anomaly.

Milner: Is the diabetic/non-diabetic ratio for sacral agenesis factorially many times higher than it is for any of the other congenital anomalies?

Bennett: As far as I know, no full-blown cases have been described in a non-diabetic.

Pedersen: It is not specific but it is very characteristic, with 'red spots' in the eyes and microangiopathy.

Deuchar: We have seen rat fetuses in which the sacral vertebrae are incompletely ossified. This is completely eliminated when we treat the mothers with insulin and keep the blood sugar level, which we check daily, below 100 mg/100 ml (5.5 mmol/l).

Hoet: Would you like to comment, Dr Deuchar, on why sacral defects are reported in infants of diabetic mothers?

Deuchar: This could be due to high insulin levels in the fetus. Insulin itself may lead to abnormalities when it is present in very high concentrations.

Histological pictures of fetal rat pancreases from diabetic animals indicate that the islets are larger than normal. But the β cells appear insulin-depleted. So perhaps at a critical moment, at 17 to 18 days of gestation, which is when ossification should be starting in the sacrum, a high level of insulin in the fetal blood might affect osteogenesis. There is a great deal of work *in vitro* which shows that insulin can derange osteogenesis.

Hoet: But it would be endogenous insulin?

Deuchar: Yes, from the fetus, in this case.

Battaglia: When did you start treating these diabetic animals?

Deuchar: On the first day that I check the blood glucose, which is always day 4. The animals are not stably diabetic until about four days after the streptozotocin injection. From then on they are treated once daily with insulin at 0.4–1.0 unit per rat according to what the blood sugar level showed.

Pedersen: I am surprised that your results are so good, completely abolishing the defect.

Hoet: Horii *et al.* (1966) showed the same.

Deuchar: We have not looked for every possible abnormality in all the organs of these fetuses, but in the streptozotocin-diabetic animals, the defects that I had observed at 20 days are completely eliminated.

Stowers: Dr Bennett, you did glucose tolerance tests 24–72 hours after delivery. Have you any evidence whether the recent pregnancy had an effect on glucose tolerance at that stage?

Bennett: We did some tests six weeks *post partum* in the same women. We also compared their biennal test with the post-partum test. The 24–72-hour tests differ slightly from either the six-week or the biennial tests. They are slightly worse but it is a matter of a few milligrams difference on average.

Gillmer: The study of Lind & Harris (1976) showed that although plasma glucose levels after a glucose load were similar in the immediate post-partum period and late pregnancy, the plasma insulin concentrations returned to non-pregnant values within 48 hours of delivery.

Bennett: We haven't done systematic insulin measurements during pregnancy and *post partum.*

References

CHUNG, C. S. & MYRIANTHOPOULOS, W. C. (1975) Factors affecting risks of congenital malformations. Report from the Collaborative Perinatal Project, in *Birth Defects Orig. Article Series* (Bergsma, D., ed.), vol. 11, No. 10, pp. 23–38, The National Foundation-March of Dimes Symposia Specialists, Miami

DURAISWAMI, P. K. (1950) Insulin induced skeletal abnormalities in developing chickens. *Br. Med. J. 2,* 384–390

HORII, K., WATANABE, G. & INGALLS, T. H. (1966) Experimental diabetes in pregnant mice. Prevention of congenital malformations in offspring by insulin. *Diabetes 15,* 194–204

KUČERA, J. (1971) Rate and type of congenital anomalies among offspring of diabetic women. *J. Reprod. Med. 7*, 73–82

LANDAUER, W. (1945) Rumplessness of chicken embryos produced by injection of insulin and other chemicals. *J. Exp. Zool. 98*, 65

LIND, T. & HARRIS, V. G. (1976) Changes in the oral glucose tolerance test in the puerperium. *Br. J. Obstet. Gynaecol. 83*, 460–463

PEDERSEN, J., MØLSTED-PEDERSEN, L. & ANDERSEN, B. (1974) Assessors of fetal perinatal mortality in diabetic pregnancy. Analysis of 1332 pregnancies in the Copenhagen series, 1946–1972. *Diabetes 23*, 302–306.

PUCHE, R. C., ROMANO, M. C., LOCATTO, M. E. & FERRETTI, J. L. (1973) The effect of insulin on bone resorption. *Calcif. Tissue Res. 12*, 8–15

STEHBENS, J. A., BAKER, G. L. & KITCHELL, M. (1977) Outcome at ages 1, 3, and 5 years of children born to diabetic women. *Am. J. Obstet. Gynecol. 127*, 408–414

TUCHMAN-DUPLESSIS, H. G. (1970) The effect of teratogenic drugs, in *Scientific Foundations of Obstetrics* (Philipp, E.E. *et al.*, eds.), pp. 636–648, Heinemann Medical, London

The outcome of diabetic pregnancies: a prospective study

RICHARD L. NAEYE

Department of Pathology, M.S. Hershey Medical Center, The Pennsylvania State University College of Medicine, Hershey, Pennsylvania

Abstract   In a large prospective study of pregnancy the perinatal mortality rate was 141/1000 births for diabetic gestations in which the onset of labour was spontaneous, 33/1000 for diabetic gestations in which labour was induced or the infant delivered by Caesarean section and 34/1000 for the non-diabetics.   Forty per cent of the perinatal mortality excess in the diabetics was due to the conse-quences of maternal vascular lesions, i.e. large placental infarcts and marked retardation of placental growth.   Seventeen per cent of the perinatal mortality excess was related to maternal acidosis or to insulin shock, 12% to severe congenital anomalies, 12% to the complications of Caesarean sections and the remainder to other disorders.   Mothers with diabetes mellitus had more than twice the frequency of atheromata, fibrinoid change and thrombi in decidual arteries as non-diabetic mothers.

Histological grading revealed that overweight newborns of diabetic mothers had immature lungs by comparison with the lungs of normally grown infants of diabetic mothers and infants of non-diabetic mothers.   Low IQ values and an excess of neurological abnormalities in children of diabetic mothers who were ketotic during pregnancy were found to be due to amniotic fluid bacterial infec-tions and their complications rather than to the maternal ketosis.

Each major advance in the management of diabetes mellitus has opened up new issues about the course and outcome of diabetic pregnancies.   Insulin made successful pregnancy possible in diabetic women but it uncovered the fact that maternal vascular lesions and congenital anomalies as well as keto-acidosis were responsible for many of the stillbirths and neonatal deaths in diabetic gestations (Pedersen *et al.* 1974; Drury *et al.* 1978).   The present study re-examined the consequences of these vascular lesions and determined the frequency of other disorders responsible for the excessive perinatal morta-lity rates in diabetic gestations.   Data from a large prospective study of pregnancy were used in the analyses.

An increased frequency of respiratory distress, due to hyaline membrane disease, has often been reported in the neonates of diabetic mothers (Robert *et al.* 1976). If the reported increase in respiratory distress is due solely to the consequences of late gestational or intrapartum hypoxia, lungs of the involved neonates might be expected to show a normal histological maturation. On the other hand, if chronic metabolic abnormalities predispose neonates to the hyaline membrane disease, their lungs might show histological evidence of retarded maturation. The present study examined this question by comparing the lungs of neonates of diabetic mothers with those of non-diabetics for their stage of maturation.

Finally, there has been uncertainty about the long-term intellectual development of children of diabetic mothers. Both Churchill *et al.* (1969) and Stehbens *et al.* (1977) have reported that diabetic mothers with gestational acetonuria have offspring with lower IQ values than do non-diabetic mothers or diabetic mothers without acetonuria. The present study re-examined this question, taking into consideration factors not known to be neurotoxic at the time the previous studies were conducted.

PATIENTS

The Collaborative Perinatal Project of the National Institute of Neurological and Communicative Disorders and Stroke provides a unique opportunity to study placental lesions and the causes of fetal and neonatal death associated with maternal diabetes mellitus. It prospectively followed the course of 53 518 pregnancies in 12 US hospitals between 1959 and 1966 and systematically recorded events of gestation, labour, delivery and the subsequent course of the infants to eight years of age (Niswander & Gordon 1972; Collaborative Study etc. 1966). Autopsy material was available for histological evaluations of fetal lung maturation and follow-up tests were undertaken for long-term assessments of psychomotor development.

METHODS

I reviewed the clinical and post-mortem material, including microscopic sections, from the fetal and neonatal deaths in the Collaborative Study to standardize the recognition of abnormalities and the assignment of diagnoses. Four specially trained technicians reviewed microscopic sections from the 48 975 available placentas to standardize the recognition and recording of abnormalities. I also checked non-routine abnormalities. Only single-born infants were used in the present analyses. Mothers were considered diabetic if their glucose tolerance curves during pregnancy met the criteria set forth by

Somogyi-Nelson or if the patient was clearly known as diabetic and was treated with more than 20 units of insulin daily (Churchill *et al.* 1969). Ketoacidosis was recorded when it was severe enough to be considered clinically significant (Churchill *et al.* 1969). The duration of pregnancy was represented in completed weeks of gestation as calculated from the last menstrual period. The Stanford-Binet IQ test was administered at four years of age and neurological examinations were done at regular intervals (Collaborative Study etc. 1966).

The following were excluded from analyses of IQ values: children with neurological abnormalities, any major congenital malformation, Down syndrome, hydrocephalus, lead intoxication, a fractured skull, any recognized inborn error of metabolism (including hypothyroidism), meningitis or evidence of any other central nervous system infection including cytomegalic inclusion disease, toxoplasmosis, congenital syphilis and rubella. Also excluded were infants whose mothers or fathers were mentally retarded or whose mothers were known alcoholics, drug addicts or who had experienced anaesthetic or hypovolaemic shock during labour or delivery.

Primary and secondary diagnoses were assigned to each fetal and neonatal death. The primary diagnosis was intended to identify the disorder that initiated the course to death. For example, hypoxia may have caused an intrapartum death but the death was ascribed to abruptio placentae if this latter disorder caused the hypoxia. Cases were ascribed to *amniotic fluid infections* when acute funisitis and inflammation of the plate of the placenta were associated with congenital pneumonia (Naeye & Peters 1978). For this diagnosis, membranes had to be intact at the onset of labour. Cases were placed in the *abruptio placentae* category when gross inspection showed an adherent retroplacental clot with depression or disruption of the underlying placental tissue or when there were otherwise classical clinical findings including external or occult bleeding and fetal or neonatal death with evidences of hypoxia including aspirated squames in the lungs and petechiae on the serosal surfaces of the visceral organs (Naeye *et al.* 1977).

Premature rupture of the fetal membranes was diagnosed when the membranes ruptured without known cause before the onset of labour before 37 weeks of gestation. The fetuses and neonates in this category died of infection or of the consequences of premature delivery. Death was ascribed to *congenital anomalies* when such anomalies were severe and incompatible with fetal or neonatal survival. Cases were placed in the category of *large placental infarcts* when 25% or more of the placenta was involved by one or more infarcts greater than 3 cm in diameter and there was no other explanation for death (Naeye 1977*a*). All infants in this category had evidences of antenatal hypoxia, i.e. aspirated squames. Death was ascribed to *Caesarean section* when

TABLE 1

Classification of fetal lung maturation based on light microscopy; classification system is derived from Platt (see Naeye *et al.* 1974).

Lung	Stage
Continuous layer of cuboid cells, abundant mesenchyme, few capillaries	1
Continuous layer of cuboid cells, abundant mesenchyme, increased numbers of capillaries, some adjacent but not penetrating the cuboid layer	2
Cuboid layer continuous in some alveoli but in others a few capillaries have encroached between the cuboid cells and are in contact with the lumen, abundant mesenchyme	3
Cuboid layer not continuous and moderate numbers of capillaries penetrate and contact lumen, mesenchyme reduced	4
Few cuboid cells still present: numerous capillaries and mesenchyme reduced to 3 to 6 cells thick	5
Mature form; no cuboid cells, numerous capillaries and mesenchyme reduced to 3 or less cells in thickness; alveolar duct development complete	6

the operation delivered an infant younger than the gestational age estimated before surgery and the infant died of the complications of immaturity. Cases were placed in the category *placental growth retardation* when the placenta was 40% or more below normal weight for gestational age and there was no other explanation for perinatal death (Naeye 1978*a*). All such infants had aspirated squames as evidence of antenatal hypoxia. The criteria for other diagnoses have recently been published (Naeye 1977*b*).

Platt's histological classifications were used to grade the structural maturity of the lungs of neonates (Naeye *et al.* 1974) (Table 1). Histological grades were assigned to cases without knowledge at the time of examination of the infants' gestational ages or clinical diagnoses. Neonates were placed in various percentiles of fetal growth by comparing their body weights with recently published fetal growth standards (Naeye & Dixon 1978). χ^2 was the statistical method used in the study.

RESULTS

Perinatal mortality rates were more than twice as great in diabetic as in non-diabetic gestations and increased fourfold in diabetic gestations in which labour and delivery were spontaneous (Table 2). Five categories of disorders were responsible for the mortality excess in diabetics: (a) disorders resulting from reduced uteroplacental perfusion, i.e. large placental infarcts and growth-retarded placentas, (b) Caesarean section, (c) specific metabolic com-

TABLE 2

Primary causes of fetal and neonatal death in offspring of diabetic and non-diabetic mothers.

	Perinatal mortality rates (fetal + neonatal deaths/1000 births)			
	Non-diabetic mothers	Mothers with diabetes mellitus		All diabetic mothers
		Labour induced or Caesarean section	Spontaneous onset of labour	
Amniotic fluid infection syndrome	5.9 (282)	0	22.0 (5) $P < 0.01$	7.7 (5) $P > 0.1$
Abruptio placentae	3.8 (181)	4.7 (2) $P > 0.1$	0	3.1 (2) $P > 0.1$
Premature rupture of membranes	3.5 (167)	0	22.0 (5) $P < 0.001$	7.7 (5) $P > 0.1$
Congenital anomalies	3.2 (153)	2.4 (1) $P > 0.1$	17.6 (4) $P < 0.002$	7.7 (5) $P < 0.1$
Large placental infarcts	2.1 (100)	7.1 (3) $P < 0.1$	13.2 (3) $P < 0.005$	9.2 (6) $P < 0.001$
Placenta markedly growth-retarded	0.9 (43)	2.4 (1) $P > 0.1$	17.6 (4) $P < 0.001$	7.7 (5) $P < 0.001$
Caesarean section	0.3 (14)	7.1 (3) $P < 0.001$	0	4.6 (3) $P < 0.001$
Maternal ketoacidosis	0	2.4 (1) $P > 0.1$	8.8 (2) –	4.3 (3) –
Insulin shock	0	0	4.4 (1) –	1.5 (1) –
Other disorders	6.9 (330)	2.4 (1) $P > 0.1$	13.2 (3) $P > 0.1$	6.1 (4) $P > 0.1$
Diagnosis unknown	7.2 (344)	4.7 (2) $P > 0.1$	22.0 (5) $P < 0.05$	10.7 (7) $P > 0.1$
Totals	33.8 (1614)	33.2 (14) $P > 0.1$	140.8 (32) $P < 0.001$	70.3 (46) $P < 0.001$
Number of infants born	(47 745)	(425)	(227)	(652)

Number of cases in parentheses.   P values are compared with non-diabetic gestations.

plications of maternal diabetes, i.e. ketoacidosis and insulin shock, (d) congenital anomalies and (e) amniotic fluid infections (Table 2). The mean duration of gestation for pregnancies that ended with spontaneous labour were: non-diabetics 39.1 ± 3.4 weeks, diabetics 36.4 ± 4.9 weeks ($P < 0.001$).

There was an excess of vascular lesions in the superficial decidua of diabetic mothers, i.e. atheromata, fibrinoid change and thrombi in arteries and arterioles (Table 3). Acute funisitis and acute inflammation of the plate of the placenta, which are characteristic consequences of amniotic fluid bacterial

TABLE 3

The relationship between maternal diabetes mellitus and findings in the placenta, umbilical cord and fetal membranes.

| | Non-diabetic mothers | Mothers with diabetes mellitus | |
| | | Labour induced or Caesarean section | Spontaneous onset of labour |
	%	% P	% P
Umbilical cord			
Infiltration by neutrophils	12.4	3.8 < 0.001	14.7 > 0.1
Single umbilical artery	1.1	2.6 < 0.02	3.5 < 0.005
Extraplacental membranes			
Amnion nodosum	0.2	0.8 < 0.05	1.4 < 0.05
Infiltration by neutrophils	18.6	5.8 < 0.001	16.5 > 0.1
Subchorionic plate of placenta			
Infiltration by neutrophils	12.3	3.3 < 0.001	13.3 > 0.1
Decidua (superficial)			
Atheromata, arteries	0.6	1.8 < 0.005	1.8 < 0.1
Fibrinoid change arteries	2.1	5.0 < 0.002	4.9 < 0.01
Thrombi in blood vessels	1.0	1.7 > 0.1	3.1 < 0.001
Basalis			
Infiltration by neutrophils	7.5	2.8 < 0.001	7.6 > 0.1
Necrosis	2.6	0.8 < 0.04	3.6 > 0.1
Capsularis			
Infiltration by neutrophils	25.4	16.1 < 0.001	17.0 < 0.01
Necrosis	10.9	2.8 < 0.001	7.1 < 0.1
Villi			
Nucleated red cells in blood vessels	2.9	21.0 < 0.001	13.2 < 0.001
Excessive syncytial nuclear knots	4.2	3.9 > 0.1	3.7 > 0.1
Retained cytotrophoblast	1.5	9.1 < 0.001	5.7 < 0.001
Micro infarcts	13.0	5.4 < 0.001	15.4 > 0.1

P values compare diabetics with non-diabetics.

TABLE 4

Fetal lungs reached full histological maturity at 32 weeks of gestation in the offspring of non-diabetic mothers and in the infants of diabetic mothers who were normally grown at birth. Lung maturation was retarded in overweight newborns of diabetic mothers

Gestational age (weeks)	All infants of non-dia-betic mothers	Infants of diabetic mothers	
		Birth weight percentile	
		< 90	90 & over
20-24	2.4 ± 1.1 (105)	2.6 ± 0.6 (4)[a]	1.0 ± 0 (5)[b]
25-27	3.8 ± 0.6 (97)	3.5 ± 0.5 (4)[a]	–
28-32	4.1 ± 1.4 (109)	4.1 ± 1.5 (8)[a]	3.5 ± 1.0 (6)[a]
Over 32	5.9 ± 0.2 (114)	6.0 ± 0 (10)[a]	5.3 ± 1.1 (11)[b]

[a] $P > 0.1$ compared with non-diabetic controls, [b] $P < 0.005$. Mean ± S.D., number of cases in parentheses.

infections, had a slightly greater frequency in spontaneously delivered diabetic than in non-diabetic pregnancies. These infections were mainly responsible for the shorter duration of spontaneously delivered diabetic than of non-diabetic gestations. Amnion nodosum was several times more frequent in diabetic than in non-diabetic pregnancies (Table 3).

Fetal lungs reached full histological maturity at 32 weeks of gestation in the offspring of non-diabetic mothers (Table 4). There was a similar rate of maturation in infants of diabetic mothers who were normally grown at birth for gestational age, whereas lung maturation was retarded in those offspring who were overweight for their gestational age.

Children whose diabetic mothers had one or more episodes of ketoacidosis during pregnancy had lower mean IQ values and more neurological abnormalities than children whose diabetic mothers had no overt ketoacidosis (Table 5). This was true in infants born at term as well as preterm, the poor and non-poor, blacks and whites. These signs of psychomotor impairment disappeared when infants who had evidences of amniotic fluid infections at birth, i.e. acute inflammation in the plate of the placenta, were excluded from the analyses (Table 5). Values for head circumference were not much affected by gestational ketoacidosis (Table 5).

DISCUSSION

All of the perinatal mortality excess associated with maternal diabetes in the present study was in patients permitted to go into spontaneous labour. Forty

TABLE 5

Neurological abnormalities and low IQ values decreased in frequency in children of diabetic mothers who had gestational ketoacidosis when infants who had evidence of amniotic fluid infections before birth were excluded from the analyses

	IQ values at age 4 yr	Cases with neurological abnor- malities at age 7 yr (%)	Head circumference at age 7 yr (cm)
Infants born at gestational ages 28 - 36 weeks Maternal diabetes with ketoacidosis			
With amniotic fluid infections	97.9 ± 18.8 (11) [a]	44.4 [b]	51.0 ± 1.3 [a]
Without amniotic fluid infections	102.3 ± 16.1 (7)	0	51.0 ± 0.8
Diabetes without ketoacidosis			
With amniotic fluid infections	102.0 ± 20.2 (158) [a]	22.8 [a]	51.4 ± 1.7 [a]
Without amniotic fluid infections	102.2 ± 21.2 (68)	16.2	51.6 ± 2.2
Infants born at gestational ages 37 - 43 weeks Maternal diabetes with ketoacidosis			
With amniotic fluid infections	90.6 ± 16.1 (10) [c]	42.1 [a]	51.3 ± 1.6 [a]
Without amniotic fluid infections	103.7 ± 10.2 (9)	33.0	51.3 ± 1.1
Diabetes without ketoacidosis			
With amniotic fluid infections	99.6 ± 17.6 (69) [a]	15.9 [a]	51.3 ± 1.6 [a]
Without amniotic fluid infections	99.3 ± 18.1 (203)	17.2	51.4 ± 1.5

[a] $P > 0.1$ compared with no amniotic fluid infections; [b] $P < 0.05$; [c] $P < 0.03$.
Mean ± S.D., number of cases in parentheses. The category of neurological abnormalities includes infants with suspicious and definite abnormalities.

per cent of the perinatal mortality rate excess associated with the diabetes was due to large placental infarcts and to marked placental growth retardation. These two disorders are characteristic consequences of uteroplacental underperfusion (Naeye 1977a, 1978a). The superficial decidua from the diabetics in the study had more than twice the frequency of arterial atheromata, fibrinoid change and thrombi than did the decidua of non-diabetics. Such vascular lesions presumably restrict uteroplacental perfusion. Most of these vascular and placental lesions can be produced by maternal hypertension but the diabetic mothers in the present study had no greater frequency of gestational hypertension than did the non-diabetic mothers (Driscoll 1965; Fox 1975). Such vascular lesions presumably have a cumulative effect because class C, D and F diabetics are more apt to have undergrown placentas and neonates than class A diabetics (Driscoll 1965).

It has been postulated that hereditary influences are partially responsible for the great variations in the rate at which vascular lesions develop in various diabetics (Siperstein *et al.* 1977). There is evidence that rigid glucose control during pregnancy only partially prevents the development of lesions in the spiral arteries of diabetic mothers (Jones & Fox 1976). Some of the fibrinoid material which develops in such arteries is due to the deposition of fibrin (Emmrich *et al.* 1975). Fibrinogen and platelet survival are usually shorter in diabetics than in non-diabetics, presumably due to the increased sensitivity of platelets in diabetics to spontaneous and induced aggregation (Breddin *et al.* 1976; Colwell *et al.* 1976). It is possible that some of the fibrinoid lesions and thrombi that develop in the spiral arteries of diabetics might be prevented by drugs that reduce platelet aggregation.

There was a slightly greater frequency of amniotic fluid infections in diabetic than in non-diabetic gestations in which the onset of labour was spontaneous. These infections were partially responsible for the most frequent preterm deliveries and the perinatal mortality excess in diabetic gestations. Much has recently been learned about the pathogenesis of these infections. Invasion of the fetal membranes near the cervical os by bacteria appears to be a common event in pregnancy, particularly in late gestation (Naeye & Peters 1978). When the bacteria spread and grow in the amniotic fluid, the fetal membranes, subchorionic plate of the placenta and umbilical cord become inflamed. Poor maternal nutrition during pregnancy appears to have a major role in such infections by retarding or preventing the development of antimicrobial activity in the amniotic fluid (Tafari *et al.* 1977).

These infections also appear to have a role in the increased frequency of psychomotor impairment found in children of diabetic mothers. In previous studies, such impairment has been attributed to maternal gestational acetonuria (Stehbens *et al.* 1977; Churchill *et al.* 1969). Findings in the present study indicate that amniotic fluid infections rather than ketosis may be responsible for the psychomotor impairment. Non-infected infants of ketotic gestations had normal IQ values and no excess of neurological abnormalities at 4 and 7 years of age. Another analysis of data from the Collaborative Perinatal Project recently found that infants with antenatal amniotic fluid infections had an increased frequency of subsequent mental, motor, visual and hearing impairment (Naeye 1978*b*). Such infections also markedly potentiated the neurotoxicity of neonatal hyperbilirubinaemia and such hyperbilirubinaemia is more frequent in neonates of diabetic than of non-diabetic mothers.

The present study found an increased frequency of amnion nodosum in the diabetic gestations, a probable consequence of oligohydramnios. We have no ready explanation for this finding. Infants of diabetic mothers had three times the expected frequency of a single umbilical artery, an anomaly associated with diabetes mellitus by previous investigators (Driscoll 1965). Most previous authors have reported an increased frequency of congenital anomalies in the offspring of diabetic mothers (Day & Insley 1976; Soler et al. 1976; Gabbe 1977) The present study found an increase in the frequency of such diabetes-associated anomalies.

Infants of diabetic mothers are several times more likely to develop the newborn respiratory-distress syndrome (RDS) than matched infants of non-diabetic mothers (Robert et al. 1976). This appears to be due to both an increased frequency of low lecithin/sphingomyelin (L/S) ratios in amniotic fluid late in gestation and a significant increase in RDS in neonates who have a mature L/S ratio (Mueller-Heubach et al. 1978; Cruz et al. 1976; Dahlenburg et al. 1977). Some recently published findings and results of the present study provide some explanations. Smith et al. (1975) reported that insulin added to rabbit lung monolayer cell cultures abolishes the stimulatory effect of cortisol on lecithin synthesis. More recently, Neufeld et al. (1977) found that insulin had no effect on the incorporation of glucose into phosphatidylcholine and other lipids but did inhibit its incorporation into lysolecithin. This would help to explain why some fetuses of diabetic mothers have inhibited surfactant production with normal L/S ratios. The present study found that the histological maturation of fetal lungs was retarded in overweight infants of diabetic mothers but not in those normal in size for gestational age. Previous studies from our laboratory found that such histological maturation was more rapid in overnourished than in undernourished gestations of non-diabetic mothers (Naeye et al. 1974; Naeye 1975). The exact nutritional or other factors responsible for these differing rates of structural maturation have not been determined.

Other organs besides the lungs may be retarded in their fetal maturation by maternal diabetes mellitus. Brain growth may be somewhat retarded in such fetuses (Naeye 1965). Erythropoietic activity often appears to be greater in neonates of diabetic than of non-diabetic mothers and it is far from certain that this increased erythropoiesis is entirely due to a greater degree of hypoxaemia in the offspring of the diabetics. Placentas in diabetics often appear histologically immature for their gestational age, with retained cytotrophoblast and an excess of Hofbauer cells (Driscoll et al. 1961). This was confirmed by the present study. It is not known whether fetal hyperinsulinaemia plays a role in any of these maturational delays.

Finally, there has been great emphasis over the years on the role of fetal hyperinsulinaemia in promoting fetal overgrowth in diabetic gestations. This overgrowth has most often been defined in terms of excess lipogenesis. In fact, much of the excess growth in such fetuses is in the visceral organs, which characteristically have parenchymal cells with a greater volume of cytoplasm than similar cells in infants of non-diabetic mothers (Naeye 1965). Cell number is more nearly normal in the organs of newborns of diabetic mothers than is cell size, which probably explains their normal long-term growth (Haworth et al. 1976; Naeye 1965).

ACKNOWLEDGEMENTS

Informed consent was obtained before data were collected in these studies. Mr J.B. Dixon performed most of the statistical analyses. These studies were supported by US Public Health Service Contract NOI-NS-3-2311.

References

BREDDIN, K., GRUN, H., KRZYWANEK, H. R. & SCHREMMER, W. P. (1976) On the measurement of spontaneous platelet aggregation: the platelet aggregation test. III. Methods and first clinical results. *Thromb. Haemostasis 35,* 669–691

CHURCHILL, H. A., BERENDES, H. W. & NEMORE, J. (1969) Neuropsychological deficits in children of diabetic mothers. *Am. J. Obstet. Gynecol. 105,* 257–268

Collaborative Study on Cerebral Palsy, Mental Retardation and Other Neurological and Sensory Disorders of Infancy and Childhood Manual (1966) US Dept Health, Education & Welfare, Public Health Service, Bethesda

COLWELL, J. A., HALUSHKA, P. V., SARJI, K., LEVINE, J., SAGEL, J. & NAIR, R. M. G. (1976) Altered platelet function in diabetes mellitus, *Diabetes 25, Suppl. 2,* 826–831

CRUZ, A. C., BUHI, W. C., BIRK, S. A. & SPELLACY, W. N. (1976) Respiratory distress syndrome with mature lecithin/sphingomyelin ratios: diabetes mellitus and low Apgar scores. *Am. J. Obstet. Gynecol. 126,* 78–82

DAHLENBURG, G. W., MARTIN, F. I. R. & JEFFREY, P. E. (1977) Amniotic fluid lecithin/sphingomyelin ratio in pregnancy complicated by diabetes. *Br. J. Obstet. Gynaecol. 84,* 294–299

DAY, R. E. & INSLEY, J. (1976) Maternal diabetes mellitus and congenital malformation. Survey of 205 cases. *Arch. Dis. Child. 51,* 935–938

DRISCOLL, S. G. (1965) The pathology of pregnancy complicated by diabetes. *Med. Clin. N. Am. 49,* 1053–1067

DRISCOLL, S. G., BENIRSCHKE, K. & CURTIS, G. W. (1961) Neonatal deaths among infants of diabetic mothers. *Am. J. Dis. Child. 100,* 818–835

DRURY, M. I., GREENE, A. T. & STRONGE, J. M. (1978) Pregnancy complicated by clinical diabetes mellitus, a study of 600 pregnancies. *Obstet. Gynecol. 49,* 519–522

EMMRICH, P., BIRKE, R. & GODEL, E. (1975) Beitrag zur Morphologie der myometrialen und dezidualen Arterien bei normalen Schwangerschaften, EPH-Gestosen und mutterlichem Diabetes mellitus. *Pathol. Microbiol. 43,* 38–61

FOX, H. (1975) Morphologic pathology of the placenta, in *The Placenta* (Grunewald, P., ed.), pp. 218, University Park Press, Baltimore

GABBE, S. G. (1977) Congenital malformations in infants of diabetic mothers. *Obstet. Gynecol. Surv. 32,* 125–131

HAWORTH, J. C., McRAE, K. N. & DILLING, L. A. (1976) Prognosis of infants of diabetic mothers in relation to neonatal hypoglycaemia. *Dev. Med. Child Neurol. 18,* 471–479

JONES, C. J. P. & FOX, H. (1976) Placental changes in gestational diabetes, an ultrastructural study. *Obstet. Gynecol. 48,* 274–280

MUELLER-HEUBACH, E., CARITIS, S. N., EDELSTONE, D. I. & TURNER, J. H. (1978) Lecithin/sphingomyelin ratio in amniotic fluid and its failure for the prediction of neonatal respiratory distress syndrome in pregnant diabetic women. *Am. J. Obstet. Gynecol. 130,* 28–34

NAEYE, R. L. (1965) Infants of diabetic mothers: a quantitative morphological study. *Pediatrics 35,* 980–988

NAEYE, R. L. (1975) Fetal lung and kidney maturation in abnormal pregnancies. *Arch. Pathol. 99,* 533–535

NAEYE, R. L. (1977*a*) Placental infarction leading to fetal or neonatal death. *Obstet. Gynecol. 50,* 583–588

NAEYE, R. L. (1977*b*) Causes of perinatal mortality in the U.S. collaborative perinatal project. *JAMA (J. Am. Med. Assoc.) 238,* 228–229

NAEYE, R. L. (1978*a*) Perinatal death due to placental growth retardation, a prospective study. *JAMA (J. Am. Med. Assoc.), 239,* 1145–1147

NAEYE, R.L. (1978*b*) Amniotic fluid infections, neonatal hyperbilirubinemia and psychomotor impairment. *Pediatrics 62,* 497–503

NAEYE, R. L. & DIXON, J. B. (1978) Distortions in fetal growth standards. *Pediatr. Res. 12,* 987–991

NAEYE, R. L. & PETERS, E. C. (1978) Amniotic fluid infections with intact membranes leading to perinatal death; a prospective study. *Pediatrics 61,* 171–177

NAEYE, R. L., FREEMAN, R. K. & BLANC, W. A. (1974) Nutrition, sex and fetal lung maturation. *Pediatr. Res. 8,* 200–204

NAEYE, R.L., HARKNESS, W. L. & UTTS, J. (1977) Abruptio placentae and perinatal death: a prospective study. *Am. J. Obstet. Gynecol. 128,* 740–746

NEUFELD, N. D., SEVANIAN, A. & KAPLAN, S. A. (1977) Mechanisms of production of respiratory distress syndrome (RDS) in infants of diabetic mothers: inhibition of surfactant synthesis by insulin. *Diabetes 26,* 371

NISWANDER, N. R. & GORDON, M. (1972) *The Women and Their Pregnancies,* Saunders, Philadelphia

PEDERSEN, J., MØLSTED-PEDERSEN, L. & ANDERSEN, R. (1974) Assessors of fetal perinatal mortality in diabetic pregnancy. *Diabetes 23,* 302–305

ROBERT, M. F., NEFF, R. K., JUBBELL, J. P., TAEUSCH, H. W. & AVERY, M.E. (1976) Association between maternal diabetes and the respiratory-distress syndrome in the newborn. *New Engl. J. Med. 294,* 357–360

SIPERSTEIN, M. D., FOSTER, D. W., KNOWLES, H. C. JR., LEVINE, R., MADISON, L. L. & ROTH, J. (1977) Control of blood glucose and diabetic vascular disease. *New Engl. J. Med. 296,* 1060–1062

SMITH, B. T., GIROUD, C. J. P., ROBERT, M. & AVERY, M. E. (1975) Insulin antagonism of cortisol action on lecithin synthesis by cultured fetal lung cells. *J. Pediatr. 87,* 953–955

SOLER, N. G., WALSH, C. H. & MALINS, J. M. (1976) Congenital malformations in infants of diabetic mothers. *Q. J. Med. 45,* 303–313

STEHBENS, J. A., BAKER, G. L. & KITCHELL, M. (1977) Outcome at ages 1, 3 and 5 years of children born to diabetic women. *Am. J. Obstet. Gynecol. 127,* 408–413

TAFARI, N., ROSS, S. M., NAEYE, R. L., GALASK, R. P. & ZAAR, B. (1977) Failure of bacterial growth inhibition by amniotic fluid. *Am. J. Obstet. Gynecol. 128,* 187–189

Discussion

O'Sullivan: Were the pathology examinations done locally in each clinic?

Naeye: The autopsies were done at 12 different academic affiliated hospitals throughout the United States. All of the autopsy material came to us. In 3½ years I personally reviewed all the autopsy material including the microscopic slides to standardize the recording of abnormalities and criteria used to make diagnoses. Technicians in our laboratory were specially trained to recognize and record abnormalities in the placenta.

O'Sullivan: Were they aware of the study category of the patients?

Naeye: They had no such information at the time they examined the placentas.

Räihä: What is your definition of amniotic fluid infection? At least in our hospital amniotic fluid infection is fairly unusual.

Naeye: We ascribed cases to the amniotic fluid infection syndrome when acute funisitis and inflammation of the subchorionic plate of the placenta were associated with congenital pneumonia. To date, only bacteria have been shown capable of producing the infections (Lauweryns *et al.* 1973). Invasion of the fetal membranes near the cervical os by bacteria appears to be a frequent event, particularly in late gestation. The frequency with which the bacteria spread and grow in the amniotic fluid varies greatly among various population groups. Many obstetricians have become sceptical about the bacterial origin of the disorder because they so often fail to culture bacteria from patients with the characteristic anatomical features of the syndrome. The proportion of patients from whom bacteria are recovered tends to be proportionate to the efforts expended in the bacteriology laboratory. For example, mycoplasma and a wide variety of anaerobic bacteria are often responsible for the infections. Appropriate tests to recover these agents are often not undertaken. When such tests are performed, bacteria are recovered from more than three-quarters of patients in whom the anatomical evidences of amniotic fluid infections are present (Naeye *et al.* 1977).

Räihä: If the adverse effects of hyperbilirubinaemia are so high, we should really in our clinical work try to look very hard for this infection.

Dr Bennett said that the Pima Indians had a frequency of diabetes in the mothers of 3% and that was 10 times higher than in the US population, which must be 0.3%. In your study you gave a figure of 652/47 740, which is 1.3%, or four times higher than in the US population.

Naeye: Our cases are not a cross-section of the US population but rather women who came to academic medical centres for prenatal medical care and delivery. They include a disproportionate number of women in high-risk categories.

Brudenell: You listed spontaneous deliveries amongst 227 of your 652 diabetic cases. Did those 227 have spontaneous onset of labour?

Naeye: Yes.

Brudenell: It is surprising that a third of your women went into labour spontaneously at an average duration of 36 weeks.

Naeye: That was almost entirely due to an excess of amniotic fluid infections. Such infections usually induce labour within 72 hours of their onset.

Brudenell: What is the evidence in humans that excessive syncytial knots represent underperfusion of the placenta?

Naeye: Excessive syncytial knots are characteristic findings in several disorders in which restrictive lesions are found in the spiral arteries, e.g. chronic maternal hypertension.

Brudenell: But you are not measuring placental perfusion – this is inferred?

Naeye: Studies in the 1950s correlated these vascular lesions with reduced uteroplacental blood flow (Dixon & Robertson 1958; Morris *et al.* 1955).

Pedersen: Presumably the amniotic fluid infection can go unrecognized by a clinician?

Naeye: Most such infections are unrecognized.

Beard: We have compared the incidence of infection during labour in women who had intrauterine catheters put in and those who did not have them. If the criterion of infection is a single recording of a temperature of over 38 °C, we find that the incidence is 3% if the labour is less than 12 hours and 9% if it is over 12 hours. None of those cases were recorded as having clinical amniotic fluid infection. The pyrexial episode may be due to a transient bacteraemia which the body overcomes by natural means.

Naeye: I am not certain that all the adverse clinical effects in the infant are due to sepsis. For example, the fetus presumably aspirates the toxic products of leucocyte breakdown along with the bacteria in the amniotic fluid. Some of these leucocyte breakdown products may cause clinical complications.

Räihä: Amniotic fluid infection seems to me a very important question. We are now getting rid of exchange transfusions for Rh babies. If we have to start to exchange hyperbilirubinaemic babies at 10 mg/100 ml (170 μmol/l) in 9% of the cases, we are really getting back to a very frequent exchange rate again.

Naeye: It also worries us. There is a strong correlation between the anatomical evidences of the amniotic fluid infections in the plate of the placenta and hyperbilirubinaemia. Thus, a substantial proportion of neonates with hyperbilirubinaemia have been exposed to amniotic fluid infections.

Räihä: Can we get the diagnosis as soon as 24 hours?

Naeye: We are struggling with this problem. At present the only certain criterion we have is the anatomical evidence from the placenta. That poses a problem because most pathologists won't be available at 3 a.m. to examine placentas. We need other criteria. Some proposed tests, like the examination of gastric aspirate for leucocytes, yield too many false positive results.

Hull: You said that the brain is small. Is it not possible that a baby with larger organs might have accelerated maturation in some areas? Can you be sure that the brain is small?

Naeye: I am not personally convinced that many newborn infants of diabetic mothers have subnormal-sized brains.

Gillmer: When analysing autopsy studies it is necessary to consider why the infant died if we are to avoid bias resulting from the cause of death. What we require at present is a prospective study of brain volumes using modern techniques.

Battaglia: Has anyone shown that cellular changes can be induced in the placenta by a whole variety of causes, among which infection is one?

Naeye: No one has ever shown that acute inflammation in the subchorionic plate of the placenta is produced by anything but bacteria.

Battaglia: Most of the neurological data were collected to see whether these tests meant anything in newborns, not as an application of the tests to see if the infants were normal. Therefore, one should not be surprised to find that in some cases 40% of the babies examined were found to be 'abnormal'.

References

DIXON, H. G. & ROBERTSON, W. B. (1958) A study of the vessels of the placental bed in normotensive and hypertensive women. *J. Obstet. Gynaecol. Br. Emp.* 65, 803–809

LAUWERYNS, J., BERNAT, R., LERUS, A. & DETOURNAY, G. (1973) Intrauterine pneumonia, an experimental study. *Biol. Neonate* 22, 301–318

MORRIS, N., OSBORN, S. B. & WRIGHT, H. P. (1955) Effective circulation of the uterine wall in late pregnancy. *Lancet 2*, 323–325

NAEYE, R. L., TAFARI, N., JUDGE, E., GILMOUR, E. & MARBOE, C. (1977) Amniotic fluid infections in an African city. *J. Pediatr. 90*, 965–970

General discussion III

Chez: We have been doing some work on the acute regulation of glucose concentrations in the monkey fetus and therefore some aspects of glycogen metabolism. Clinically and physiologically there are two separate concepts. We are curious to know whether the fetus can regulate its own glucose levels and whether it has any acute responsivity when it is exposed to either hyperglycaemia or hypoglycaemia. We perfused the liver of the monkey fetus *in situ* at 92% gestation. The liver was isolated and the perfusate started within 60 seconds of birth. In the presence of hyperglycaemia the normal fetus does not remove glucose from the perfusate, it does not synthesize glycogen, and it does not activate liver glycogen synthetase. When hypoglycaemia is present there is a slow release of glucose from the liver, reaching levels of about 1 mg/ml. This release is enhanced if glucagon or cyclic AMP is added to the perfusate. If insulin is present as well as glucose, there is some retardation of the release of glucose, but these numbers are not very significant (Glinsmann *et al.* 1975).

Using fetal livers from streptozotocin-treated pregnancies in the same hypoglycaemic situation, we compared normal two-week-old newborns with a fetus of a glucose-intolerant mother. The full-term fetus of a streptozotocin pregnancy with fetal hyperinsulinaemia present during the latter part of pregnancy has a release in an aglycaemic perfusate which is very similar to the normal. In fact it would appear that the streptozotocin conceptus releases more glucose in these conditions. We cannot explain why that occurs but at least we can say there is no evidence of an intrinsic defect in glucose mobilization in this particular liver (Sparks *et al.* 1976).

Lactose is present in breast milk and supplies 40% of the newborn caloric requirements. Therefore, galactose supplies 20%. The question is, does galactose have a role in glycogen synthesis separate from glucose? In the

243

normal fetal liver, hyperglycaemia does not seem to affect either glycogen synthetase activity or glycogen uptake.   The percentage of active synthetase is about 4 % in the normal.   When the glucose concentration in the perfusate was increased, the percentage of the active form did not change.   When insulin was added, there was a slight change, to about 8 %.   When galactose and glucose and insulin were all added, there was a linear relationship to percentage active form which was not related to the concentration of glucose in the perfusate.   This went as high as 40 %.   Galactose levels in the *in vitro* perfusion were calculated to be analogous to the concentration that might be found in the portal vein after breast feeding.

I would also like to comment on the net uptake of hexose.   When glucose is released slowly into the perfusate from the liver, galactose in the perfusate is being taken up at the same time.   There is actually a net hexose uptake because the amount of galactose taken up is greater than the amount of glucose which has been released.   If we then add the variable of streptozotocin we get some interesting findings.   The first is that the percentage of active glycogen synthetase in the fetal liver is 16 % in the streptozotocin-perfused liver compared with 4 % in the normal.   Secondly, the glycogen content which is normally about 3 % of the weight of the liver rises to around 9 %.   Furthermore, in the streptozotocin-perfused liver, when there is hyperglycaemia there is no stimulation of glucose uptake, and there is no further increase above 16 % in the percentage of the active form.

In the presence of galactose, again with streptozotocin, as with the normal there is also net hexose uptake.   The only thing that is different in these studies with streptozotocin in the presence of galactose is that this sugar does not further stimulate the percentage active form of the glycogen synthetase.   It stays at 16 % and does not go up to 40 % as I showed you in the normal.   We believe that galactose may be necessary for substrate regulation of glycogen synthesis via the UDP-glucose pathway.

Girard: Have you looked at the effect of an amino acid mixture in addition to glucose on liver glycogen synthesis?

Chez: No.

Girard: That would be interesting, since it has been shown in isolated rat hepatocytes that addition of amino acids markedly increases glycogen synthesis from glucose (Katz *et al.* 1976).   This could have a physiological significance for the glycogen storage in the liver of the mammalian fetus.

Williamson: Did you show that in the infant of the diabetic mother there was increased total hexose uptake by the liver?

Chez: No, there was no increased total uptake.

Naismith: In experiments with adult rats we have shown that enzymes that are induced by corticosterone show a fall in activity if progesterone is administered simultaneously with the corticosterone (Naismith 1977). Progesterone appears therefore to negate the effect of corticosterone. This might explain the failure of fetal enzymes to respond to steroid hormones. Whether there is enough progesterone in the fetal circulation, I am not sure.

Hoet: There should not be much progesterone in the fetus.

Kalkhoff: My understanding is that progesterone is turned over extremely rapidly in maternal blood. Nevertheless, Professor Young has just shown me literature that indicates placental transfer of progesterone into the fetus. This is most interesting in view of Dr Naismith's remarks.

Räihä: We haven't added progesterone *in vitro* but in experiments on prolonging pregnancy by injecting progesterone into the rat mother we examined the fetal liver for urea cycle enzymes. There was no change in these enzymes. Whether progesterone went from mother to fetus I can't answer. This was a control for our other experiments.

Kalkhoff: Dr Naismith has observations that are very relevant to what is going on in the maternal liver. As we showed in our rat studies, and as he has so beautifully shown, progesterone does have an effect on hepatic gluconeogenesis. It also impairs the effects of cortisol on induction of gluconeogenic enzymes. I don't know whether this is a direct effect or is mediated in part by the hyperinsulinaemia that we see during progesterone administration.

Battaglia: Physiologists tend to think about plumbing a good bit. This may have some relevance when we try to compare fetal studies of the effects of hormones. In reproductive biology it was thought that catecholamines produced vasoconstriction in the vasculature of the non-pregnant uterus at lower concentrations than in the pregnant uterus. The error was in the experimental design, in that the catecholamines were being given to pregnant animals on a weight basis and the concentrations were not being expressed per millilitre of blood going to that vascular bed. Barton *et al.* (1974) demonstrated that when dose-response curves for the effect of catecholamines upon uterine blood flow were expressed in terms of uterine blood concentrations, the pregnant and non-pregnant dose-response curves were identical. Thus, there was no difference in sensitivity of the uterine bed to catecholamines in the pregnant and non-pregnant states.

Oestradiol is as potent a vasodilator on the uterine vascular bed as any compound. One microgram will produce a 15- or 18-fold increase in blood flow in ovariectomized non-pregnant ewes. W. Clewell *et al.* (unpublished work, 1978) have shown that the manner in which oestradiol is given makes a tremendous difference. The effect is very marked when it is given as a pulsatile dose and is just about absent if the same amount is given as a continuous infusion. The plumbing, the way hormones are given, and the way the hormone concentrations are expressed make big differences in the effects one sees and in the proper interpretation of the data. Sparks *et al.* (1976) have pointed out that glucose and galactose uptake by fetal rhesus monkey liver is quite different. Segal *et al.* (1963) reported that fetal rat liver slices took up galactose much more than glucose. Essentially the same observations were made by Ballard & Oliver (1964) for fetal sheep liver. Here we have a number of different studies which suggest that as glucose comes into the fetal umbilical circulation it may by-pass the liver and go on to be used by other tissues in the fetus. Thus, the differences in results we see among several studies might be due to differences in plumbing reflecting differences in where the substrates or hormones were delivered.

Kalkhoff: We heard earlier that the infant of the diabetic mother had higher insulin concentrations and more sluggish responses of glucagon to the fall in blood sugar than infants of non-diabetic mothers. In the *post partum* state, when the infant is often treated with glucose, this will ameliorate the low blood sugar but it will also stimulate insulin secretion even more and suppress glucagon release appreciably. This leads to some questions. Why is glucagon suppressed in infants of diabetic mothers? Is it because of the high fetal glucose concentrations before birth? Where is the glucagon measured in fetal blood coming from? Is it coming from the α cell of the pancreas or is it elaborated by the gastroduodenal segment or what?

Although we have talked about the possibility of increasing enzyme induction in the fetal liver of the diabetic mother with hormones, what about nutrients and enteric hormones? Are we giving the wrong thing *post partum* to these infants? Should we be giving something as a nutrient or agent that would help to raise glucagon as well as perhaps hold insulin in abeyance? This is defining a very practical problem: can we improve our care of the neonate of the diabetic mother?

Girard: In the adult it has been shown that glucagon contributes significantly to hyperglycaemia only when there is an insulin deficiency. The situation in the newborn of the diabetic mother is not the same. The blunted increase of glucagon in the newborn of the diabetic mother could be due to the chronic increase in glucose and insulin levels during gestation. Perhaps insulin plays a role in the maturation of the sensitivity of α_2 cells to glucose.

Kalkhoff: Do nutrients affect the stimulation of glucagon release in the newborn period, Dr Blázquez?

Blázquez: From *in vitro* studies we know that the pancreatic α_2 and β cells of the rat fetus release their hormonal products in response to a specific stimulus in a different form than cells from adult animals. In this way, high glucose concentrations cannot stimulate insulin secretion (Asplund *et al.* 1969) and α_2 cells are not able to discriminate between high or low glucose levels (Blázquez *et al.* 1974).

In nursing rats an oral glucose load produces a marked intolerance to glucose and a more modified insulin secretion than in the fetus, suggesting that factors other than developmental ones may be involved in the regulation of pancreatic hormone release.   As well as these factors the diet may be very important.   From the last third of pregnancy to the end of weaning three metabolic phases can be distinguished in the fetus and the newborn rat, which are defined, at least in part, by the different routes for acquiring nutrients.   During intrauterine life the main source of energy is the glucose the fetus receives from the mother, but after birth the animal changes to a diet rich in fat (69 % of the calorie intake) and protein but poor in carbohydrate (only 8 % of the calorie intake), from mother's milk.   On about the 20th postnatal day the rats start to ingest a standard laboratory diet, rich in carbohydrates and poor in fats.

These dietetic changes are accompanied by different responses of the tissues and by marked modifications in the metabolism of both of the pancreatic hormones.   In adult humans (Böttger *et al.* 1973) and laboratory animals (Blázquez & López Quijada 1968) the ingestion of diets rich in carbohydrates, fat or proteins profoundly changes the secretory, biosynthetic and biological effects of insulin and glucagon, which suggests that the nutrients may play a similar role during development in the rat.   At present, we are trying to find out which environmental or developmental factors are responsible for modifying insulin and glucagon metabolism during perinatal life; artificial diets with different amounts of fat, carbohydrates or proteins may help us to differentiate the influence of the two kinds of factors.

Girard: It has been shown that the secretion of glucagon is increased by milk-feeding in the young calf (Bloom *et al.* 1975) and that plasma glucagon is very high in suckling rats (Blázquez *et al.* 1974; Girard *et al.* 1977).   Gut hormones and the autonomic nervous system could be important modulators of glucagon secretion during the suckling period.

Hoet: Tejning (1947) about 30 years ago showed that in rats on a high fat diet the number and the volume of the islets were definitely reduced.   This was even more apparent in females than in males.   There was a correlation between these changes and pancreatic insulin content which may have many functional consequences.

Blázquez: Glucagon is widely distributed in the body and after the pancreas the fundus of the stomach is the main source of this hormone.   On the other hand, the ingestion of different types of diets significantly modifies the immunoreactive concentrations of circulating glucagon, but we do not know what is the exact contribution of pancreatic and extrapancreatic glucagon to these levels. Since the diet changes dramatically from one metabolic period to another during rat development, I am wondering what effect nutrients have on glucagon release and also what the relationships are between nutrients, glucagon and gastrointestinal hormones.

Kalkhoff: A lot of interesting enteric hormones are present immediately after birth. Many of them have an effect on the α and β cells. This might be relevant to the infant of the diabetic mother if there is any immaturity or dysfunction of the cell types in the gastrointestinal tract that secrete enteric hormones and influence the endocrine pancreas. This might be relevant to the question about enzyme induction in liver and other tissues.

Stowers: Professor W. Gepts (personal communication, 1973) says there is some increase in α_2 cells in the islets of diabetic mothers, although of course the specific increase is in β cells. The right background is present for the possibility of increased pancreatic glucagon. This was found by Dr Heding (Stowers *et al.* 1979) in plasma samples that we sent her, but it doesn't agree with Bloom & Johnston's data (1972). Our observations and Bloom's were made before feeding, about two hours after birth.

Pedersen: What kind of infants were they?

Stowers: We studied infants of mothers with no potential diabetes or Rh incompatibility. We also studied infants of chemically diabetic mothers treated with diet or with a small dose of chlorpropamide, and a few infants of insulin-dependent mothers. The more diabetic the mother, the more pancreatic glucagon we found in her infant's plasma at and shortly after birth.

Pedersen: When we measured concentrations of pancreatic glucagon in the infants of diabetic mothers, we found the opposite at two hours after birth, i.e. a decrease in glucagon concentration through White classes A–F.

Williamson: There is an ongoing study in Oxford on the metabolic and hormonal responses of normal infants to the first feed of either human milk or glucose (Aynsley-Green *et al.* 1977). The study is continuing on infants of diabetic mothers. In the normal infants with moderate respiratory distress but not the respiratory distress syndrome the changes in metabolites are very unimpressive. Glucose only rises very little in the first hour in response to human milk. There is a very small change in insulin. However the enteric hormones, which were measured by Stephen Bloom, responded quite dramatically. There was no change in pancreatic glucagon.

Gillmer: We (Gillmer *et al.,* unpublished observations) have looked at the change in plasma glucagon concentrations during the first two hours after birth in a small group of untreated chemical diabetics and a group of controls. The assay was done for us by Dr Stephen Bloom.   We found considerable individual variation, with a rise in plasma glucagon levels in about half the control infants and most of the infants of the chemical diabetic women but with no significant difference between the groups either at birth or two hours after delivery.

Pedersen: We found glucagon secretion in all classes of diabetics.   The concentrations were, absolutely and relatively, very low in all classes of neonates at birth.

Gillmer: As you said earlier, you have no control groups and this makes it rather difficult to interpret the data.

Pedersen: We compare the 30 infants of diabetic mothers in three groups: class A, B + C, D + F.

Gillmer: The infants of the chemical diabetic women in our study had raised concentrations of plasma insulin and the insulin: glucagon ratio was therefore higher in this group than in the controls.   In this respect I agree with you.

Girard: The type of glucagon circulating in the newborn is not well known.   Studies by I. Valverde (unpublished data, 1977) have shown that hyperglucagonaemia in the suckling newborn dog is primarily due to the fraction of 3500 molecular weight.   Sperling *et al.* (1977) have shown that suppression of glucagon secretion, by infusion of somatostatin into the newborn sheep, produced hypoglycaemia.   Glucagon infusion in physiological amounts reversed hypoglycaemia.   This shows that glucagon is very important for glucose homeostasis during the neonatal period.

Milner: The discussion on perinatal changes in plasma glucagon has so far referred to infants of diabetic mothers versus controls of different kinds.   It is worth commenting also on the potential but as yet unproven importance of the autonomic nervous system in stimulating pancreatic glucagon release at the time of birth.   Clamping of the umbilical cord of the newborn lamb is associated with a sharp rise in plasma glucagon (Sack *et al.* 1976).   The mechanism by which the two events are linked is open to speculation; it may have a neuronal component.

Gillmer: In addition, Bloom (1973) has reported that splanchnic nerve stimulation in the calf produces a very marked acute glucagon release.   This is also in keeping with the idea that the autonomic nervous system has a major role in the control of glucagon release.

Blázquez: Valverde & Matesanz (1977) have already reported that the hyperglucagonaemia of newborn dogs is in part due to the immunoreactive component with a molecular weight of 350.   We have observed the same results in newborn rats (unpublished work), but these findings do not demonstrate that circulating glucagon is only of pancreatic origin.   At present we know that the gastrointestinal tract (Sasaki *et al.* 1975) and the salivary glands (Silverman & Dunbar 1974; Lawrence *et al.* 1975) can synthesize a polypeptide with the same immunological, physicochemical and biological properties as pancreatic glucagon.   Also we have found (A. Perez Castillo & E. Blázquez, unpublished work) that the salivary glands, thymus, thyroid and adrenal glands of the rat can synthesize, from radioactive tryptophan, a polypeptide of 3500 molecular weight which has the same immunological, secretory and biological characteristics as pancreatic glucagon.

Kalkhoff: Dr Beard, you have always emphasized that vaginal delivery is much preferred to Caesarean section in a diabetic pregnancy.   Could the stress of pregnancy have beneficial effects not only on breathing but also on the insulin/glucagon molar concentration ratio?

Beard: We have not looked at that but we looked at catecholamines as an index of stress that might effectively induce enzyme activity.   There is a fourfold increase in plasma catecholamines, simply as a result of delivery.   So stress may have a beneficial effect.   Obstetricians who do Caesarean sections regularly and claim they never have any problems are generally dealing with healthy babies. Usher *et al.* (1971) showed quite clearly that Caesarean section increases the risk of respiratory distress, and Robert *et al.* (1975) showed that the addition of maternal diabetes to a Caesarean section further increased the risk of respiratory distress developing.

Girard: Dr Blázquez and I have shown that whether the rat is delivered at term by Caesarean section or vaginally there is a rise in plasma glucagon (Girard *et al.* 1973; Blázquez *et al.* 1974).   So it is independent of the type of delivery.   This is also independent of the nutrition, since it occurs if the newborn rat is starved or is suckling.

Kalkhoff: Did you use ether?

Girard: No.   We kill the rats by cervical dislocation which is less stressful than ether for the newborns.

Freinkel: You are absolutely correct.   We encountered enormous differences between the two methods and therefore have been relying on decapitation of unanaesthetized animals with a guillotine (Metzger *et al.* 1974).

Girard: Sherwood *et al.* (1974) have reported the case of a newborn infant with pancreatic agenesis.   No insulin and no glucagon were found at autopsy in the vestigial organ.   The newborn was hypotrophic, hypoglycaemic and showed an impairment of gluconeogenesis.   So glucagon is essential for the development of gluconeogenesis, not only in the rat but also in the human newborn.

Hoet: The noradrenaline content per gram of pancreas is very definitely reduced in fetuses from rats with streptozotocin-induced diabetes compared with fetuses from non-diabetic animals.   The reduction is related to the severity of the diabetes.

Streptozotocin was given in doses of 30, 40 and 50 mg/kg body weight.   With severe diabetes after 40 and 50 mg/kg body weight the noradrenaline content was the lowest.   The experiments were carried out by de Gasparo and will be published in the report of the Aberdeen meeting (Reusens *et al.* 1979).   The lack of catecholamines may mean that these neurotransmitters have no inhibitory effect upon the endocrine pancreas, leaving the β cells with an unabated insulin secretion.

Kalkhoff: Is there any information about adrenaline or the total catecholamine content?

Hoet: No, not yet.

Naeye: Does anyone have any information about neurotransmitter levels including noradrenaline (norepinephrine) in the brains of these experimental animals?

Freinkel: We have been very interested in the implications of the changes in amino acids for neurotransmitter function in the brains of the fetuses of streptozotocin-treated mothers (L. Airoldi *et al.*, unpublished observations, 1977–1978).   Diabetes has been established with streptozotocin 11 days before mating and animals have been killed on day 20 and 21 of pregnancy.   We have been comparing such pregnant diabetic animals to pregnant animals with normal carbohydrate metabolism and pregnant diabetic animals in whom treatment with insulin has been instituted.   Despite very radical changes in the amino acid profiles in the diabetic mothers and their fetuses, the maturation of brain noradrenaline (norepinephrine), dopamine, and serotonin does not appear to have been altered.   Steady-state levels of these neurohumours remain very immature and not appreciably influenced by the maternal diabetes.

Absolute concentrations in the fetal brain are extremely low.   Maturation of the enzymes that regulate the synthesis of neurohumours is apparently still the rate-limiting step and not accelerated by diabetes.

References

ASPLUND, K., WESTMAN, S. & HELLERSTRÖM, C. (1969) Glucose stimulation of insulin secretion from the isolated pancreas of fetal and newborn rats. *Diabetologia 5,* 260–262

AYNSLEY-GREEN, A., BLOOM, S. R., WILLIAMSON, D. H. & TURNER, R.C. (1977) Endocrine and metabolic response in the human newborn to first feed of breast milk. *Arch. Dis. Child. 52,* 291–295

BALLARD, F. J. & OLIVER, I.T. (1964) Ketohexokinase, isoenzymes of glucokinase and glycogen synthesis from hexoses in neonatal rat liver. *Biochem. J. 90*, 261–269

BARTON, M. D., KILLAM, A.P. & MESCHIA, G. (1974) Response of ovine uterine blood flow to epinephrine and norepinephrine. *Proc. Soc. Exp. Biol. Med. 145*, 996–1003

BLÁZQUEZ, E. & LÓPEZ QUIJADA, C. (1968) The effect of a high-fat diet on glucose, insulin sensitivity and plasma insulin in rats. *J. Endocrinol. 42*, 489–494

BLÁZQUEZ, E., SUGASE, T., BLÁZQUEZ, M. & FOA, P. P. (1974) Neonatal changes in the concentration of rat liver cyclic AMP and of serum glucose, free fatty acids, insulin, pancreatic and total glucagon in man and in the rat. *J. Lab. Clin. Med. 83*, 957–967

BLOOM, S. R. (1973) Glucagon, a stress hormone. *Postgrad. Med. J. 49*, 607–611

BLOOM, S. R. & JOHNSTON, D. J. (1972) Failure of glucagon release in infants of diabetic mothers. *Br. Med. J. 4*, 453–454

BLOOM, S. R., EDWARDS, A. V., HARDY, R. N., MALINOWSKA, K. & SILVER, M. (1975) Cardiovascular and endocrine responses to feeding in the young calf. *J. Physiol. (Lond.) 253*, 135–155

BÖTTGER, I., DOBBS, R., FALOONA, G. & UNGER, R. H. (1973) The effects of triglyceride absorption upon glucagon, insulin and gut glucagon-like immunoreactivity. *J. Clin. Invest. 52*, 2532–2541

GIRARD, J. R., CUENDET, G. S., MARLISS, E. B., KERVIAN, A., RIEUTORT, M. & ASSAN, R. (1973) Fuels, hormones and liver metabolism at term and during the early postnatal period in the rat. *J. Clin. Invest. 52*, 3190–3200

GIRARD, J. R., FERRE, P., KERVRAN, A., PEGORIER, J. P. & ASSAN, R. (1977) Influence of insulin-glucagon ratio in the change of hepatic metabolism during development of the rat, in *Glucagon: its Role in Physiology and Clinical Medicine* (Foa, P. P. *et al.*, eds.), pp. 563–581, Excerpta Medica, Amsterdam

GLINSMANN, W. H., EISEN, H. J., LYNH, A. & CHEZ, R. A. (1975) Glucose regulation by isolated near term fetal monkey liver. *Pediatr. Res. 9*, 600–604

KATZ, J., GOLDEN, S. & WALS, P. A. (1976) Stimulation of hepatic glycogen synthesis by amino acids. *Proc. Natl. Acad. Sci. U.S.A. 73*, 3433–3437

LAWRENCE, A. M., KIRSTEINS, L., HOJUAT, S., RUBIN, L. & PALOYAN, V. (1975) Salivary gland glucagon: a potent extrapancreatic hyperglycemic factor. *Clin. Res. 23*, 563A

METZGER, B. E., PEK, S., HARE, J. & FREINKEL, N. (1974) Relationships between glucose, insulin, and glucagon during fasting in late gestation in the rat. *Life Sci. 15*, 301–308

NAISMITH, D. J. (1977) Protein metabolism during pregnancy, in *Scientific Foundations of Obstetrics and Gynaecology*, 2nd edn. (Philipp, E.E. *et al.*, eds.), pp. 503–510, Heinemann Medical, London

REUSENS, B., DE GASPARO, M., KUHN & HOET, J. J. (1979) Controlling factors of fetal nutrition, in *Carbohydrate Metabolism in Pregnancy and the Newborn* (Sutherland, H.W. & Stowers, J. M., ed.), Springer Verlag, Berlin

ROBERT, M. F., NEFF, R. K., HUBBELL, J. P., TAEUSCH, H. W. & AVERY, M. (1975) Association between maternal diabetes and the respiratory distress syndrome in the newborn. *New Engl. J. Med. 294*, 357

SACK, J., GRAJWER, L. A., SPERLING, M. A. & FISHER, D. A. (1976) Umbilical cord cutting: the stimulus to the glucagon surge in newborn lambs. *Pediatr. Res. 10*, 880 (abstr.)

SASAKI, H., RUBALCAVA, B., BAETENS, D., BLÁZQUEZ, E., SRIKANT, C. B., ORCI, L. & UNGER, R. (1975) Identification of glucagon in the gastrointestinal tract. *J. Clin. Invest. 56*, 135–145

SEGAL, S., ROTH, H. & BERTOLI, D. (1963) Galactose metabolism by rat liver tissues: influence of age. *Science (Wash. D.C.) 142*, 1311–1313

SHERWOOD, W. G., CHANCE, G. W., TOEWS, C. J., MARTIN, J. M. & MARLIS, E. B. (1974) A new syndrome of familial pancreatic agenesis: essential role of glucagon in neonatal gluconeogenesis. *Pediatr. Res. 8*, 438 (abstr.)

SILVERMAN, H. & DUNBAR, J. C. (1974) The submaxillary gland as a possible source of glucagon. *Bull. Sinai Hosp. Detroit 22*, 192–193

SPARKS, J. W., LYNCH, A., CHEZ, R. A. & GLINSMANN, W. H. (1976) Glycogen regulation in isolated perfused near-term monkey liver. *Pediatr. Res. 10,* 51–56

SPERLING, M. A., GRAJWER, L., LEAKE, R. D. & FISHER, D. A. (1977) Effects of somatostatin (SRIF) infusion on glucose homeostasis in newborn lambs: evidence for a significant role of glucagon. *Pediatr. Res. 11,* 962–967

STOWERS, J. M., HEDING, L. G., FISHER, P. M., TREHARNE, I. A. L., ROSS, I. S., SUTHERLAND, H. W., BEWSHER, P.D., RUSSELL, G. & PRICE, H. V. (1979) The relationship between glucagon and hypocalcaemia in infants of diabetic mothers, in *Carbohydrate Metabolism in Pregnancy and the Newborn* (Sutherland, H. W. & Stowers, J. M., eds.), Springer Verlag, Berlin

TEJNING, S. (1947) Dietary factors and quantitative morphology of the islets of Langerhans. *Acta Med. Scand. Suppl. 198,* 1–150

USHER, R. H., ALLEN, A. C. & MCLEAN, F. (1971) Risk of respiratory distress syndrome related to gestational age, route of delivery and maternal diabetes. *Am. J. Obstet. Gynecol. 6,* 826

VALVERDE, I. & MATESANZ, R. (1977) High levels of plasma 'Proglucagon' in early life. *Diabetes 26,* 421

The influence of preconceptional glucose values on the outcome of pregnancy

N.A.M. BERGSTEIN

Department of Obstetrics and Gynecology Streekziekenhuis, Zevenaar, The Netherlands

Abstract A relationship between maternal diabetes and fetal malformations has been recognized for a long time, but there has been considerable difference of opinion about the size of the risk.

Several defects of the pelvis and lower limbs appear to be relatively common in offspring of diabetic mothers. In experimental studies a dose relationship has been shown between some drugs (insulin-Trypan blue) and lower limb malformations. Three patients are described with congenital malformations with diabetes or prediabetes during pregnancy. Is the caudal regression syndrome a part of a larger syndrome caused by a disturbance of glucose homeostasis?

One of the few metabolic disorders which change the environment in which the fetus develops is diabetes mellitus during pregnancy. The percentage of malformations, macrosomia, hyperinsulinism and stillbirth is increased, which may be the result of a relatively minor disturbance of glucose homeostasis.

The relationship between diabetes mellitus during pregnancy and congenital malformations in the resulting infants has interested paediatricians and obstetricians for many years. The incidence of congenital malformations seems to be about three times as high in the newborn infants of diabetic mothers as in control series. Table 1 shows that there is a striking similarity between four series in percentages of malformations and it reveals that the problem of congenital abnormalities among diabetics is far from resolved.

The object of this study is to investigate whether there are particular patterns of typical congenital malformations in newborn infants born to diabetic mothers and the influence of the preconceptional glucose values on these malformations. The following three cases are from our clinic.

255

TABLE 1

Summary of studies of congenital abnormalities occurring among the infants of diabetic mothers and control groups (adapted from Beard & Oakley 1976)

Study	No. of infants	Malformations (%)		
		Major	Minor	Total
Mølsted-Pedersen *et al.* (1964)				
Diabetic	864	5.2(2.1)	1.2	6.4
Normal	1212	1.2(0.3)	0.9	2.1
Watson (1972)				
Diabetic	240			9.6
Normal				5.9
Pedersen (1975)				
Diabetic	1332	6.1(2.4)	1.9	8.0
Normal	8789	1.6(0.4)	1.2	2.8
Malins (1975)				
Diabetic	205	7.6(4.4)	5.0	12.6
Normal	205	0.0(0.0)	5.7	5.7

Figures in parentheses refer to incidence of fetal malformations

Case 1:Kl A

This woman has had seven pregnancies with four abortions and three infants delivered.   She has been diabetic since the age of 11 years.   Her sister had diabetes mellitus since the age of 12 years.   The mother and grandmother did not have diabetes.   Some of her mother's brothers and nephews have diabetes.

Her first pregnancy ended with an intrauterine death in the 32nd week of gestation.   The child was normal.   After this pregnancy she had two abortions, both in the eighth week of gestation.   Her fourth pregnancy was controlled from the 9th week of gestation.   Glucose levels in the blood were then sometimes high and sometimes very low.   From the 10th week of gestation the blood glucose levels were stable (around 100–120 mg/100 ml; 5.5–6.7 mmol/l).   Oestriol excretion was measured regularly.   In the 37th week of gestation a Caesarean section was done because the oestriol values were decreasing.   A girl was born (weight 2360 g, length 40 cm).   There was hypoplasia of both femora and the humerus was strongly connected with the radius in both arms.   There were fistulae on the sacrum and both tubercula majus, hypoplasia of the under-jaw, and pes equinovarus adductus on both sides.   The girl had a caudal regression syndrome.

After this gestation the patient had two more abortions (ninth and tenth weeks of gestation).   Before her seventh pregnancy the patient was advised that before she became pregnant again her blood glucose values had to be normal and around 100 mg/100 ml for at least three months before conception.   This pregnancy was controlled from the sixth week of gestation and the blood glucose values at that time and during the previous three months were around 100 mg/100 ml.   The patient was very cooperative.   Oestriol excretion and the fetal heart rate pattern were measured regularly.   In the 38th week of gestation she delivered a healthy girl by Caesarean section (weight 3330 g, length 50 cm).   The child had no congenital malformations.

Case 2 U-M

This patient is a primigravida, no abortions.   She became pregnant after ovulation was induced with clomiphene.   Her grandmother has severe diabetes mellitus which is difficult to control.   One year after our patient's child was born, the patient's mother was also discovered to have diabetes.   During her pregnancy our patient had a borderline response to the oral glucose tolerance test but after a diabetic pregnancy diet her three-hour day and night curve was normal.   In the 40th week of gestation she delivered a boy with an extrophia vesicae totalis and an epispadias totalis.   There were no other congenital malformations.   One year after the birth a uterus bicornis unicollis was found on salpingography.   After a cortisone load the oral glucose tolerance test was disturbed.

Case 3 vW-E

This patient has had two pregnancies, no abortions, one liveborn infant.   She had diabetes mellitus since the age of 12 years. Her first pregnancy was at the age of 18 years.   Her diabetes was always difficult to control because the patient was not very cooperative and not very intelligent.   She came for control of the first pregnancy in the 14th week of gestation.   At that time she had several diabetic comas.   In the 35th week of gestation the oestriol excretion decreased sharply and she delivered a boy by Caesarean section (weight 2000 g, length 40 cm).

At four months the child died of a great ventricular septum defect.   No other malformation was found.   In her second pregnancy the patient came under control from the 10th week.   The advice that she should not get pregnant again before the blood glucose values were reduced and well regulated was neglected by her and by her husband, who was also not very cooperative or intelligent.   In the 26th week there were some signs indicative of an anencephalus.   The patient had a hydramnion and ultrasonic investigation showed the criteria and signs of a pregnancy complicated by an anencephalus.   In the 29th week the picture by ultrasonic investigation gave a definitive diagnosis.   The α-fetoprotein was increased from 22 ng/ml in the 15th week to 435 ng/ml in the 28th week of gestation.   In the 30th week the pregnancy was terminated and she delivered an anencephalic girl (weight 1560 g, length 3.5 cm).   There were no other malformations and neither the lower limbs nor the internal genitalia were affected.

Congenital skeletal deformities have been experimentally produced in animals by various methods, including X-rays, heavy metals, vitamin deficiency, viruses and certain drugs.   Several studies have clearly demonstrated that developing organs have particular periods of sensitivity to damaging factors during gestation.   Zwilling found in 1952 that when insulin was injected into the yolk sac of chicken embryos during the first three days of incubation, caudal anomalies were especially frequent, consisting of either partial suppression or total absence of tail structures.   He suggested that these abnormalities were due to interference with normal carbohydrate metabolism during a critical phase in morphogenesis.   In 1955 Duraiswami published studies similar to Zwilling's and reported a consistent relationship between the time of injection, the dose of the drug and the part of the body primarily affected.   Landauer (1947) injected insulin into incubating chicken eggs and produced a syndrome of shortened legs, hypoplastic maxillae and other malformations bearing a close resemblance to the diabetic embryopathy syndrome in the human being.   Brinsmade et al. (1956) and Brinsmade (1957) administered insulin to pregnant rabbits and produced embryos with numerous defects, including absent and hypoplastic limbs, spina bifida occulta and agnathia.   Three types of caudal anomalies were demonstrated by Lendon (1968) after Trypan blue was injected intraperitoneally in the rat:
(1) embryos with a myelocoele accompanied by minimal vertebral defects and later by a normal tail;
(2) short-tail embryos with a myelocoele underlain by a notochord and vertebral row exhibiting abnormal ventral deflection;
(3) short-tailed embryos with premature termination of spinal cord accompanied by ventral deflection of the vertebral row and notochord.
From their study Kaplan & Johnson (1968) suggested that the teratogenic action with Trypan blue results from deprivation of the oxygen required for normal growth and differentiation in a tissue with high metabolic requirements.   Trypan blue perhaps acts as an uncoupling agent in oxidative phosphorylation, thereby increasing the oxygen consumption of embryonic tis-

sues. Grabowski (1964) produced malformations of the neural tube in chickens by inducing various degrees of hypoxia. Warkany & Schaffenberger (1943) demonstrated that limb abnormalities, micrognathia, cleft palate and other congenital defects could be produced in rats given a riboflavin-deficient diet during gestation.

The glucose values of the chicken embryo are not correlated to the glucose values of the mother since the egg is a separate unit. However the same malformations have been seen in the rat embryo after the same injections. The glucose values of the rat embryo are correlated to the glucose values of the mother as has been found in all mammals.

Whether by destruction of cells, by interference with the normal developmental sequences or by some other mechanism, the teratogens mentioned above cause these developmental defects. Duhamel (1961) summarized the more constant findings in monsters with the caudal regression syndrome (Table 2).

The 50 cases described by Blumel et al. (1959) had sacral and coccygeal agenesis. Only seven mothers had diabetes mellitus. In spite of this Blumel et al. thought that diabetes could possibly be the aetiological factor. In their study Mølsted-Pedersen et al. (1964) found that about 1% of infants of diabetic mothers had severe bone malformations, especially of the limbs. Passarge & Lenz (1966) observed that the caudal regression syndrome occurred in 1% of infants born to diabetic mothers and 16% of infants reported to have the syndrome of caudal regression had diabetic mothers. One of the most impressive studies is that by Osler (1961). He compared the length of the long bones on X-ray films in a small series of infants of

TABLE 2

Characteristic elements in siren monsters (adapted from Duhamel (1961)

Lower limb anomalies	Flexion, external rotation: union (symelia) and often atrophy
Vertebral anomalies	Increased in number (epistasis), or sacral agenesis
Anorectal agenesis	
Urinary tract anomalies	Bilateral renal agenesis: ureteral, vesical and urethral agenesis
Genital anomalies	Wolffian or Müllerian duct agenesis (gonads present in all cases)

diabetic women and normal children of identical birth weight.   He demonstrated that the mean tibial and femoral diaphyses are shorter in the diabetic
group.

Many of the published case reports are very brief and not well documented.   The obstetrical history, especially the family history of diabetes, is not
mentioned.   There are publications describing children with the caudal regression syndrome whose mothers had no sign of diabetes at the time of
delivery.   However, those women developed diabetes mellitus some years
later.   These published findings are not a coincidence.   We also found in our
case 2, one year after delivery, that the mother of the patient had diabetes and
the patient herself had a pathological oral glucose tolerance test after a
cortisone load.   McCracken (1965) described an infant with unilateral absence of the femur whose mother had no sign of diabetes at the time of
delivery.   She developed diabetes mellitus six years later.   Kalitzki (1965)
found a persistent hyperglycaemia one year after a woman gave birth to a child
without a sacrum and without lumbar vertebra 5.

In the published work we found the following groups of malformations in
children born to mothers with metabolic disorders (caused by diabetes?):

Caudal regression syndrome (caudal dysplasia)

Limb abnormalities   Both femora short or hypoplasia of one leg
                        Very small and poorly developed legs

Urogenital system   Double ureters
                        No ureters
                        No anus
                        Rectovaginal fistula
                        Lack of urethra in penis
                        Poor testis differentiation

Renal   Aplasia of left or right kidney
                        Two calyces
                        Kidney cysts
                        Renal agenesis
                        Neurogenic bladder
                        One kidney not functioning

Uterus   Uterus bicornis
                          Uterus unicornis
                          Uterus duplex

There are some reports of children with one or two or more of these malformations, all in the lower half of the body.   More localized lesions can also be found in which the lower limbs, the Wolffian system and the vertebral column all escaped damage and malformations occurred only in the cloacal region (our case 2).

Surveying all these findings, Mølsted-Pedersen *et al.* (1964) concluded that in pregnant diabetic women there is an unusual combination of circumstances which tend to favour the development of congenital malformations:

(1) A divergent gene pattern which in any event predisposes to congenital malformations;

(2) An abnormal intrauterine environment of the fetus manifesting as diabetic changes in the uterine mucosa, an altered composition of the maternal blood, and late diabetic changes in the maternal vessels.

There are many reports of insulin coma in the first months of pregnancy without any malformation of the delivered child.   Therefore hypoglycaemia cannot be the only cause of malformation.   Perhaps there is no relationship with hypoglycaemia or hyperglycaemia.

Kučera (Kučera *et al.* 1965) mentioned that he found six cases of caudal regression syndrome only in babies born to mothers who were working in a factory producing acetone.   B. Vedra (personal communication) found no caudal regression syndrome in a large group of diabetic pregnant women in Prague.   He found a caudal regression syndrome only among a group of women working in an acetone factory.

Navarrete *et al.* (1966, 1970) sent all their patients who had clinical features suggestive of glucose metabolic disorders to a diabetic clinic.   These women were submitted to a triamcinolone glucose tolerance test (T-GTT) and a standard glucose tolerance test (GTT).   Those patients with an abnormal T-GTT and a normal GTT were classified as 'early glucose metabolic disorders' and received tolbutamide (125 mg) at each meal.   A new T-GTT was done after four and eight months of treatment, with the drug being stopped five days before the new test.   They studied two groups of patients: those in group 1 were treated and started their pregnancy with a normal T-GTT test, while group 2 started pregnancy with an abnormal T-GTT test.   In group 1 they observed no congenital malformations, pre-eclampsia, stillbirth, over-sized babies, polyhydramnion or glycosuria, and about 80% of pregnancies and babies were normal.   In group 2 they observed that the incidence of materno-fetal complications was comparable to that observed in the pregnancy before treatment.   From these interesting findings they concluded that bringing the T-GTT back to normal achieves a better glucose homeostasis on the basis of the disappearance of several materno-fetal complications.

The work of Vallance-Owen (1962), Vallance-Owen and Ashton (1963), Vallance-Owen *et al.* (1967, 1973), Wilson & Vallance-Owen (1966) is of great interest.   Is there a relationship between insulin antagonists and malformations of the fetus?   The presence of antagonists is interpreted as indicating a prediabetic state and is detectable before there is any disturbance of carbohydrate metabolism.   Those substances associated with plasma albumin were found more frequently in the mothers of some groups of deformed babies than in controls.

A disturbance of glucose metabolism before conception or during the first trimester of gestation can produce a caudal regression syndrome, as has been demonstrated in experimental studies and also in the carefully investigated groups of patients reported from many countries.   The similarity between the deformities seen in the chicken, rabbit and rat studies and the malformations seen in babies born to diabetic mothers is striking.   Since both hyperinsulinism and intrauterine hypoglycaemia (probably!) occur in those infants, one or both of these factors seems likely to be implicated in the causation of these anomalies. Reid (1970) has proposed that certain fetal cells may be especially sensitive to exogenous glucose levels.   He hypothesizes that fluctuating glucose levels could carry a greater risk of fetal deformity than persistent hyperglycaemia.   High blood glucose levels might switch sensitive cells to a glycolytic pattern of metabolism.   Reversion to normal blood glucose levels could further widen the energy gap by reducing the rate of glycolysis before restoration of aerobic metabolism.

Our first case is difficult to understand.   Of her three children only one had a caudal regression syndrome.   The first child was an intrauterine death and no pathological investigation was possible as maceration was too far advanced.   Were the four abortions caused by a metabolic disorder or a chromosomal anomaly?   Before the last pregnancy the blood glucose values were low before conception and in the first trimester of pregnancy.   But her sister also had severe diabetes and delivered three healthy children.   If we had not regulated the blood glucose values before conception patient 1 might also have delivered two children with congenital malformations, as did patient 3.   Our case 3 is one of a small group of patients who had delivered two children with congenital malformations.   Both malformations have been described in mothers whose pregnancy has been complicated by diabetes.

Mestwert (1961, 1964) found a higher percentage of congenital malformations in diabetics who are badly controlled. Our case 3 was not very cooperative and it was very difficult to control her blood glucose levels. Case 2 had a prediabetic glucose tolerance curve and delivered a child with congenital malformations only in the region of the bladder. One year after the delivery we found a pathological GTT after a cortisone load.

We sometimes find uterine anomalies in women who during their pregnancies had prediabetic or diabetic GTT. In their family history there were some diabetic relatives: mothers, grandmothers or aunts. Were these anomalies of the uterus also caused by diabetic disturbances of glucose metabolism in the first trimester of the pregnancies of the mothers of those patients?

CONCLUSION

If we wish to lower the percentage of congenital malformations we must treat our diabetic patients before conception. If these women are using the contraceptive pill they will have to stop taking it three months before conception. During those three months the glucose values must be controlled. The women may become pregnant again when the blood glucose values are around 100 mg/100 ml, as Pedersen has prescribed (1977). If they are prediabetic, the therapy schedule described by Navarrete *et al.* (1966, 1970) can be followed.

I should like to pose the following question:

Is the caudal regression syndrome one part of a whole spectrum of congenital malformations (ureter duplex–situs viscerorum inversus–spina bifida–uterus anomalies) *that are all seen more often in pregnancies complicated by diabetes mellitus than in normal pregnancies?*

References

BEARD, R. W. & OAKLEY, N. W. (1976) The fetus of the diabetic mother, in *Fetal Physiology and Medicine* (Beard, R. W. & Nathanielsz, P. W., eds.), Saunders, London & Philadelpia

BLUMEL, J., EVANS, E.B. & EGGERS, G. W. N. (1959) Partial and complete malformation of the sacrum with associated anomalies: etiologic and clinical study with special reference to heredity. A preliminary report. *J. Bone Joint Surg. Am. Vol. 41*, 497–518

BRINSMADE, A. B. (1957) Entwicklungsstörungen am Kaninchenembryo nach Glucosemangel beim trächtigen Muttertier. *Beitr. Pathol. Anat. Allg. Pathol. 117*, 140–153

BRINSMADE, A. B., BÜCHNER, F. & RÜBSAAMEN, H. (1956) Missbildungen am Kaninchenembryo durch Insulininjectionen beim Muttertier. *Naturwissenschaften 43*, 259

DUHAMEL, B (1961) From the mermaid to anal imperforation: the syndrome of caudal regression. *Arch. Dis. Child. 36*, 152–155

DURAISWAMI, P. K. (1955) Comparison of congenital defects induced in developing chickens by certain teratogenic agents with those caused by insulin. *J. Bone Joint Surg. 37*, 277–294

GRABOWSKI, C. T. (1964) The etiology of hypoxia-induced malformations of the chick embryo. *J. Exp. Zool.* 157, 307–326

KALITZKI, M. (1965) Congenital malformations and diabetes. *Lancet 2,* 641–642

KAPLAN, S. & JOHNSON, B. M. (1968) Oxygen consumption: normal and trypan blue treated chick embryos. *Teratology 1,* 369–373

KUČERA, J., LENZ, W. & MAIER, W. (1965) Missbildungen der Beine und caudalen Wirbelsäule bei Kindern diabetischer Mutter. *Dtsch. Med. Wochenschr. 90,* 901–905

LANDAUER, W. (1947) Insulin induced abnormalities of back, extremities and eyes in chickens. *J. Exp. Zool. 105,* 145–172

LENDON, R. G. (1968) Studies on the embryogenesis of spina bifida in the rat. *Dev. Med. Child Neurol. Suppl. 16,* 54–61

MALINS, J. M. (1975) Cited by Beard & Oakley (1976)

McCRACKEN, J. S. (1965) Absence of foetal femur and maternal prediabetes. *Lancet 1,* 1274

MESTWERT, G. (1961) Die Bedeutung der Prophylaxe bei Diabetes und Schwangerschaft. *Arch. Gynäkol. 195,* 334

MESTWERT, G. (1964) Geburtshilfliche Komplikationen beim Diabetes mellitus und ihre Verhütung. *Ther. Ggw. p.* 1420

MOLSTED-PEDERSEN, L., TYGSTRUP, I. & PEDERSEN, J. (1964) Congenital malformations in newborn infants of diabetic women. *Lancet 1,* 1124–1126

NAVARRETE, V. N., TORRES, I. H., AYALA, L. C., ALGER, C. R. & FLORES, H. V. (1966) Modification of response to the triamcinolone glucose tolerance test by treatment with oral hypoglycemic agents. *Diabetes 15,* 726–729

NAVARRETE, V. N., PAIAGUA, H. E., ALGER, C. R. & MANZO, P. B. (1970) The significance of metabolic adjustment before a new pregnancy. Prophylaxis of congenital malformations. *Am. J. Obstet. Gynecol. 107,* 250–253

OSLER, M. (1961) *The Body Composition of Newborn Infants of Diabetic Mothers.* Thesis, Medical Faculty, University of Copenhagen

PASSARGE, E. & LENZ, W. (1966) Syndrome of caudal regression. *Pediatrics 37,* 672–675

PEDERSEN, J. (1975) *The Pregnant Diabetic and her Newborn,* Munksgaard, Copenhagen

PEDERSEN, J. (1977) *The Pregnant Diabetic and her Newborn,* 2nd edn., Munksgaard, Copenhagen

REID, R. A. (1970) Diabetes and congenital abnormalities. *Lancet 1,* 1030

VALLANCE-OWEN, J. (1962) Diabetes mellitus. Causation. *Proc. R. Soc. Med. 55,* 207–210

VALLANCE-OWEN, J. & ASHTON, W. L. (1963) Inheritance of essential diabetes mellitus from studies of the Synalbumin insulin antagonist. *Diabetes 12,* 356

VALLANCE-OWEN, J., BRAITHWAITE, F. & WILSON, J. S. P. (1967) Cleft lip and palate deformation and insulin antagonism. *Lancet 2,* 912–914

VALLANCE-OWEN, J., McMASTER, D. & BAJAJ, J. S. (1973) Maternal Synalbumin antagonism and large babies. *Lancet 2,* 358

WARKANY, J. & SCHAFFENBERGER, E. (1943) Congenital malformations induced in rats by maternal nutritional deficiency: effects of a purified diet lacking riboflavin. *Proc. Soc. Exp. Biol. Med. 54,* 92–94

WATSON, C. (1972) Late prognosis of children born to diabetic mothers. M. D. thesis, University of London

WILSON, J. S. P. & VALLANCE-OWEN, J. (1966) Congenital deformities and insulin antagonism. *Lancet 2,* 940–942

ZWILLING, E. (1952) The effects of some hormones on development. *Ann. N.Y. Acad. Sci. 55,* 196–202

For discussion of this paper, see pp. 273–281

Congenital malformations: the possible role of diabetes care outside pregnancy

JØRGEN PEDERSEN* and LARS MØLSTED-PEDERSEN

Diabetes Centre, Department of Obstetrics and Gynecology Y (B), Rigshospitalet, University of Copenhagen

Abstract A consecutive and prospective series comprising 949 newborn infants of diabetic mothers treated during pregnancy and delivery in the period 1966–1977 has been analysed. The malformation rate was 8.2%.

As compared to infants of mothers (White classes B–F alone) controlled *outside* pregnancy elsewhere, the rate of malformations was significantly reduced (from 14.1 to 7.4%) in infants whose mothers attended two hospitals specializing in the treatment and ambulatory control of diabetics.

For diabetics not controlled at a diabetic centre *outside* pregnancy the malformation rate was 9% in classes B + C and 19.4% in classes D + F, compared to 6.2 and 8.5%, respectively, for those who were controlled. The rates of malformation (total as well as severe alone) were significantly reduced in infants of White's classes D + F, and insignificantly reduced in classes B + C (in class A no comparison could be made).

The findings indicate that poor diabetic control outside pregnancy is teratogenic, although the 'disastrous malformation factor' of diabetes appears not to be totally dependent on the degree of compensation of the diabetic metabolism, as measured by the variables usually applied.

In 1964 we proposed the view that congenital malformations in infants of diabetic mothers were due in particular to the presence of maternal vascular complications with an insufficient blood supply to the uterus and placenta. The hypothesis was based upon the positive correlation of malformation rate with White's classification A–F (Tables 1, 2)(Pedersen *et al.* 1964; Pedersen 1977; White 1965).

The 'metabolic' hypothesis – a natural 'first-choice' guess – that incomplete metabolic compensation at nidation and during the first trimester might also be important has so far been based only on sparse circumstantial evidence. For example:

* Professor Dr Jørgen Pedersen died on 21 November 1978.

265

TABLE 1
White's classification as applied in the Rigshospital

A	Chemical diabetes (diet ±oral drugs)				
	Age of onset (years)		*Duration (years)*		*Retino-pathy*
B	≥ 20	and	< 10		Absent
C	10-19	or	10-19		Absent
D	< 10	or	≥ 20	or	Benign
F	Nephropathy and/or proliferative retinopathy				

TABLE 2
Rate of congenital malformation (CM) in relation to White's classification in Copenhagen series 1926–1972 (adapted from Pedersen 1977).

White classes	Total no. of infants	Infants with CM	
		No.	%
A	182	7 ⎫	3.9 ⎫
B	398	22 ⎬ 47	5.5 ⎬ 4.9
C	368	18 ⎭	4.9 ⎭
D	424	55 ⎫ 69	13.0 ⎫ 13.7
F	80	14 ⎭	17.5 ⎭

A strong *negative* tendency exists between insulin reactions, including insulin coma, in the first trimester and the incidence of malformations, and generally it is more difficult to compensate for diabetes in White's classes D + F with a high malformation rate than it is in classes A + B + C.   Seven women in the Rigshospital series had an infant with a fatal malformation (White class B + C: 2; D + F: 5), but in subsequent pregnancies one to six years later eight normal babies were born.   No prophylactic measures to compensate for the diabetic state had been taken; but the maternal complications, if altered, could only have worsened.   Finally four women in class F had babies with fatal malformations.   At their request we controlled their diabetes just before and after the start of the new pregnancy and each had a normal baby.

PLAN OF THE PRESENT STUDY

As there is a lack of direct measurements of the degree of compensation we have been looking for several indirect criteria which would allow a division of the Rigshospital series into two groups, one of which might be considered to have had a more normal metabolism, just before pregnancy and/or over the first trimester, than the other group.   As explained below, there is a natural division of the series into women attending or not attending a centre for the care of diabetics outside pregnancy.

The Rigshospital in Copenhagen has no Diabetes Department like those known in other countries, but its Obstetrics Department has a Diabetes Centre for pregnant diabetics.   In the Copenhagen area, however, the Hvidøre and the Steno Memorial hospitals care for diabetics, and both hospitals have a large clientèle.   The Rigshospital series includes the pregnant diabetics from the Steno Memorial and Hvidøre hospitals.   During pregnancy these patients and the remainder of the Rigshospital series follow the same regimen as inpatients and outpatients at the Diabetes Centre at the Obstetric Department.   Beforehand it was felt that the patients attending the two hospitals for diabetics, most of whom have been cared for over a span of years, might have a more normal metabolism generally than the remainder of the Rigshospital series, who were women living in or outside Copenhagen, especially in provincial cities and in the countryside, few of whom were attending any hospital department, never mind a diabetes department.   The malformation rate in the Steno Memorial + Hvidøre material was therefore compared with the remainder of the Rigshospital series in the expectation that we would find a lower rate in the Steno Memorial + Hvidøre material.

MATERIAL, METHOD AND DEFINITIONS

The Rigshospital series 1966–1977 has been analysed.   The investigation is prospective, consecutive and conducted by very few persons over the years.   The series comprises 949 infants with a birth weight of 1000 g and over.   Only malformations detected in the course of the first 10 neonatal days were included.   Congenital malformations were defined as structural abnormalities present at birth and detected by clinical examination or by X-ray examination performed on a clinical indication.   Some malformations were diagnosed only *post mortem.*

Poly- and syndactyly represent the mildest degree of malformation in the series.   *Severe malformations* comprise *partly* the fatal malformations (those responsible for intrauterine death or incompatible with extrauterine life for more than 10 days) and *partly* malformations causing death or necessitating major operations (e.g. cardiac surgery) within the first six months of life.   In the applied terminology thus, 'severe' is more severe than 'major', which we usually apply to malformations (see Pedersen 1977).

RESULTS

The malformation rate of 8.2% is similar to that usually found in the

TABLE 3
Rigshospital series 1966–1977: rate of CM in relation to White's classification

White	No. of	Rate of CM	
class	infants	No.	%
A	302	11	3.7
B	145	13	9.0
C	177	11	6.2
D	274	34	12.4
F	51	9	17.7
Total	949	78	8.2

Rigshospital series (Table 3).   The positive correlation between malformation rate and classes A–F is seen, but it is more distinct in the next few tables in which – owing to a lack of material – the five classes have been reduced to three.

The differences between the three groups of classes are statistically significant with the exception of that between classes A and B + C in severe malformations (Table 4).   No less than half of the malformations were severe, and the proportion of severe cases was the same in each White class.

Next, it is of more than local interest to note the similar malformation rates (total rate as well as the rate in White classes) for patients from either the Steno Memorial or the Hvidøre hospital (Table 5).   Furthermore, the increase in malformation rate between classes B + C and D + F in these patients was insignificant.

The malformation rate in White classes B–F was lower in the Steno Memorial + Hvidøre material compared with the remainder of the Rigshospital series, though for severe congenital malformations only insignificantly so (Table 6).

The more detailed analysis in Tables 7 and 8 shows that the difference in the

TABLE 4
Rigshospital series 1966–1977: rate (%) of total and severe CM in relation to White's reduced classification

White	No. of	Rate (%)	
class	infants	Total CM	Severe CM
A	302	3.7	2.0
B+C	322	7.5	3.7
D+F	325	13.2	7.1
Total	949	8.2	4.3

TABLE 5

Rate (%) of CM in the Steno Memorial and Hvidøre Hospital series

White class	Hvidøre		Steno Memorial	
	No. of infants	Rate	No. of infants	Rate
B+C	66	6.1	111	6.3
D+F	91	8.8	958.4	
Total	157	7.6	206	7.3

TABLE 6

Rate (%) of CM in the Hvidøre +Steno Memorial Hospital material and the remainder of the Rigshospital series 1966–1977: White classes B–F

Total CM		Severe CM	
Steno Mem. and Hvidøre material (363 infants)	Remainder of series (284 infants)	Steno Mem. and Hvidøre material (363 infants)	Remainder of series (284 infans)
7.4	14.1	4.4	6.7

TABLE 7

Rate (%) of CM in the Hvidøre + Steno Memorial Hospital material and the remainder of the Rigshospital series 1966–1977

White class	Steno Memorial and Hvidøre		Remainder of series	
	No. of infants	Rate	No. of infants	Rate
A	7	0	295	3.7
B + C	177	6.2	145	9.0
D + F	186	8.6	139	19.4

TABLE 8

Rate (%) of severe CM in the Hvidøre + Steno Memorial Hospital material and the remainder of the Rigshospital series 1966–1977

White class	Steno Memorial and Hvidøre		Remainder of series	
	No. of infants	Rate	No. of infants	Rate
A	7	0	295	2.0
B + C	177	4.5	145	2.7
D + F	186	4.3	139	10.8

rate of malformations between the Hvidøre + Steno Memorial material and the remainder of the Rigshospital series *is limited exclusively to White classes D + F,* while class A contains too few cases for a comparison. Only the difference in class D + F is significant (Table 7). This also applies to the rate of *severe* malformation alone (Table 8).

In summary we found that the rate of malformations in White classes B–F was significantly reduced from 14.1 to 7.4% in infants whose mothers attended the two hospitals (Steno Memorial and Hvidøre) which specialize in the treatment and ambulatory control of diabetics.

The rates of malformation (total as well as severe) were significantly reduced in infants of White's classes D + F alone, in which the maternal vascular complications are manifest, and the malformation rate is the highest.

The observations might be taken as demonstrating the importance of procuring constant care for diabetic women *outside* pregnancy in order to decrease the malformation rate. The case for teratogenicity being due primarily to maternal vascular complications has also been weakened.

Although several factors (e.g. chronological age of the mothers, their socioeconomic class, geographical birth places and residences) remain to be analysed, the new circumstantial evidence supports the plausible notion that poor diabetic control is teratogenic. Unfortunately, we have to stress the fact that at present with the 'best' care outside and inside pregnancy the rate of *severe* malformations is regrettably as high as 4.4% in White classes B–F.

We also found that the rate of severe, including fatal, malformations is increased in any White class in which severe malformation constitutes about half of the total malformation rate.

Several observations point to the presence of a 'disastrous malformation factor' in connection with maternal diabetic metabolism (Pedersen & Mølsted-Pedersen 1979).

The mechanism of the teratogenicity of the diabetic state seems to be not simply a question of good or poor compensation of the diabetic metabolism in the usual meaning, e.g. of blood glucose control. Since there is a low malformation rate in pregnancies with hypoglycaemic reactions, a fluctuating blood glucose level, as speculated by Reid (1970), is also not a probable mechanism. The unknown 'disastrous malformation factor' may be present or not, or in a high or low concentration, and the factor is to some extent, but not totally, dependent on the degree of compensation of the diabetes. Such a factor seems necessary to explain (1) the presence of very severe malformations in White's classes A and B, e.g. the caudal regression type, (2) the birth of completely normal babies to diabetics who notoriously have never had a compensated metabolism, and (3) why diabetic women can have fatally malformed infants one year and the next year a completely normal baby, although the metabolic compensation is not normal, yet is possibly better.

Although the 'malformation factor', alias the unknown mechanism of the teratogenicity of diabetes, appears *not* to be totally dependent on the degree of compensation of the diabetic metabolism, as measured by the variables usually applied, constant good compensation and care must be provided for any diabetic woman liable to become pregnant. But, even so, the increased risk of severe malformations will probably not be eliminated.

The enigma of the often disastrously severe malformations in infants of diabetic women remains to be further investigated.

References

PEDERSEN, J. (1977) *The Pregnant Diabetic and Her Newborn.* 2nd edn., pp. 191–197, Munksgaard, Copenhagen

PEDERSEN, J. & MOLSTED-PEDERSEN, L. (1979) Congenital malformations in newborns of diabetic mothers, in *Carbohydrate Metabolism in Pregnancy and the Newborn* (Sutherland, H. & Stowers, J., eds.) *(2nd Aberdeen Int. Colloq.)* Springer-Verlag, Berlin

PEDERSEN, L. MOLSTED, TYGSTRUP, I. & PEDERSEN, J. (1964) Congenital malformations in newborn infants of diabetic women. *Lancet 1,* 1124–1126

REID, R. A. (1970) Diabetes and congenital abnormalities. *Lancet 1,* 1030–1031

WHITE, P. (1965) Pregnancy and diabetes. Medical aspects. *Med. Clin. N. Am. 49,* 1015–1024

For discussion of this paper, see pp. 273-281

Discussion of the two preceding papers

Gillmer: Professor Pedersen, one problem is how one assesses control. Can you quantify control as opposed to giving a qualitative estimation? Where the patients had intensive care for their diabetes how would you define control?

Pedersen: I cannot give a figure. It is only one speculation that control may be better for those patients. The socioeconomic conditions may be better too. At present we don't know.

Gillmer: I was very interested in the recent reports of Sönksen *et al.* (1978) and Walford *et al.* (1978) concerning the value of Dextrostix-type analysers for assessing control in pregnant and non-pregnant diabetics. These instruments may provide the means for doing a prospective epidemiological study. Tattersall's group (Walford *et al.* 1978) have shown that non-pregnant patients, who are probably less highly motivated than pregnant diabetics, will do their own plasma glucose measurements as many as 11 times a day twice a week. This technique would provide a much better quantitative estimate of plasma glucose control than any in current use and could be used to determine how good the control is during the first trimester in groups of patients with and without fetal malformations.

Pedersen: I agree on the need for quantitative estimation of control but I don't think that that could be an acceptable way.

Beard: At King's College Hospital they consistently have a lower incidence of malformations than you see, Professor Pedersen. The only difference is that they appear to have more patients whose diabetes is already well controlled when they become pregnant, which suggests that metabolic control is important. Until we can assess the effect of diabetic control achieved during the first trimester in a prospective type of study we cannot say whether it is in any way a factor that can be implicated in the causation of fetal anomalies. Haemoglobin A_{1c} is still a rather general index of control that we are not sure about.

Pedersen: Unfortunately the malformation rate at King's College Hospital is not much different from ours (Gamsu 1978). The malformation rate is not as low as I expected in looking for support of the 'metabolic' hypothesis.

Beard: That is the point I am trying to make. Both the Steno Memorial patients and the King's patients are well controlled when they become pregnant so it looks as though preconceptual control has something to do with it.

Pedersen: I think we can agree on 'something'.

Williamson: Have you compared the rates of malformation for non-diabetic mothers in urban and non-urban populations?

Pedersen: Not yet. We should be very open-minded about what I call the

273

malformation factor.   It must be something that occurs in the general population but is much more frequent in diabetics, without being simply diabetes, e.g. too slow a passage of the ovum through the tube, or a noxious, non-insulin-dependent, secondary product of diabetes.

Battaglia: We may be focusing too much on glucose here.   There might be changes in metabolism, for instance of relatively minor carbohydrates. Myoinositol, for example, is the sugar in highest concentration in CNS as a free carbohydrate.   Calcium concentration may be important in regulating cell division.   People seem to agree now that paternal diabetes has no association with the anomaly rate and that gestational diabetes in the mother has no association with it.

Pedersen: It depends on your definition of gestational diabetes.

Beard: You mean gestational and not prediabetes?

Battaglia: Yes.   There is also agreement that the degree of control at least reduces the severe congenital anomaly rate but there is still a residual increased anomaly rate; even in well-controlled groups it is higher than normal.   Do we know anything about how well the daughters of diabetic mothers do as reproducing females?   A number of interesting leads in both humans and animals show that what is done to the female fetus *in utero* affects performance when that female reaches the reproductive age.   Were your diabetic patients who had a high congenital anomaly rate and were well controlled the daughters of diabetic mothers?   Damage to the ovary of the fetus of a diabetic mother may not be associated with changes in body proportions at birth but it is possible that a crucial organ (the ovary) in the female infant of the diabetic mother was affected.   After all, there is already cell death in the ovary at the time of birth which continues through childhood into the reproductive age.

Pedersen: I don't know anything specifically about the anomaly rates in such women.   They are very few.

Beard: The congenital anomaly rate for non-diabetic women whose mothers were diabetics would be important too, wouldn't it?

Battaglia: Yes.

Kalkhoff: What about the non-diabetic women who have babies with congenital anomalies?   Are there clues from the environment or drugs and other things?   Is there a difference in the incidence of congenital anomalies in people who live in rural areas versus urban areas?   This is a very broad epidemiological question, with all sorts of variables.

Pedersen: We know there are such differences.   We have the material from about 2000 cases from 1946 on and it remains to see whether there is any clustering to special regions of Denmark.

Beard: One of the major factors in the incidence of congenital anomaly is the social class of the individual.   It would be valuable to know the social class distribution in your series.

Pedersen: We will do that in a more extensive study, with many more cases.

Dr Bergstein, among those malformations of your patients should some have been spontaneous abortions?

Bergstein: We have in our clinic some women who had a high rate of abortions and who had diabetes.   In this group we also found a high rate of uterine anomalies.   There is a group of obstetricians in Holland who believe that many women who have diabetes or prediabetes also have anomalies of the uterus.   J. L. Mastboom from the University of Nijmegen is using an unusual method of therapy for patients with diabetes who have had many failed pregnancies.   They are divided into groups with manifest, latent and potential diabetes (Table 1).

The 14 patients with manifest diabetes had lost eight conceptuses before 17 weeks and 27 after the 16th week of pregnancy.   The 135 patients in the latent group between them had 286 pregnancies with abortions before the 17th week and 167 pregnancies which lasted more than 16 weeks.   So the total of 205 patients had 684 failed pregnancies, 439 of which were abortions and 255 of which were deliveries after the 16th week of pregnancy.   Mastboom treated all these patients with insulin very early in pregnancy, sometimes immediately after ovulation and before pregnancy was diagnosed.   On this regimen the 14 patients with manifest diabetes produced 14 healthy child-

TABLE 1 (Bergstein)
Repeated failures of pregnancy in relation to diabetes (data from J. L. Mastboom, University of Nijmegen)

Diabetes	No. of patients	Previous failures (n = 684)		After treatment	
		<17 wk	>16 wk	Live children	Failed pregnancies
Manifest	14	8	27	14	0
Latent	135	286	167	128	8
Potential	56	145	51	51	4
	205	439	245	193	12
		684		(95%)	

N.B. *Manifest* diabetes: relatively frequent fetal death > 16 wk
Latent/potential diabetes: relatively frequent fetal death < 16 wk

ren.   The 135 in the latent group had 128 healthy children and eight unsuc-cessful pregnancies.   The 56 potential diabetics gave birth to 51 healthy children and only four unsuccessful pregnancies.   Mastboom is at present giving 12–16 units of insulin and stops this therapy in the 32nd week of pregnancy.   Then after one week he does a glucose tolerance test.   He told me that he found pathological glucose tolerance tests in those cases.   Early in these pregnancies, the glucose tolerance test was not disturbed after a glucose load.   He treated those patients and the outcome of pregnancy was mostly very successful.   He defines a potential diabetic as a woman who will develop mild diabetes later in her life, because there is diabetes in the family and/or disturbance in her obstetrical history which could be caused by diabetes (intrauterine death or neonatal death, habitual abortions, habitual premature parturition, congenital malformations of the child, hydramnios, macroso-mia).   However, all these women have a normal oral GTT before the pregnancy.   The latent diabetic, he says, is a woman who had a normal oral GTT before the pregnancy but has a pathological oral glucose tolerance test in the second or third trimester.   So with insulin treatment in the early part of pregnancy he gets this improvement in full-term deliveries with healthy child-ren.   As far as I know, these children have no congenital malformations.

Stowers: In Treharne & Sutherland's (1979) study of chemical gestational diabetes in Aberdeen one of the reasons for testing is obesity.   They were able to look at the birth weights of many of these women because they were born in the same hospital and recorded there.   They found that 86% of those obese women shown to have chemical diabetes when tested in pregnancy were in the top quartile of birth weight themselves, whereas this was true in only 24% of those with normal intravenous glucose tolerance.   We also know that glucose intolerance is positively associated with congenital anomalies.   If we test mothers of infants with congenital anomalies there is an increased inci-dence of glucose intolerance, looking at it the other way.

Kalkhoff: Were the mothers of these heavy babies diabetic or don't you know?

Stowers: They were not known to be diabetics.

Freinkel: Quite clearly, with glucose we are talking about an insulin-dependent fuel.   As we discussed earlier, we should broaden this to include a variety of fuels which contribute to anabolism in an integrated fashion and which are also insulin-dependent, i.e. amino acids and fats.   One could go further and consider a series of phenomena due to metabolic changes which are not insulin-dependent by themselves but which arise via derangements in insulin-dependent fuels.   Haemoglobin A_{1c} is a prototypic example (Bunn *et al.* 1978).   Herein, a change supervenes which is not affected by insulin but which depends upon a fuel which has gone awry due to insulin lack.   In other words, the hyperglycaemia *per se* is the culprit.   Such post-translational changes in protein structure need not necessarily be confined to haemoglobin.   It is quite conceivable that glucose-dependent glycosylations could equally affect a variety of proteins, including the placenta, the lens of the eye, basement membranes and a whole spectrum of structures with appropriately reactive groupings.   Other possibilities also warrant consideration.   For example, whenever the ambient fuel mixture is varied, preferential substrate selections become operative.   As we discussed earlier, many tissues seem to oxidize ketones and/or fatty acids in place of glucose or amino acids when the former are added to artificial substrate mixtures (Shambaugh *et al.* 1977*a, b*).   The precise implications of such oxidative substitutions remain to be clarified.   Conceivably, the sparing of some fuels in preference to others might effect changes in structure as well as function.

Finally, there are certain reactions which arise in a non-insulin-dependent fashion.   The polyol pathway has always been cited as one of the best examples (Winegrad *et al.* 1972; Gabbay 1973).   Herein, pathways of glucose disposition become operative in cells which contain the appropriate enzymes whenever they are confronted with a plethora of glucose.   The consequent intracellular accumulation of polyols such as sorbitol and fructose has been invoked as a classical explanation for consequent cellular pathology.   We have only recently begun to appreciate that the defects may not be due to the accumulation of polyols but rather to the concurrent depletion of myoinositol.   In other words, it would appear that intracellular myoinositol may become depleted whenever there is concurrent competition for non-insulin-dependent glucose entry.   The levels of free myoinositol in most tissues (Dawson & Freinkel 1961) are already close to the K_m for biosynthesis of phosphatidylinositol (Paulus & Kennedy 1960; Lucus *et al.* 1970).   One can speculate that formation of this phospholipid may be compromised in any situation in which intracellular myoinositol depletion occurs (Freinkel *et al.* 1975).   Could this have pathophysiological significance?   There is an excellent example from recent studies by Winegrad's group of nerve conduction defects in streptozotocin-diabetic rats (Greene *et al.* 1975).   They showed that when hyperglycaemia occurred in these animals, not only did sorbitol and fructose accumulate in the sciatic motor nerves, but free myoinositol also decreased.   Complete amelioration of the nerve conduction defect occurred when 1% myoinositol was included in the diet and tissue inositol was repleted even though hyperglycaemia was not attenuated and the accumulation of sorbitol and fructose within the nerve was not diminished (Greene *et al.* 1975).   Here then, again, a secondary metabolic lesion, i.e. the depletion of intracellular myoinositol, which had been triggered by an insulin-dependent fuel, i.e. hyperglycaemia, was perpetuated quite independently of our conventional concepts of insulin-mediated mechanisms.

Our own recent preoccupation with amino acids of the central nervous system has been prompted by the same type of consideration (L. Airoldi *et al.* unpublished observations, 1977–1978). Insulinopenia gives a distorted profile for plasma amino acids. The altered pattern of circulating amino acids can, in turn, initiate an intracellular realignment of neurohumoral precursors. The latter can sustain pathophysiological changes independent of continuing mediation by insulin lack.

Beard: From an epidemiological point of view we must always remember that it may not be diabetes *per se* which is responsible for congenital anomaly. Otherwise every diabetic woman would have an abnormal baby. It is likely that it is diabetes plus some other factor such as low social class which is responsible.

Freinkel: I would suggest that the 'something else' could be linked to a self-perpetuating spiral of metabolic derangements which no longer requires insulinopenia to sustain itself. Obviously, however, interruption of that spiral would require rectification of the insulinopenia or repletion of the specific moiety through which the cycle is sustained (as with the myoinositol to which I alluded earlier).

Deuchar: Could the something else be in the genetic make-up of the fetus? In the rat sometimes only one or two fetuses out of a whole litter are abnormal yet they have all been subjected to the same kind of metabolic abnormality of the mother. Why aren't they all affected?

Freinkel: In Harvey Knowles's study of juvenile diabetics (1971) about 20% seemed to have some genetic resistance to vascular complications. In these patients after 30 years or more of 'poorly controlled' juvenile onset diabetes, clinically significant retinopathy and nephropathy could not be demonstrated.

Battaglia: You can't say that it is due to genetic factors without doing proper breeding experiments in polytocous species. The idea that the environment is the same because they are in the same litter is naive. The placentas could be different and the environment to which each fetus is exposed could be quite different in a polytocous species. You put it very strongly when you said that if it was diabetes that produced anomalies then every diabetic mother must produce a baby with anomalies. I don't know that we should put it that way. If toxins that we know are teratogenic are given to animals they rarely produce anomalies in every fetus. Yet if you remove that toxin you don't get the anomalies. It seems that one is searching for the background factors in a fetus which, when the additional multiple factors of diabetes are introduced, may lead to anomalies.

There are other ways in which one could produce anomalies through diabetes that would not be directly glucose-dependent. Inositol is the carbohydrate in highest concentration in the water phase of neural tissue, skeletal muscle, heart (Battaglia *et al.* 1961) and a number of tissues that we know may develop anomalies in these infants. At some conferences people have discussed environmental hazards that produce anomalies. In those areas also people don't often study the ovaries of fetuses that are exposed to hazards such as diabetes and environmental toxins. I think we all ought to be encouraged, where appropriate, to look at those cells.

Kalkhoff: Dr Freinkel, have you been able to relate your studies of maternal amino acid metabolism to the outcome of pregnancy? Do you or anyone else know of any instances in which amino acids in maternal blood are abnormal in association with an abnormal outcome of pregnancy?

Chez: There is the example of phenylketonuria which is not recognized in the heterozygous or carrier mother. Apparently she has enough excess phenylalanine to affect the otherwise normal fetus adversely.

Hoet: It has been suggested that a low phenylalanine diet during pregnancy may prevent the brain damage occurring in the non-phenylketonuric children (Mabry *et al.* 1963; Perry & Tischler 1966). This is another important example of maternal nutrients influencing the performance of the child's brain. The phenylalanine levels were not remarkably high in the mother.

Young: Phenylketonuria is rather an extreme case because the plasma levels of phenylalanine are at least 1 mM in the untreated homozygous mother and much higher in the fetal plasma. Maternal hyperphenylalaninaemia, in which the plasma levels are not high enough to exceed the renal threshold might give us more clues. Homozygous phenylketonuria infants born of heterozygous mothers have quite normal plasma phenylalanine levels at birth, presumably due to excretion of the amino acid by the placenta. There is some foreshadowing of the metabolic disorder because these infants are light for their gestational age at birth and have a high incidence of prematurity and perinatal problems (Scriver & Rosenberg 1973).

Hull: With the possible exception of sacral agenesis, the congenital abnormalities in the infants of diabetic mothers appear to be the same as those found in the rest of the community. We need to know the incidence of those abnormalities in the community from which a study is made if we are to conclude that there has been an increase. I would like to hear a distinction made between those congenital abnormalities that are known to be polygenically inherited, with accepted inheritance risks, and those congenital abnormalities which have not got a strongly established polygenic inheritance and in which environmental factors may be important in producing that disturbance. It would be very interesting to know whether those defects in which no strong genetic trend has been demonstrated are increased or decreased in frequency.

Beard: It is important to make the point that diabetes is a general metabolic disturbance for which one particular component may take a greater share of the disturbance in one individual compared with another.

Hull: That is on the assumption that diabetes is a single disorder and that it is polygenically inherited. The statement that there is no link between the genetic pattern of the diabetic and the genetic pattern of the abnormality is very difficult to make with confidence, because of the relative infrequency of the two conditions. That is why I think one has to distinguish between the abnormalities we are talking about rather than say that glucose has a blanket influence on the incidence of all abnormalities.

Bennett: You are absolutely correct. Presumably a lot more information might come out if it were possible to get large enough numbers to do the sorts of comparisons you are talking about. Even the largest series reported so far are hopelessly small for that type of analysis.

Hull: But until you get the numbers you can't start drawing the kinds of conclusions that are being made at the moment.

Beard: Dr Deuchar may have had some luck finding that the administration of a single agent may constantly induce fetal anomaly.

Hull: In sacral agenesis the position is a lot clearer. It seems that diabetes is a major factor in the genesis of that abnormality. That is why I don't despair quite so much on the epidemiological approach. It would be interesting to know in Professor Pedersen's series just what sorts of congenital abnormalities were less frequent in the group that had the lower incidence. In other words, did you reduce the number of infants with spina bifida or anencephaly, or did you actually reduce some of the other abnormalities which don't have such a strong genetic trend? It would be interesting to know whether the distribution of the individual abnormalities was the same in the two groups, if they came from the same population.

Pedersen: We will do that. But we will have groups of only 35 to 50 cases, so it will be a little difficult. However, a comparison between the 32 and 28 congenital malformations of the heart found in the Copenhagen series, 1926–1972, and in the non-diabetic control series, respectively, did not disclose any significant difference in type of malformation. The types were similar, only more severe in the diabetic series (Pedersen 1977).

References

BATTAGLIA, F. C., MESCHIA, G., BLECHNER, J. N. & BARRON, D. H. (1961) The free myo-inositol concentration of adult and fetal tissues of several species. *Q.J. Exp. Physiol. Cogn. Med. Sci. 46*, 188–193

BUNN, H. F., GABBAY, K. H. & GALLOP, P. M. (1978) The glycosylation of hemoglobin: relevance to diabetes mellitus. *Science (Wash. D.C.) 200*, 21–27

DAWSON, R. M. C. & FREINKEL, N. (1961) The distribution of free *myo*inositol in mammalian tissues, including some observations on the lactating rat. *Biochem. J. 78*, 606–610

FREINKEL, N., EL YOUNSI, C. & DAWSON, R. M. C. (1975) Inter-relations between the phospho-lipids of rat pancreatic islets during glucose stimulation and their response to medium inositol and tetracaine. *Eur. J. Biochem. 59*, 245–252

GABBAY K. H. (1973) The sorbitol pathway and the complications of diabetes. *New Engl. J. Med. 288*, 831–836

GAMSU, H. R. (1978) Neonatal morbidity in infants of diabetic mothers. *J. R. Soc. Med. 71*, 211–222

GREENE, D. A., DEJESUS, P. V. Jr. & WINEGRAD, A. (1975) Effects of insulin and dietary myoinositol on impaired peripheral motor nerve conduction velocity in acute streptozotocin diabetes. *J. Clin. Invest. 55*, 1326–1336

KNOWLES, H. C. Jr. (1971) Long term juvenile diabetes treated with unmeasured diet. *Trans. Assoc. Am. Phys. 84*, 95–101

LUCUS, C. T., CALL, F. L. II, & WILLIAMS, W. J. (1970) The biosynthesis of phosphatidylinositol in human platelets. *J. Clin. Invest. 49*, 1949–1955

MABRY, C. C., DENNISTON, J. C., NELSON, I. L. & SON, C. D. (1963) Maternal phenylketonuria: cause of mental retardation in children without metabolic defect. *New Engl. J. Med. 269*, 1404–1408

PAULUS, H. & KENNEDY, E. P. (1960) The enzymatic synthesis of inositol monophosphatide. *J. Biol. Chem. 235*, 1303–1311

PEDERSEN, J. (1977) *The Pregnant Diabetic and Her Newborn*, 2nd edn., pp. 191–197, Munks-gaard, Copenhagen

PERY, Th. L. & TISCHLER, B. (1966) Phenylketonuria in a woman of normal intelligence and her child. *New Engl. J. Med. 274*, 1018–1019

SCRIVER, C. R. & ROSENBERG, L. E. (1973) *Amino Acid Metabolism and its Disorders*, p.306, Saunders, Philadelphia

SHAMBAUGH, G. E. III, MROZAK, S. C. & FREINKEL, N. (1977*a*) Fetal fuels. I. Utilization of ketones by isolated tissues at various stages of maturation and maternal nutrition during late gestation. *Metabolism 26*, 623–636

SHAMBAUGH, G. E. III, KOEHLER, R. A. & FREINKEL, N. (1977*b*) Fetal fuels. II. Contributions of selected carbo fuels to oxidation metabolism in the rat conceptus. *Am. J. Physiol. 233*, E457–E461

SÖNKSEN, P. H., JUDD, S. L. & LOWY, C. (1978) Home monitoring of blood-glucose. *Lancet 1*, 729–733

TREHARNE, I. A. L. & SUTHERLAND, H. W. (1979) Reproduction in obese women, in *Carbohy-drate Metabolism in Pregnancy and the Newborn* (Sutherland, H. W & Stowers, J. M., eds.), Springer-Verlag, Berlin

WALFORD, S., GALE, E. A. M., ALLISON, S. P. & TATTERSALL, R. B. (1978) Self-monitoring of blood-glucose. *Lancet 1*, 732–735

WINEGRAD, A. I., CLEMENTS, R. S. Jr. & MORRISON, D. A. (1972) Insulin-independent path-ways of carbohydrate metabolism, in *Handb. Physiol.* Sect. 7: *Endocrinology*, Vol. 1: *The Endocrine Pancreas* (Steiner, D. & Freinkel, N., eds.), pp. 457–471, Williams & Wilkins, Baltimore

Clinical perspectives in the care of the pregnant diabetic patient

J.J. HOET and R.W. BEARD*

*Université Catholique de Louvain, Brussels and *St Mary's Hospital Medical School, London*

Abstract Despite the considerable improvement in the care of the diabetic mother and the prognosis for her baby, a number of clinical problems remain unresolved.   Apart from the increased incidence of major and minor fetal anomalies, morbidity amongst the newborn and the high incidence of diabetes in later life of women who have had relatively minor carbohydrate intolerance during pregnancy are a cause for concern.   In this paper the outstanding clinical problems and their possible solutions are considered.   The elucidation of the origin of congenital malformations is discussed.

   The prevention of congenital anomalies in the diabetic requires a precise knowledge of their aetiology which is currently not available.   However, on the hypothesis that diabetes creates an abnormal biochemical environment which may well disturb embryogenesis, it is logical to try and control maternal blood sugar as soon as possible in pregnancy or even before conception.   To extend this argument further, it follows naturally that the maintenance of normoglycaemia throughout pregnancy until delivery is also desirable.   The practicalities of various methods of screening for diabetes in pregnancy and new approaches in the medical and obstetric problems of the pregnant diabetic are also considered.   Finally, the question of contraception and its implications for the woman who is known to have carbohydrate intolerance in pregnancy is discussed.

The care of the pregnant diabetic patient continues to have important clinical implications.   With the increasing safety to mother and fetus that results from good antenatal care, young diabetic women are less inclined to accept the advice that they should limit their families.   In addition, the incidence of diabetes in the population is said to be increasing.   For these reasons it would be wrong to believe that the major clinical problems of the pregnant diabetic have been solved and to adopt an attitude of complacency.   The fact that the incidence of congenital malformation amongst diabetic mothers remains unchanged and the morbidity of the newborn is still high (Gabbe *et al.* 1977) is a clear indication of how little we understand of the influence on the developing fetus of the environment provided by the mother.

It seems likely that diabetes interferes with the normal physiological metabolic adaptation of the mother to the needs of the developing fetus.   Biochemical changes may well affect placental function, embryogenesis and organogenesis, as a result of which the normal adaptive mechanisms of the fetus which ensure that growth and development proceed smoothly, may be interrupted at critical stages.   The fetus of the diabetic is known to have a tendency to the premature release of more insulin than is normal which, amongst the many effects on the fetus, is probably responsible for excessive growth, abnormal maturation of pulmonary tissue (Smith *et al.* 1975) and inhibition of hepatic enzyme activity (Räihä, this symposium).   The studies of Deuchar (1979), showing how maternal diabetes can produce skeletal anomalies in the fetus, reveal how seriously normal development can be disorganized.

The perinatal mortality associated with diabetes in pregnancy has shown a consistent fall, especially during recent years, in the major centres with a special interest in this subject (Essex *et al.* 1973; Hare & White 1977; Pedersen 1977). One might be tempted to think that pregnancy for the diabetic is no longer a major obstetric problem, until one looks closely at the criteria of successful outcome other than perinatal mortality.   Not only is the incidence of congenital malformations still significantly higher amongst diabetics compared with non-diabetics but morbidity amongst the newborn from hypoglycaemia, hyperbilirubinaemia, and respiratory distress has been reported to be as high as 25% (Gabbe *et al.* 1977).   In addition, Persson (1979) has emphasized the considerable difference in results between hospitals with a special interest in the subject and hospitals that manage diabetes as part of their routine obstetric service.   In a nearby hospital that apparently applied the same principles of management as his own, Persson found that the perinatal mortality was very much higher.

This paper deals with some of the recent developments in the care and management of the pregnant diabetic.   Consideration is also given to the potential of these developments and some of the practical problems they pose.

THE PREVENTION OF CONGENITAL MALFORMATIONS

For the future, the critical question for clinicians caring for the pregnant diabetic is how to reduce the incidence of congenital malformations.   To do this, they must have more knowledge than is at present available on the origin of these malformations and, in particular, the influence of diabetes on the ovum and developing embryo.   It seems probable that information of this nature is more likely to come, not from the human, but from experimental studies such as those of Horii *et al.* (1966) using alloxan to induce diabetes, or Deuchar (1979) using streptozotocin.

These experiments revealed that the abnormal environment resulting from uncompensated diabetes can influence both the preimplantation and implantation stages. Fertility is diminished and, in those animals that do become pregnant, resorptions are increased. However, we need to know the specific metabolic insults to the fertilized ovum before and after implantation which induce abnormal cell division. For example, do the changes in the mucopolysaccharides of cell membranes, which are a feature of diabetes in the nonpregnant, occur in the oocyte? Equally, since the oocyte allows the passage of nutrients and makes food reserves in its cytoplasm, is the trypsin-digestible material on the membrane affected by the disease? Are these particular functions under passive or active environmental control? Does the ovum after fertilization become in some manner more sensitive to environmental changes? It is well known that the fertilized ovum is metabolically very active, having an increased oxygen consumption, protein synthesis and monophosphate shunt. The fact that protein synthesis is likely to be dependent on RNA formed in the oocyte before ovulation underlines the possible importance of good diabetic control before conception.

Chapman (1976) showed that the rate of cleavage is determined by the mother. The differentiation of the blastocyst is also dependent on the external environment which can influence the differentiation of cells into trophoblasts. However, it is the inner cells which will eventually become the embryo proper. Protein synthesis at this stage depends on the messenger RNA transmitted from the embryogenome. Up to the stage of implantation the life of the embryonic cells is dependent on their own protein synthesis. Micromolecules can be exchanged between cells, and glucose is transferred by means of a carrier system. At implantation the cellular contacts and exchange of micromolecules are initiated between the mother and her embryo. At any of these stages of development diabetes may interrupt or disorganize these delicate interactions. Deuchar (1979) has shown that, although the fertilized ovum of the diabetic can survive, it may not achieve implantation at the blastocyst stage or may be subsequently resorbed. The factor influencing these changes may well be in the red blood cells. Dr Deuchar was able to show that the characteristic effects of diabetes were not seen when maternal serum, from which the RBC's had been removed, was used. A possible explanation for this observation might be the effect of reduced oxygenation due to the presence of glycosylated haemoglobin. However, little is known about the sensitivity of the early embryo to hypoxia.

It seems unlikely that the many kinds of congenital malformations associated with maternal diabetes have the same origin. For example, fetal skeletal anomalies may well be induced relatively late in pregnancy. The maturation of fetal bone which is characterized by ossification and resorption of cartilage occurs late in intrauterine life and is a slow process. It has been shown, *in vitro,* that certain types of malformations, in particular skeletal, can be produced by injecting insulin into chick embryos (Duraiswami 1959). *In vitro* experiments on bone preparations of the early embryonic phase also indicate that the effect of insulin is dose-related (Chen 1954). In addition, it has been shown in animals with experimentally induced diabetes that good control of the blood sugar, apart from preventing fetal hyperinsulinism, also prevents fetal skeletal anomalies, in particular sacral agenesis (Horii *et al.* 1966; Deuchar 1979). In the human, hyperinsulinaemia is often found in the mature fetus of the diabetic (Oakley *et al.* 1972), but whether the increase occurs early enough and is of sufficient severity to induce skeletal malformations still has to be determined.

What is the influence of diabetes on the intellectual development of the fetus? Persson & Gentz (1977) could find no evidence of intellectual impairment in the offspring of women whose diabetes had been well controlled throughout pregnancy, whereas the Copenhagen group (Yssing 1975) found, in a group whose control was not stated, definite evidence of an increase. It may well be that once again diabetic control is the critical factor. If this is so then to what feature of poor diabetic control can the effect on intellect be ascribed? The possibility that ketone bodies may be implicated has been suggested (Berendes 1975). However, this work has been challenged by Naeye (this symposium), who discussed the many other possible aetiological factors known to be associated with poor intellectual performance of the offspring. He made the point that when women with complications known to be associated with intellectual impairment of the offspring were excluded, the association with ketosis could not be demonstrated. This is a question that needs to be resolved because of the considerable anxiety it has induced.

The foregoing discussion reveals how little is known about the origin of congenital anomalies in diabetes. However, it does seem likely that the key to the problem lies in good diabetic control at the time of conception. How can this be achieved? At present, diabetics are rarely seen before the end of the first trimester of pregnancy. Characteristically their control is poor at that time and many present for the first time with a hyperglycaemic or hypoglycaemic crisis – they are often taking oral hypoglycaemic agents and have no knowledge about the effect that pregnancy will have on their diabetes or on their baby. Undoubtedly the single most effective way of dealing with the problem is to educate young diabetic women well before they become pregnant. The importance of planning their pregnancy so that as good control as possible is obtained before they attempt to become pregnant must be stressed.   This education can be provided by general practitioners and diabetologists, but it would be much more effective if approached as a campaign by an organization with a particular interest in diabetes, such as the British Diabetic Association or the International Diabetic Federation.

Finally, good control of the diabetic whose pregnancy has advanced beyond the period of gestation when organogenesis is thought to be critical may also reduce the incidence of children with defects.   The results of Roversi *et al.* (1977) are of considerable interest because they suggest that, even if good control of the diabetes is not achieved until the second or third trimester, the incidence of malformations expected from the past history of malformations and the fact that the mothers had diabetes, is reduced.

Further epidemiological research is needed into the factors responsible for congenital defects in diabetics and the means of reducing them.   For instance, it could be that diabetes increases the predisposition to congenital malformations in individuals known to be at risk, such as those who have had a baby with a neural tube defect.   No mention has been made in this review of haemoglobin A_{1c}, but it may prove to be a useful index of the pre-existing diabetes and thereby provide a guide to the likely risk of congenital malformation.   The place of α-fetoprotein and ultrasound screening for defects also needs to be considered for the future.

SCREENING FOR DIABETES IN PREGNANCY

It is well recognized that pregnancy increases insulin resistance and in those with borderline carbohydrate tolerance this may lead to transient chemical diabetes.   The follow-up studies of O'Sullivan (1979) suggest that as many as 60% of these women become insulin-requiring diabetics 10 years later.   Of more immediate consequence is the effect on the fetus of the metabolic disturbance which characterizes diabetes.   There is good epidemiological evidence, reviewed by Beard & Oakley (1976), that the incidence of congenital malformations is about three times the normal.   Pregnant women have a variable degree of carbohydrate intolerance and it is still a matter of opinion at what point it should be regarded as 'diabetic'.   However, it does seem sensible to try to detect those who are clearly abnormal, in an attempt to reduce the incidence of congenital abnormalities and so that they can be treated.   How effective this is in reducing the incidence of congenital abnormalities still has to be demonstrated, but for the time being it is the only approach that is available which is likely to be effective.

Diagnostic criteria

Successful detection of diabetes clearly depends on the condition being diagnosed early enough in pregnancy for the patient to be able to benefit from therapy.   Many physicians apply criteria for diagnosing diabetes which may be suitable for the non-pregnant individual but have little relevance to the problems that arise when the disease is associated with pregnancy.   Although advancing pregnancy tends to increase carbohydrate intolerance in the mother, thereby making management more difficult, of greater significance is the fact that even minor degrees of carbohydrate intolerance may influence fetal development.   O'Sullivan & Mahan (1964) and Guttorm (1975) have defined an abnormal value in an oral glucose tolerance test (OGTT) as being more than two standard deviations above the mean from a group of pregnant women with no features of potential diabetes.   O'Sullivan & Mahan (1964) have stated precisely that 'the diagnosis should be made on a 3-hour GTT after the oral administration of 100 g of glucose after preliminary dietary preparation and with Somogyi Nelson glucose determination on venous whole blood.   A diagnosis of carbohydrate intolerance can only be made if two or more values equal or exceed 90 mg/100 ml [5 mmol/l] fasting, 165 mg/100 ml [9.2 mmol/l] one hour, 145 mg/100 ml [8.1 mmol/l] two hours, and 125 mg/100 ml [6.9 mmol/l] three hours after the start of the test.'   This definition is soundly based on results obtained from a large, well-conducted study.   Its defect, as far as pregnancy is concerned, is that it is not based on the effect of maternal carbohydrate intolerance on the developing fetus.

Gillmer *et al.* (1975*a,b*), using a standard 50 g oral load in normal and chemical diabetic pregnant women, compared the results with the plasma glucose concentration of their babies two hours after delivery.   A highly significant correlation was found between these variables, demonstrating that the glucose regulation in the mother is reflected in the fetus.   From these data, using a glucose value of 30 mg/100 ml (1.7 mmol/l) as evidence of neonatal hypoglycaemia, we determined critical diagnostic criteria for the OGTT in pregnancy (Beard 1976).   Critical values for the fasting, one- and two-hour values and 'area of the curve' of maternal OGTT were determined that correctly predicted whether the baby was likely to become hypoglycaemic two hours after delivery.   It was found that the critical OGTT values in this study differed little from those of O'Sullivan & Mahan (1964).   This is of interest when one remembers that these authors used a 100 g rather than a 50 g glucose load, suggesting that while their relative values are correct, the absolute values are a little high if normoglycaemia in the newborn is the end-point used for determining the significance of the OGTT.   Gillmer *et al.* (1975*a,b*) observed that the best correlation was found between the total area under the OGTT curve and the two-hour neonatal glucose concentration.   Plasma glucose values above 43 units (mmol/l) or 755 units (mg/100 ml) were considered abnormal.

Screening in pregnancy

Numerous methods of screening for diabetes in pregnancy are in use.   The generally accepted method is to test a random sample of urine in the antenatal clinic, and glycosuria on two consecutive occasions is an indication to perform a GTT.   Sutherland *et al.* (1970) have demonstrated how insensitive this system is.   The incidence of glycosuria among 1418 pregnant women was 11%, yet the incidence of chemical diabetes among these glycosuric women was less than 1%.   In contrast, the incidence of diabetes was 7% amongst a group of potential diabetic women with no glycosuria.

If every case of carbohydrate intolerance is to be picked up, then logically all women should have a GTT in early and late pregnancy.   This would ensure not only that all diabetics would be picked up as early as possible in pregnancy, but also that the diabetogenic effect of pregnancy would be detected.   Such a policy, although ideal, is unrealistic.   If the expected incidence of previously unrecognized abnormal OGTT values amongst pregnant women is accepted as being about 2.5% (O'Sullivan *et al.* 1973) then it is clear that the majority of pregnant women would be subjected to an unnecessary and expensive test.   A greater degree of selection needs to be applied that is not easy to administer but also maintains a reasonable balance between success of detection and expense.   This has long been recognized by those who have attempted to devise practical screening tests.

Many screening systems have been advocated but two are particularly worthy of consideration.   O'Sullivan *et al.* (1973) have proposed the oral administration of a 50 g glucose load without prior fasting by the patient.   All patients with a value of 130 mg/100 ml (7.2 mmol/l) or more, one hour after drinking the glucose, have a full three-hour OGTT.   They showed that this test picked out about 80% of those with an abnormal GTT, that is, 20% of those with an abnormal GTT had a screening blood sugar of less than 130 mg/100 ml and so were missed.   A similar study done at St Mary's Hospital, London (unpublished study), using a screening value of 140 mg/100 ml (7.8 mmol/l) plasma glucose revealed that, of the 948 women screened, 74 (7.8%) had a positive screening value and of these 14 (1.5%) had an abnormal GTT.   Of the 14, five had no features of potential diabetes, nor did they develop glycosuria at any time during their pregnancies, confirming the conclusions of O'Sullivan *et al.* (1973).   O'Sullivan and co-workers suggested that, since 84% of these women with abnormal OGTT values were aged 25 or over, there would be a saving in time and money if screening was confined to women in this age group, who represented less than 50% of their pregnant population. They also suggested that all those with potential diabetic features or an abnormal screening value with a normal OGTT should be screened again at 28 weeks of gestation.

The Copenhagen group have proposed a different screening system which depends on the presence of glycosuria and certain features of potential diabetes (Guttorm 1975; Pedersen 1977). They showed that the incidence of abnormal OGTT in a group of 514 pregnant women was 5% amongst the glycosuric women and 1% in those without glycosuria. The subdivision of the glycosuric women into those with and without potential diabetic features doubled the detection rate. However, the numbers were small and neither glycosuria nor potential diabetic features showed a degree of diagnostic specificity comparable to that of the O'Sullivan system.

The use of 'fasting glycosuria' as the screening determinant for a full GTT has been reported by Sutherland et al. (1970). Their figures show that only 0.8% of pregnant women have fasting glycosuria, of whom only 17% have chemical diabetes, i.e. 0.05% of the total. This figure is well below the 2.5% of O'Sullivan et al. (1973) and the 1.5% figure from St Mary's Hospital (unpublished study), suggesting that while fasting glycosuria is a good discriminant for selecting diabetics presenting with glycosuria, it does not reliably pick up all women with chemical diabetes. This may be because many women with chemical diabetes never develop glycosuria at any time during the day.

The justification for any screening system is that it should be cost-effective and also acceptable to the patient. A comparison of specificity rates and the relative costs of materials used for the tests is shown in Table 1. A full OGTT

TABLE 1
Estimate of specificity and cost of various screening systems based on data provided on 752 women by O'Sullivan et al. (1973)

	Specificity	Relative cost (%)		
	(%)	Screen	OGTT	Total
OGTT for whole population	100	–	100	100
OGTT on potential diabetics only[a]	64	–	49	49
O'Sullivan screen on whole population	79	14	16	30
O'Sullivan screen on women aged 25 years	74	7	7	14

[a] Estimated from the unpublished study at St Mary's Hospital.

is clearly time-consuming and disagreeable to pregnant women, apart from being expensive, while equally limiting the test to potential diabetics only is not justified because of the relatively lower pick-up rate. The system proposed by O'Sullivan *et al.* (1973) and in the St Mary's Hospital study, whereby an OGTT is done only on women with a blood sugar above a certain critical level one hour after a 50 g glucose load, has the advantage that it is easy to administer at the first visit to the clinic as part of the overall haematological screening procedure. It is also reasonably specific (79%) and inexpensive. The cost can be halved by confining the screening test to women aged 25 or over, with only a small reduction in diagnostic specificity from 79 to 74%. The saving in time, patient and staff involvement, and cost, would seem to justify this modification and it seems likely that it will become the screening method of choice for the future.

MANAGEMENT OF THE PREGNANT DIABETIC

Karlsson & Kjellmer (1972) observed that the lower the maternal blood sugar, the better the outcome for the baby. They reported that perinatal mortality and neonatal complications were lowest amongst women whose mean blood sugar had been below 100 mg/100 ml (5.5 mmol/l) in pregnancy. These authors noted, however, that there was no relationship between the maternal blood sugar concentration and the birth weight of the baby. This is not surprising, since the more effective treatment is in normalizing the blood sugar of the mother, the more likely are the influences to operate that determine the considerable variation in birth weight of the baby of the non-diabetic. The evidence simply adds further support to the concept that fetal development is likely to be optimal in a well-regulated physiological environment, and for blood sugar this requires a mean diurnal value of less than 100 mg/100 ml (Gillmer *et al.* 1975 *a,b*).

Antenatal diabetic control

The method of treating the pregnant diabetic still remains controversial. There seems to be general acceptance of the view that oral hypoglycaemic agents should not be used in pregnancy, although the Aberdeen group (Sutherland *et al.* 1973) have demonstrated that a low dose of chlorpropamide (100 mg daily) does not affect the baby adversely. However, the general view is that, because these drugs cross the placenta, some are teratogenic (albeit in large doses) and that as they act by stimulating increased secretion of insulin, their use is precluded, provided a satisfactory alternative is available. Diet alone or insulin and diet are the two therapeutic options that are currently in regular use, the former tending to be the choice for mild chemical diabetics. However, it is remarkable how commonly the babies of chemical diabetics treated with diet alone are significantly heavier for gestational age than those of the normal and of the insulin-treated mothers. O'Sullivan (1975) has shown quite clearly that treatment of the Class A diabetic with insulin normalizes the weight of their babies as compared with those treated with diet alone. It is tempting to suggest that the use of insulin for the treatment of all Class A diabetics might have a beneficial effect on the fetus by reducing the increased incidence of neonatal complications. Physicians are reluctant to accept that a mild deviation of metabolism from normal, which temporarily requires the administration of insulin, should be labelled as 'diabetes'. However, it should be remembered that in pregnancy it is the fetus that is of major concern rather than the mother.

Reference has already been made to the need to normalize maternal blood sugar as early as possible during, and preferably before, pregnancy. The practicability of achieving control in early pregnancy and the benefit in terms of a reduction in congenital defects still has to be demonstrated. In later pregnancy it seems likely that good diabetic control will benefit the fetus and reduce the incidence of complications of pregnancy such as pre-eclamptic toxaemia and hydramnios (Pedersen 1977).

Physiological glycaemia

The demonstration of how constant blood sugar is in normal as compared with diabetic pregnancy (Gillmer *et al.* 1975 *a,b;* Persson 1974) has encouraged a more radical approach to the normalization of blood sugar.

Three approaches have been used:

(i) The method in routine use in the UK, as advocated by Essex *et al.* at King's College Hospital, London, in 1973, is to maintain random blood sugar levels measured in the antenatal clinic at less than 150 mg/100 ml (8.3 mmol/l). After 32 weeks' gestation in-patient care begins and attempts are made to keep the blood sugar below 100 mg/100 ml (5.5 mmol/l). It has been argued that admission to hospital reduces the physical activity of the mother, making her diabetes more difficult to control. Cassar *et al.* (1978) have reported on 101 women treated throughout pregnancy as outpatients whose blood sugar levels were maintained from 12 weeks onwards at a mean value of 6.7 mmol/l (120 mg/100 ml) in the second trimester. Although these women spent a mean period of 29 days in hospital, which is not so different from the five to six weeks spent by women admitted routinely at 32 weeks' gestation, the important point these authors make is that 55% of the women were in hospital for less than 21 days.   Cassar *et al.* were thus exercising a more discriminating approach, only admitting for prolonged in-patient care those women with serious complications such as diabetic retinopathy. With the use of more reliable methods for assessing fetal wellbeing, it seems likely that diabetics will be treated as outpatients as long as their pregnancy remains quite free of complications.

(ii) Recently two groups in the UK have reported on the monitoring of blood sugar by the patient herself at home (Sönksen *et al.* 1978; Walford *et al.* 1978).   Both groups found that better control could be obtained by the patient on short and medium-acting insulin when the dosage was based on the result of the blood sugar profile obtained at home.   Postprandial peaks of blood sugar were generally eliminated and hypoglycaemic attacks were less frequent than when the more usual regimen of management is used.   Blood sugar values at home were generally lower than those obtained in the clinic.   This approach is particularly relevant to the pregnant diabetic for whom strict control is very important.   The benefit of providing all young diabetic women with glucose meters, and persuading them to use these reliably, still has to be proven, but the potential value to such women certainly makes this approach persuasive.   For the woman who is planning to become pregnant, there may be a possibility of reducing the risk of congenital malformation by careful regulation of blood glucose immediately before conception.   For the woman who is already pregnant there is the likelihood that, with good diabetic control at home, she will reduce the amount of time she has to spend in hospital before delivery.

(iii) The third approach to diabetic control in pregnancy is that described by Roversi *et al.* (1977).   In essence, they advocate that as much insulin should be given as the patient will tolerate without developing persistent, troublesome symptoms of hypoglycaemia.   They describe a series of 479 patients (237 White Class A and 242 Class AB-R).   The uncorrected perinatal mortality was 29 per 1000 births and the incidence of total malformations was 1.6%, which is well below that commonly reported in association with diabetic pregnancy (Beard & Oakley 1976).   The excellence of these results indicates that this approach to diabetic control, which is popular throughout Europe, should be given careful consideration.   The theoretical disadvantage is that the maternal blood sugar is kept below the physiological norm, and this may reduce the availability to the developing fetus of essential energy-producing substrates.   This, in theory, could result in fetal growth retardation with a selective effect on organs such as the liver and the brain.   The mean diurnal values reported ranged between 55 and 75 mg/100 ml (3.0–4.2 mmol/l), with the exception of a peak of 95–100 mg/100 ml (5.3–5.5 mmol/l) at 20.00 hours. In addition, there is the practical disadvantage of the unpleasant effects of hypoglycaemia which most patients experience when they are first started on the regimen.

Antenatal diabetic control complicated by administration of hyperglycaemic agents

Diabetic control is complicated when β-sympathomimetic agents, either alone or in conjunction with steroids, are used to treat premature labour (Borberg *et al.* 1978; Beard 1978). Hyperglycaemia results and insulin requirements are greatly increased. On these occasions the blood glucose is best controlled by the simultaneous intravenous administration of insulin and glucose. Doses of up to 10 i.u. of insulin per hour have been reported to be necessary to maintain normoglycaemia in a diabetic whose control is difficult (Borberg *et al.* 1978).

Intrapartum diabetic control

The maintenance of normoglycaemia should be attempted regardless of the method of delivery of the diabetic. In the past, when most women were delivered by Caesarean section, little consideration was given to diabetic control in labour. Then, as it became clear that vaginal delivery was safer with fetal monitoring, increasing numbers of women were allowed to attempt a vaginal delivery. Brudenell & Beard (1972) described a method of dietary restriction and regulation of insulin based on serial measurement of blood glucose in labour. However, the method was dependent on the subcutaneous administration of insulin. More recently West & Lowy (1977) have described the administration of a low-dose insulin-glucose infusion to 15 diabetic women in labour. The mean rate of infusion of insulin ranged between 1.4 and 2.0 U/h, and a mean blood glucose, determined by hourly Dextrostix or Eyetone reflectance meter measurements, of 5.0–6.6 mmol/l (90–120 mg/100 ml) was achieved. None of the patients developed ketonuria in labour and none of the infants became hypoglycaemic. This is clearly a highly effective method of regulating blood glucose in women whose diabetic control is likely to be very variable because of parenteral glucose administration and the stress of labour. At present the role of the recently developed sophisticated methods of blood glucose regulation, such as the artificial pancreas, is difficult to determine because they cannot be used in daily life, but undoubtedly any system that achieves normalization of blood sugar for 24 hours a day will have a place in the management of the pregnant diabetic.

Obstetric management

While strict control of the blood glucose concentration has become the central issue in medical management of diabetic pregnancy, there have also been some major changes in thinking on obstetric management. In most centres premature delivery by Caesarean section around 37–38 weeks of gestation (Persson 1979) is practised. Beard & Brudenell (1975) reported a 50% Caesarean section rate which is similar to that of Roversi *et al.* (1977). One does, however, have to question why it is necessary to deliver so many diabetic women by this route if their diabetic control has been good. The reasons are chiefly historical. Delivery some time before term was advocated as a means of reducing stillbirths and there was also an understandable desire to avoid the stress of labour. In addition, many premature inductions of labour failed, leading inevitably to Caesarean section. The clinical situation has now changed. Stillbirth is an uncommon event and, when it does occur, is usually accompanied by clear evidence of poor diabetic control. For these reasons the need to induce labour before term has diminished and there is little justification for inducing the woman with an unfavourable cervix. Furthermore, the risk of intrapartum asphyxia has largely been overcome by the use of continuous fetal heart rate monitoring (Edington *et al.* 1975), and the necessity of repeating a Caesarean section for indications other than cephalopelvic disproportion, or malformation, is extremely doubtful. Thus, it should be possible to allow more diabetic women to have a spontaneous onset of labour and to deliver by the vaginal route. Disproportion due to the large baby still remains a hazard which must never be forgotten, particularly in the woman whose diabetes has been poorly controlled or who is seen for the first time late in pregnancy, having had no proper diabetic control.

CONTRACEPTION

The advice on contraception that should be given to the diabetic, whether insulin-requiring or sub-clinical, is far from settled. The use of contraceptive steroids carries a potential risk of exacerbating the metabolic disorder of diabetes and some authors (Oakley & Beard 1975) have concluded that it is better for diabetics to use other methods of contraception. The reasons for this are the risk of inducing a permanent deterioration in glucose tolerance with all that this implies for the woman and for the fetus if a further pregnancy is contemplated. There is also the possibility in the established insulin-requiring diabetic of an acceleration of the development of long-term vascular disease (Beck 1975). Thus, there are two separate questions that have to be considered in our discussions of the clinical perspectives relating to the use of oral contraceptives by diabetics. Firstly, are there contraceptive steroids that can be recommended to diabetics because of their minimal effect on carbohydrate and lipid metabolism? Secondly, if the pill is prescribed to a woman with a known tendency to carbohydrate intolerance, what is the possible long-term risk of such women developing clinical diabetes, and is the risk of fetal anomaly increased?

The influence of contraceptive steroids on carbohydrate and lipid metabolism in non-diabetics has recently been reviewed by Briggs & Briggs (1977). It seems certain that both the synthetic oestrogen and progestogens have some effect on CHO tolerance but individual steroids vary in their potential for disturbing CHO metabolism. The adverse effect of the 19-nortestosterone-derived progestogens has been recognized for some time (Landon et al. 1962: Spellacy et al. 1970a,b). Mestranol and probably all oestrogens appear to potentiate the hyperglycaemic effects of these nortestosterone derivatives in non-diabetic women, and Spellacy et al. (1970a,b) found that women using norethisterone and mestranol for a mean of 8.3 years had a 40% incidence of abnormal CHO tolerance whereas the incidence was much less when a compound containing a progestogen was used (Spellacy et al. 1971).

A consistent change in lipid metabolism has been difficult to detect. Oestrogens tend to increase serum triglycerides (Furman et al. 1967; Gustafson & Svanborg 1972), whereas the nortestosterone and progestogens tend to depress them (Glueck et al. 1971; Larsson-Cohn et al. 1970). Beck (1970) on the other hand considered that progesterone derivatives produce no observable effect. Briggs & Briggs (1977), reviewing the literature on the subject, stated that there is general agreement that oestrogenic oral contraceptives increase fasting triglycerides, and usually increase blood cholesterol, while progestogens on their own have no effect. The response to the combined oral contraceptive pill is variable, although the sequential oestrogen–progestogen pill is said to be free of adverse effects (Schneider et al. 1975).

Studies on the effects of contraceptive steroids on the metabolism of diabetics have been limited by ethical considerations. The knowledge that they may induce a metabolic disturbance similar to that seen in diabetes has, not surprisingly, dissuaded many doctors from prescribing them. Reliable studies give conflicting results. In one, by Goldman & Eckerling (1970), there was a significant impairment of CHO metabolism in chemical diabetic women treated with norethynodrel and mestranol for only three months, whereas Moses & Goldzieher (1970) recorded an improvement in CHO tolerance after one year of treatment with mestranol and chlormadinone. Unfortunately, pills containing chlormadinone are no longer available in the UK or the

USA. Aznar *et al.* (1976), studying 16 diabetics, reported no changes in tolerance when progestogen-only mini-pills were used, while an improvement in tolerance was noted on the sequential pills. Here again we have suggestive evidence that the selection of the correct steroid is of considerable importance if an oral contraceptive is to be prescribed for the diabetic.

Beck (1973) has questioned whether one may legitimately ask about the pathological significance of a 10 mg/100 ml (0.5 mmol/l) rise in fasting serum triglyceride. It seems reasonable at this time to say that his comment is valid for the proven non-diabetic but not when applied to those with borderline CHO intolerance. In the latter group the use of the combined pill should be contraindicated unless considered absolutely essential. However, it does seem that the progestogen-only pill and possibly some sequential oestrogen – progestogen combinations can be prescribed with caution because they are free of serious effects on carbohydrate tolerance and lipid metabolism although the sequential pill is no longer available in the UK. For the time being it is advisable to do serial glucose tolerance tests on women who have shown transitory evidence of carbohydrate intolerance in pregnancy if any oral contraceptive is prescribed.

We still do not know for certain whether the gestational diabetic is more likely to develop uncompensated diabetes if she has been taking an oral contraceptive. It is therefore probably best to recommend that these women should use either an intrauterine device or one of the barrier methods of contraception. If this is not possible then the progestogen-only mini-pill is an acceptable alternative. For the women with insulin-requiring diabetes or taking oral hypoglycaemic agents, an oral contraceptive can be used. Sterilization should not be insisted on by the clinician although the advantages of limiting the number of children should be discussed at an early stage of pregnancy.

References

AZNAR, R., LARA, R., ZARCO, D. & GONZALEZ, L. (1976) The effects of various contraceptive hormonal therapies in women with normal oral diabetic and glucose tolerance test contraception. *Contraception 13,* 299–311

BEARD, R. W. (1976). Diagnosis of and screening for diabetes in pregnancy, in *Perinatal Medicine* (Rooth, G. & Bratteby, L.-E., eds.) *(Proc. 5th. Eur. Congr. Perinatal Med., Uppsala, Sweden),* pp. 88–91, distributed by Almqvist & Wiksell International, Sweden

BEARD, R. W. (1978) The effect of beta-sympathomimetic drugs on carbohydrate metabolism in pregnancy, in *Pre-Term Labour (Proc. 5th Study Group R. Coll. Obstet. Gynaecol.)* (Beard, R.W. *et al.,* eds.), pp. 203–211, RCOG, London

BEARD, R. W. & BRUDENELL, J. M. (1975) Fetal monitoring in diabetic pregnancy, in *Early Diabetes in Early Life (Proc. 3rd Int. Symp. Madeira, 1974)* (Camerini-Davalos, R. A. & Cole, H.S., eds.), pp 523–559, Academic Press, New York

BEARD, R. W. & OAKLEY, N. W. (1976) The fetus of the diabetic, in *Fetal Physiology and Medicine* (Beard, R. W. & Nathanielsz, P. W., eds.), pp. 137–157, Saunders, London

BECK, P. (1970) Comparison of the metabolic effects of chlormadinone acetate and conventional contraceptive steroids in man. *J. Clin. Endocrinol. 30*, 785–791

BECK, P. (1973) Contraceptive steroids: modifications of carbohydrate and lipid metabolism. *Metabolism 22*, 841–855

BECK, P. (1975) The effects of oral anticonceptional drugs on diabetes mellitus, in *Early Diabetes in Early Life (Proc. 3rd int. Symp. Madeira 1974)* (Camerini-Davalos R. A. & Cole, H. S., eds.), pp. 349–352, Academic Press, New York

BERENDES, H. W. (1975) Effect of maternal acetonuria on I.Q. of offspring, in *Early Diabetes in Early Life (Proc. 3rd Int. Symp. Madeira, 1974)* (Camerini-Davalos, R. A. & Cole, H. S., eds.), p. 135, Academic Press, New York

BORBERG, C., GILLMER, M. D. G., BEARD, R. W. & OAKLEY, N. W. (1978) Metabolic effects of beta-sympathomimetic drugs and dexamethasone in normal and diabetic pregnancy. *Br. J. Obstet. Gynaecol. 85*, 184–189

BRIGGS, M. & BRIGGS, M. (1977) *Oral Contraceptives*, vol. 1 *(Annu. Res. Rev.)*, Churchill Livingstone, Edinburgh

BRUDENELL, J. M. & BEARD, R. W. (1972) Diabetes in pregnancy, in *Clinics in Endocrinology & Metabolism*, vol. 1, no. 3 (Pyke, D. A., ed.), pp. 673–695, Saunders, London

CASSAR, J., GORDON, H., DIXON, H. G., CUMMINS, M. & JOPLIN, G. F. (1978) Simplified management of diabetic pregnancy. *Br. J. Obstet. Gynaecol. 85*, 585–591

CHAPMAN, V. M. (1976) Discussion on beta-glucuronidase during early embryogenesis, in *Embryogenesis in Mammals (Ciba Found. Symp. 40)*, pp. 125–126, Elsevier/Excerpta Medica/North-Holland, Amsterdam

CHEN, J. M. (1954) The effect of insulin on embryonic limb-bones cultivated in vitro. *J. Physiol. (Lond.) 125*, 148–162

DEUCHAR, E. M. (1979) Culture in vitro as a means of analyzing the effects of maternal diabetes on embryonic development in rats, in *Carbohydrate Metabolism in Pregnancy and the Newborn* (Sutherland, H. W. & Stowers, J. M., eds.) *(2nd. Aberdeen Int. Colloq.)* Springer, Berlin

DURAISWAMI, P. K. (1959) Insulin-induced skeletal abnormalities in developing chickens. *Br. Med. J. 2*, 384–390

EDINGTON, P. T., SIBANDA, J. & BEARD, R. W. (1975) Influence on clinical practice of routine intra-partum fetal monitoring. *Br. Med. J. 3*, 341–343

ESSEX, N. L., PYKE, D. A., WATKINS, P. J., BRUDENELL, J. M. & GAMSU, H. R. (1973) Diabetic pregnancy. *Br. Med. J. 4*, 89–93

FURMAN, R. A., ALAUPOVIC, P. & HOWARD, R. P. (1967) Effects of androgens and estrogens on serum lipids and the composition and concentration of serum lipoproteins in normolipemic and hyperlipemic states. *Prog. Biochem. Pharmacol. 2*, 215–249

GABBE, S. G., MESTMAN, J. H., FREEMAN, R. K., ANDERSON, G. V. & LOWENSOHN, R. I. (1977) Management and outcome of class A diabetes mellitus. *Am. J. Obstet. Gynecol. 127*, 465–469

GILLMER, M. D. G., BEARD, R. W., BROOKE, F. M. & OAKLEY, N. W. (1975a) Carbohydrate metabolism in pregnancy. Part. I. Diurnal plasma glucose profile in normal and diabetic women. *Br. Med. J. 3*, 399–402

GILLMER, M. D. G., BEARD, R. W., BROOKE, F. M. & OAKLEY, N. W. (1975b) Carbohydrate metabolism in pregnancy, II. Relation between maternal glucose tolerance and glucose metabolism in the newborn. *Br. Med. J. 3*, 402–404

GLUECK, C. J., LEVY, R. I. & FREDRICKSON, D. S. (1971) Norethindrone acetate postheparin lipolytic activity, and plasma triglycerides in familial types I, III, IV and V hyperlipoproteinemia: studies in 26 patients and 5 normal persons. *Ann. Intern. Med. 75*, 345–352

GOLDMAN, J. A. & ECKERLING, B. (1970) Blood glucose levels and glucose tolerance in women with subclinical diabetes receiving an oral contraceptive. *Am. J. Obstet. Gynecol. 107*, 325–327

GUSTAFSON, A. & SVANBORG, A. (1972) Gonadal steroid effects on plasma lipoproteins and individual phospholipids. *J. Clin. Endocrinol. 35*, 203–207

GUTTORM, E. (1975) Practical screening for diabetes mellitus in pregnant women, in *Carbohydrate Metabolism in Pregnancy and the Newborn* (Sutherland, H. W. and Stowers, J. M., eds.), pp. 142–152, Churchill Livingstone, Edinburgh

HARE, J. W. & WHITE, P. (1977) Pregnancy in diabetes complicated by vascular disease. *Diabetes 26*, 953–955

HORRII, K., WATANABE, G. & INGALLS, T. H. (1966) Experimental diabetes in pregnant mice: prevention of congenital malformations in offspring by insulin. *Diabetes 15*, 192–204

KARLSON, K. & KJELLMER, I. (1972) The outcome of diabetic pregnancies in relation to the mother's blood sugar level. *Am. J. Obstet. Gynecol. 112*, 213–220

LANDON, J., WYNN, V., COOKE, J. N. C. & KENNEDY, A. (1962) Effects of anabolic steroid, methanedienone, on carbohydrate metabolism in man. *Metabolism 11*, 501–512

LARSSON-COHN, U., BERLIN, R. & VIKROT, O. (1970) Effect of combined and low-dose gestagen oral contraceptives on plasma lipids: including individual phospholipids. *Acta Endocrinol. 63*, 717–735

MOSES, L. E. & GOLDZIEHER, J. W. (1970) The influence of a sequential oral contraceptive on the carbohydrate metabolism of diabetics and pre-diabetics. *Adv. Planned Parent. 6*, 101–104

NAEYE, R. L. (1979) The outcome of diabetic pregnancies: a prospective study, in this symposium, pp. 227–238

OAKLEY, N. W. & BEARD, R. W. (1975) Conception control in diabetes mellitus, in *Early Diabetes in Early Life (Proc. 3rd Int. Symp. Madeira, 1974)* (Camerini-Davalos, R. A. & Cole, H.S., eds.), pp. 345–348, Academic Press, New York

OAKLEY, N. W., BEARD, R. W. & TURNER, R. C. (1972) Effect of sustained maternal hyperglycaemia on the fetus in normal and diabetic pregnancies. *Br. Med. J. 1*, 466–469

O'SULLIVAN, J. B. (1975) Prospective study of gestational diabetes and its treatment, in *Carbohydrate Metabolism in Pregnancy and the Newborn* (Sutherland, H. W. & Stowers, J. M., eds.), pp. 195–204, Churchill Livingstone, Edinburgh

O'SULLIVAN, J. B. (1979) in *Carbohydrate Metabolism in Pregnancy and the Newborn* (Sutherland, H. W. & Stowers, J. M., eds.) *(2nd Aberdeen Int. Colloq.)*, Springer, Berlin

O'SULLIVAN, J. B. & MAHAN, C. M. (1964) Criteria for the oral glucose tolerance test in pregnancy. *Diabetes 13*, 278–285

O'SULLIVAN, J. B., MAHAN, C. M., CHARLES, D. & DANDROW, R. V. (1973) Screening criteria for high-risk gestational diabetic patients. *Am. J. Obstet. Gynecol. 116*, 895–900

PEDERSEN, J. (1977) *The Pregnant Diabetic and her Newborn*, 2nd edn., Munksgaard, Copenhagen

PERSSON, B. (1974) Assessment of metabolic control in diabetic pregnancy, in *Size at Birth (Ciba Found. Symp. 27)*, pp. 247–273, Elsevier/Excerpta Medica/North-Holland, Amsterdam

PERSSON, B. (1979) in *Carbohydrate Metabolism in Pregnancy and the Newborn* (Sutherland, H. W. & Stowers, J. M., eds.) *(2nd Aberdeen Int. Colloq.)*, Springer, Berlin

PERSSON, B. & GENTZ, J. (1977) Short and long term effects of maternal diabetes on the offspring, in *Diabetes* (Bajaj, J. S., ed.) *(Int. Congr. Ser. 413)* Excerpta Medica, Amsterdam

RÄIHÄ, N. C. R. (1979) Hormonal regulation of perinatal enzyme differentiation in the mammalian liver, in this symposium, pp. 137–153

ROVERSI, G. D., GARCIULO, M., NICOLINI, U., PEDRETTI, E. & CANDIANI, G. (1977) Diabète de la mère et risque péri-natal. *Rev. Méd. Suisse Romande 97*, 401–402

SCHNEIDER, W. H. F., MATT, K., IRSIGLER, K., LAGEDER, H. & SCHUBERT, H. (1975) Gynecological hematological and metabolic studies under therapy with an estrogen-gestagen sequential drug. *Arzneim.-Forsch. 25*, 959–962

SMITH, B. T., GIROUD, C. J. P., ROBERT, M. & AVERY, M. E. (1975) Insulin antagonism of cortisol action on lecithin synthesis by cultured fetal lung cells. *J. Pediatr. 87*, 953–955

SÖNKSEN, P. H., JUDD, S. L. & LOWY, C. (1978) Home monitoring of blood glucose method for improving diabetic control. *Lancet 1*, 729–732

SPELLACY, W. N., BUHI, W. C., SPELLACY, C. E., MOSES, L. E. & GOLDZIEHER, J. W. (1970*a*) Glucose, insulin, and growth hormone studies in long term users of oral contraceptives. *Am. J. Obstet. Gynecol. 106*, 173–182

SPELLACY, W. N., MCLEOD, A.G.W., BUHI, W. C., BIRK, S. A. & MCCREARY, S. A. (1970*b*) Medroxy progesterone acetate and carbohydrate metabolism. Measurement of glucose, insulin, and growth hormone during 6 months time. *Fertil. Steril. 21*, 457–463

SPELLACY, W. N., BUHI, W. C., BIRK, S. A. & MCCREARY, S. A. (1971) Studies of chlormadinone acetate and mestranol on blood glucose and plasma insulin. II. Twelfth month oral glucose tolerance test. *Fertil. Steril. 4*, 224–228

SUTHERLAND, H. W., STOWERS, J. M. & MCKENZIE, C. (1970) Simplifying the clinical problem of glycosuria in pregnancy. *Lancet 1*, 1069–1071

SUTHERLAND, H. W., STOWERS, J.M., CORMACK, J. D. & BEWSHER, P. D. (1973) Evaluation of chlorpropamide in chemical diabetes diagnosed during pregnancy. *Br. Med. J. 3*, 9–13

WALFORD, S., GALE, E. A. M., ALLISON, S. P. & TATTERSALL, R. B. (1978) Self monitoring of blood-glucose. Improvement of diabetic control. *Lancet 1*, 732–735

WEST, T. E. T. & LOWY, C. (1977) Control of blood glucose during labour in diabetic women with combined glucose and low-dose insulin infusion. *Br. Med. J. 1*, 1252–1254

YSSING, M. (1975) Long-term prognosis of children born to mothers diabetic when pregnant, in *Early Diabetes in Early Life (Proc. 3rd Int. Symp. Madeira, 1974)* (Camerini-Davalos, R. A. & Cole, H. S., eds.), pp. 575–586, Academic Press, New York

Final general discussion

Freinkel: There are really no firm figures with regard to the proportion of all congenital anomalies that is due to diabetes. And if one had such an estimate, what would that represent in terms of the economic impact of the cost of life-time support? Public awareness of this as an economically meaningful problem would be very salutary.

Hoet: The medical research council of the EEC has decided to organize an epidemiological study on the occurrence of congenital birth defects in the countries of the EEC.

Beard: We probably won't be able to produce a figure for the UK but we can at least say that it is something that is needed.

HAEMOGLOBIN A_{1c}

Pedersen: One of the things that could easily be done in two years or so is to see whether there is any correlation between haemoglobin A_{1c} and congenital malformation.

Gillmer: I have a word of caution concerning the value of HbA_{1c} estimations in pregnancy based on the paper of Schwartz *et al.* (1976). In their non-pregnant group the HbA_{1c} concentration in normal subjects was 5.7% and in the diabetics it was 12.7%. In normal pregnant patients the value was 7.0% but that of the pregnant diabetics was only slightly higher, namely 8.5%. There is thus a much smaller difference in HbA_{1c} concentrations in normal and diabetic pregnant women than there is in non-pregnant subjects. The difference in the two pregnant groups was significant but as the two groups display a considerable overlap HbA_{1c} may not prove to be as valuable an indicator of plasma glucose control in pregnancy as it seems to be in non-pregnant patients.

Beard: As I recall, there was not a statistically significant difference between the normal and diabetic pregnant groups.

Gillmer: No, they *are* significantly different.

Pedersen: One should compare those with congenital malformations and those without congenital malformations.

Gillmer: All I am saying is that haemoglobin A_{1c} may not be such a good indicator of the degree of glycaemia as it is in the non-pregnant state.

Chez: A point which interests me is the mechanism that makes haemoglobin A_{1c} important to tissue oxygen consumption. That is, the relatively increased oxygen affinity of haemoglobin A_{1c} may mean that less oxygen is 'available' for transfer, resulting in relative hypoxaemia. That is an interesting theory but it goes back to what I consider the real importance of the quantitative approaches that Fred Battaglia presented to us. That is, what is the oxygen consumption need of the blastocyst? If there is 30% of haemoglobin A_{1c} in the total haemoglobin content, will the oxygen needed for tissue consumption still be sufficiently supplied by the remaining haemoglobin A, so that it doesn't really matter about haemoglobin A_{1c}?

The Fallopian tube fluid is an extremely interesting bath for the blastocyst. There is some evidence of active transport – in the sense that there are substrate concentrations in the tubal fluid such as hydrogen ion and carbon dioxide content (Maas *et al.* 1977; Wu *et al.* 1977) that are higher than plasma concentrations of the same substance. I am most interested in progesterone because it may be a teratogenic factor in patients who are treated with it early in pregnancy for an inadequate luteal phase or something similar. The monkey oviductal fluid has extraordinary levels of things like progesterone and perhaps other substrates. There is a period just before fertilization and then at 8 or 9 days when the egg and then the developing embryo is exposed to concentrations of substrates of which we have little knowledge. Therefore, how sensitive is the tubal oxygen environment to diffusion into the fluid from the endothelial mucosa of the tube? The possibility of a small change in haemoglobin A_{1c}, a small change in oxygen affinity, makes me think that teratogenesis might occur because of hypoxaemia, which most of us would agree is an overt teratogenic problem.

Another point is that, as opposed to the normal non-pregnant monkey, the streptozotocin non-pregnant animal has a haemoglobin A_{1c} peak. (This is work in progress in collaboration with R. Widress, R. Schwartz, and H. Schwartz.) When these same animals became pregnant the haemoglobin A_{1c} disappeared at the end of the first trimester. We do not know when or at what rate haemoglobin A_{1c} disappears. This should be a function of haemoglobin turnover or red blood cell life. This occurs in the overt streptozotocin-treated monkey that shows fetal macrosomia and a 30% stillbirth rate.

Battaglia: Why do you think it disappears at all?

Chez: I don't know.

Kalkhoff: How did you measure the A_{1c}?

Chez: H. Schwartz at Stanford used Amberlite IRC-50 with cyanide-phosphate elution.

Hoet: It is interesting that congenital malformations are not seen in the monkeys. There may be a certain correlation between your observation about HbA_{1c} and the fact that there are no congenital malformations.

Pedersen: That is because the monkeys have aborted. Diabetic women who have infants with congenital malformations perhaps ought to have had spontaneous abortions.

Battaglia: I don't know what A_{1c} is doing but I believe we have over-emphasized the effect of changes in oxygen affinity of fetal blood on fetal oxygenation. When it was recognized that diphosphoglyceric acid alters the oxygen affinity of many haemoglobins, there was great concern that if the dissociation curves were shifted to a higher affinity there might be release problems in tissues. There are many assumptions contained in that hypothesis. If blood flow to fetal tissues is kept constant, then if there is the same quantity of oxygen to unload, the same change in O_2 saturation must occur at a higher affinity in the blood. The venous blood leaving the organ would now leave at a lower Po_2. The assumption was made, though it has not been documented, that at high enough affinity there would be such a low Po_2 in the venous blood that oxygen would no longer be exchanged to the tissues and oxygen consumption would fall. In this case high A_{1c} changes by 6–12% of the total haemoglobin. The change in the mixed blood produced by adding 12% haemoglobin at a different affinity is very small. We know that we can move oxygen affinity in the sheep fetus by exchanging all of the fetal blood with homozygous B-type haemoglobin which shifts the dissociation curve 15 mm, without evidence of tissue hypoxia (Battaglia *et al.* 1969). I am not saying that a marked change in oxygen affinity couldn't, under some conditions affect oxygen release to tissues, but if it is a haemoglobin change of 10–12% I think there is every reason to doubt its clinical significance at least as it relates to tissue oxygenation.

Gillmer: There is only a 1.5% difference between the HbA_{1c} concentration of the normal and diabetic pregnant patient and this is unlikely to have any major influence on oxygen availability.

Chez: Your comment may not be pertinent for the first two weeks of conception. Those data are from mid-trimester. I think we are talking about the time just after fertilization.

Beard: We are talking about two aspects of haemoglobin A_{1c}. One is the oxygen delivery and the other is the diagnostic significance of increased concentration.

Bennett: I am not at all convinced that haemoglobin A_{1c} is going to give us any real answer to the questions about blood glucose that we are asking in terms of control. The correlation between a spot test of fasting haemoglobin and a spot test of fasting glucose is so high that the additional information that one could potentially get is very limited. I am very sceptical that it will lead us anywhere unless there is some very specific effect that is not glucose-related *per se* and that is affected by haemoglobin A_{1c}.

Beard: The problem with Bob Schwartz's paper was that he didn't know the control his diabetics had had in the preceding months. Has this matter been resolved any further?

Freinkel: We have also been securing such measurements in our pregnant diabetics and I share Peter Bennett's reservations. As an integrated epidemiological tool, it will certainly prove to have some value. However, in individual patients it is conceivable that an acute marked deterioration in metabolic regulation might have a very meaningful impact on the course of a pregnancy without exercising a significant effect on haemoglobin A_{1c} since the latter reflects the perturbations that occur during the lifetime of a red blood cell.

Bennett: We always talk about congenital malformations being formed sometime in the first trimester. Is there any better guess than that?

Deuchar: I would say it was somewhere in the first two months for gross malformations of organ systems, but for endocrine organ abnormalities probably during the third or fourth month. The metabolic maturation of organs occurs mostly during the third and fourth months of human development.

Milner: Do you date pregnancy from conception or from the first day of the last menstrual period?

Deuchar: My timing is from the time of fertilization of the ovum.

Kalkhoff: So all this is over before pregnancy is even diagnosed.

Beard: This brings us back to the point that there is a strong case for a prospective approach to management of women who *intend* to become pregnant as opposed to treating them only when they become pregnant. There is a need to emphasize this and it is something that is missing in the education of diabetic girls. It would be difficult to encourage them to go to their physicians to ensure that they are in the best possible state of control before they become pregnant.

Chez: Professor Hoet and Dr Bergstein mentioned that a woman who has been on oral contraception should wait for a specific length of time before she conceives.   Presumably this is because of the metabolic changes associated with the exogenous steroids and the suggestion that protein and carbohydrate metabolism takes about 8–9 weeks to return to normal and lipid metabolism takes about 12 weeks.   That is an interesting idea but most studies of patients who have conceived within the first month of stopping the pill show that there is no difference in the spontaneous abortion rate, the premature delivery rate, or the congenital anomaly rate at term compared with control patients who had not been taking contraceptive pills.   The only thing that can be seen in the women who have been on oral contraception is that in the first cycle the follicular phase tends to be prolonged; the latter has been correlated in humans with tetraploidy and polyploidy and those are usually lethal congenital anomalies which are spontaneously aborted.   I accept the idea emotionally that one should wait for regular menses to return after a person has been on the pill, for clearer identification of the last menstrual period and things of that sort.   But I am not sure that we have any evidence that the known changes in metabolism after women come off the pill have any adverse effect on the pregnancy.

Beard: You are referring to non-diabetics.

Chez: Yes, but there are metabolic changes.

Beard: We are talking about a group which has a certain predisposition towards congenital anomaly.

Chez: I don't think that invalidates the published data.   It is another piece of information.

NUTRITION AND METABOLISM

Garrow: When people stress the importance of a 'well-balanced' diet in pregnancy I get uneasy.   Deficiencies in the maternal diet hardly affect congenital abnormalities in the human species at all, and have remarkably little effect on growth rate.   The human species is peculiar in that the offspring at birth are only about 5% of the mother's weight and take an extraordinarily long time to grow.   It is quite likely that the mother can, at least on a one-off basis, finance the energy cost of a pregnancy entirely from her own stores.

The evidence in north-west Holland (Smith 1947; Stein *et al.* 1975) in 1944/45 was that brief but severe undernutrition in a previously well-nourished population had little effect on the fetus.   Also, if marginal malnutrition was very important, one would expect large parts of Asia to have avoided their population problems.   I would like to hear from anyone who has evidence that any dietary manipulation (other than giving toxins) in the human species could influence the prevalence of congenital abnormalities in either direction.

My own interest is in obesity, and one of the primary morbidities of obesity is a vastly increased predisposition to diabetes. If pregnancy is a closed season for the treatment of obesity, it means that some young women who weigh 80 kg at age 20–22 at their first pregnancy will weigh 90 kg with their second pregnancy and 100 kg with their third, at which stage it is very difficult to do anything useful about their obesity. A woman who is obese when she books into an antenatal clinic could, and I think should, finance the energy cost of her pregnancy from her own excess adipose tissue, rather than preserve that tissue and regard obesity as a problem which someone other than the obstetrician should worry about later.

Battaglia: If you are including changes in body size then it is partly a matter of what are 'small changes' to one investigator being 'large' to another. The Dutch women during their famine would have received almost 100 000 kilocalories over 40 weeks, as they were getting an average of 300–350 kilocalories (1260–1470 kJ) daily. The reduction in the mean birth weight of the babies was considerably greater than that associated with maternal smoking. These infants certainly were not 1200 g infants at term, so in comparison to severe intrauterine growth retardation, which occurs in some clinical situations, we can look at a 200 g reduction at term and say that it is not very big. Again, if we don't define what we will use as a reference point it is difficult to say whether an effect is small or large. It was an effect that was statistically demonstrable and larger than the impact of some other factors that we are excited about today as influencing fetal growth.

I was impressed with the INCAP studies where caloric supplementation, not necessarily protein, increased the fetal weight. They showed, as every study in humans ends up doing, a large effect on placental size. In the Dutch famine studies the babies were reduced in weight but the placenta was even more reduced. In the INCAP studies that was also true. When they gave calories the placenta increased in weight proportionately more than the baby. In some respects, however, I am very much in sympathy with your remarks, Dr Garrow. People overlook the fact that the primate has a disproportionately long gestation.

Räihä: If we assume that the newborn infant of the diabetic mother is metabolically immature for some time after birth, then we must be very much concerned about the quantity and the quality of protein intake of these infants. We know that if they are metabolically immature they have immaturities in both amino acid-synthesizing enzymes and amino acid-degrading enzymes. If we are giving them the wrong quality and amount of amino acids during a very critical period of brain development, we might affect their intellectual capacity.

Kalkhoff: In the Dutch famine study the women who were deprived of food during the last trimester as opposed to the first trimester had children who were less obese as a group.   If we are trying to prevent diabetes this tells us that overnutrition is as bad as undernutrition.   A sensible approach to maternal nutrition is very important.

I don't think any of us would recommend a 350 kcal (1470 kJ) diet for a pregnant woman.   Until the matter of ketosis and ketonaemia is settled with respect to central nervous system development, it would be very wrong to place an obese pregnant woman on such a regimen.

Garrow: It is very difficult to make a very heavy woman ketotic on a diet supplying, say, 1600 kcal (6720 kJ) with a normal proportion of carbohydrate.   There is no merit in low carbohydrate diets for fat loss.

Kalkhoff: I have seen pregnant women who have received reasonable caloric intakes who still become ketotic, particularly if they eat their last meal at 6 p.m.   The next day they are often ketonuric.   It can be reversed by increasing the carbohydrate supplementation, particularly at night before bedtime.

Hoet: Is this in pregnancy?

Kalkhoff: Yes.   I think every obstetrician has seen this.   I have taken care of diabetic pregnant women who have normal fasting blood glucose concentrations but heavy ketonuria.   This can often be reversed by increasing the carbohydrate intake.

Beard: Ketonuria doesn't necessarily mean excessive ketonaemia.

Kalkhoff: No, but if one correlates the two, one sometimes sees higher than normal ketone levels in the blood as well as in urine.

Beard: That hasn't been shown, has it?

Persson: In a previous Ciba Foundation symposium (*Size at Birth*) we demonstrated that pregnant diabetic women with ketonuria had significantly higher fasting plasma concentrations of 3-hydroxybutyrate and glucose than diabetic women without ketonuria (Persson 1974).

Milner: It is clear from the INCAP study (Lechtig *et al.* 1975) that when we start talking about a 117 g drop in mean birth weight we can easily mask something which I think is clinically important.   If a 117 g drop in birth weight occurred in every infant then I might be as sanguine about the potentially adverse effect of maternal dietetic restriction on that population of babies as Dr Garrow is. But that isn't the real story from the INCAP data.   The 117 g difference in birth weight between the two subgroups of mothers receiving low (average 43 kcal/day–180 kJ) or high (average 233 kcal/day–980 kJ) supplementation was small but significant.   But the mean is made up of a majority in whom dietary restriction had very little if any effect and a minority in whom birth weight was severely compromised.   This facet was revealed in the corollary: irrespective of the type of supplement, when the women were divided into those who had received high or low supplements, the incidence of infants weighing less than 2500 g at birth was 9% in the women getting more than 20 000 extra kilocalories (84 000 kJ) and 18% in those receiving less than 20 000 kilocalories.   That is important.   It should make us rather reserved about the implications in Guatemala of a modest caloric daily supplement to overtly malnourished women, and *pari passu* the potential effect not on mean birth weight of any population but on the incidence of small-for-dates babies that might occur within that population, if a similar overall caloric reduction was imposed.

Beard: So it is not true that the baby is well protected from maternal nutritional deprivation until an extreme state is reached?

Milner: Yes, that is my point.   Average values are misleading because the obstetrician deals with one woman at a time.   What you don't know is whether the particular woman you are dealing with is the one in whom this modest caloric restriction might produce a small-for-dates baby.

Hull: It is the associations that are important in the Guatemala study and the Dutch study.   It isn't a matter of restricting diet alone.   One group was on a different plane of nutrition before they entered the experience, and the plane of nutrition is related to a whole host of other factors which are associated with nutrition but are not 'nutrition'.   Thus with studies of this kind it is very difficult to say whether it is a nutritional factor that is the main influence or whether it is something associated with nutritional factors.   Giving food may prevent some of the harmful effects of, say, urinary tract infections and a whole host of other things.   These remarks do not establish that nutrition is the key.   Again when we are talking about nutrition we must look at what is available to the fetus rather than what is stored in the body.

Beard: Diet may have a direct effect on the fetus.   It may diminish its resistance to infections, possibly leading to problems of intrauterine growth retardation.   Or it may have an effect on the mother who then becomes perhaps more liable to infection and this is mediated through to the fetus.

Chez: We talked earlier about the possibility of controlling or treating gestational diabetes by reducing the caloric intake, and if that didn't work the next step is to give insulin.   Some clinicians believe that the diet can be modified if a patient is obese.   This is a very significant problem.   A lot of us have worked very hard to get obstetricians away from the magic number of a maximum 8 kg weight gain.   How are you going about looking at dieting, with informed consent as it were, in an experimental setting, in order to answer the question of whether total weight gain in pregnancy can be safely reduced by caloric restriction in what appears to be an obese person?

Beard: Firstly, we accepted what John Garrow had to say.   That is, obesity tends to increase with successive pregnancies and eventually has an adverse effect on the woman.   Secondly we know from obstetrical and epidemiological data that complications associated with obesity are two to three times higher than in mothers of normal weight – that is, conditions like toxaemia and problems with big babies.   It seemed to us that unless someone does the critical study of putting patients on a diet – not too severe but enough to keep their weight gain within a certain range – we are likely to remain in ignorance of what is going to happen to the babies of women who diet in pregnancy or by necessity are subjected to dietary deprivation.

Chez: Do you have women whom you are not allowing to gain even a single pound?

Gillmer: Four or five of our obese patients have gained less than 5 kg during pregnancy and thus had a total net weight loss after the delivery.   They, however, delivered babies that were not below the 50th percentile, corrected for gestational age and sex.

Chez: If the baby's weight is within the 50th percentile I don't know whether that patient would have had, and therefore should have had, a 95th percentile infant.

Gillmer: The strongest correlate between birth weight and maternal parameters on an epidemiological basis is maternal body mass.

Garrow: In what weight range?

Chez: The product for that patient is a relatively small-for-dates infant, with the implications of the pathology of small-for-dates.

Gillmer: We know that chronically undernourished mothers who are given dietary supplements deliver larger infants but do we actually know the effect of moderate carbohydrate restriction in populations who are overnourished?   In addition, there are increased obstetric hazards in obese women.   It therefore seems reasonable to determine whether diet will reduce the excess weight of the fetus delivered by obese women.

Chez: The problem with obesity in pregnancy really comes down to an intrapartum problem, with difficulty in manipulations at delivery.   What we are now talking about is an antepartum problem of metabolic derangement and you are relying on the patient's intermediary metabolism to compensate for what she is not eating.

Garrow: The question is, what sort of weight gain or what sort of diet a particular woman ought to have.   And is it right to give a pregnant woman a

1000 kcal (4200kJ) diet? The answer is that we don't know. Among pregnant women and non-pregnant women there is a very large range of individual variation in requirements (Garrow 1978). Carbohydrate restriction is not a logical way of getting them to consume roughly 200 kcal (840 kJ) of their adipose tissue. I think it is totally reasonable to expect a woman who starts off with excess adipose tissue to gain no weight at all during pregnancy (Garrow 1976).

Beard: Dieting is very much a habit in our modern society amongst women. A lot of them carry their dieting habits into pregnancy. There is a natural experiment there. We are now doing the critical experiment on the effects of limited weight reduction in pregnancy on mother and baby. Until that is done we can't advise those people. If dieting turns out to have an adverse effect, which we don't think it will from our initial experience, then we can firmly say it is a bad thing to diet in pregnancy. In my view it is essential to obtain this information.

Pedersen: We treat obese women whether they are diabetic or not by restricting them to a diet of 1200–1500 kcal (5040–6300 kJ). That is the usual way we treat these women. If you want to do anything else you must show that the babies who arrive with your assistance are better than the others. We need a controlled trial.

Chez: The point is that obstetricians tend to be meddlesome. If healthy normal primigravida are left alone they gain between 11 and 12.5 kg. There must be some reason for that and the concern that we all have is that we may be interfering with what pregnant women know, genetically or however else, has to be done. If I allow my patients to gain 11 or 12 kg I don't have to prove that I am doing right.

Beard: The figure you quote is a mean with a wide standard deviation. One can also turn to John Garrow's statement about increasing obesity being a physiological effect. In fact, is a mother keeping to her normal physiology by overeating, as these women tend to do?

Chez: I wasn't discussing obesity. A weight gain of 11 kg is balanced by the weight of the products of conception. The residue of 3 kg is for lactation.

Battaglia: There are two issues here. First an ethical one. If you wish to prescribe a change of that kind for patients, at least in the USA, it should come in the realm of clinical research with appropriate patient consent and safeguards.

The other point is that in several presentations here it wasn't just changes in glucose that were significant but changes in a whole variety of fuels, including amino acids in the mother's blood and the presumption that this might have an effect on the baby. So it is not enough to say that the mother's caloric requirement can be met by burning fat. Fat is carbon, it is not a nitrogen source. I would have to know whether other changes in substrates are induced by the restriction in calories that produces unwanted effects in the baby. That is still an open question. What happens to the amino acids when you make an adult who is pregnant start burning her fat?

Freinkel: That is precisely what I meant when I asked Mike Gillmer to specify his end-point. The end-point is very critical. We have been relying very much on anecdotal experiences and there is a calculated risk that we may be accumulating more of the same. Mothers can certainly have healthy babies on a wide range of diets. We must stop talking about qualitative phenomena but instead seek quantitative parameters which focus on the finest possible nuances. Our conference should advocate that if nutritional enquiry is initiated during pregnancy, it must be done with the most meticulous prospective indices and with yardsticks much finer than the survival and weight of the baby or the state of health of the mother. The challenge to all of us is to define such prospective indices and yardsticks. We must not only look at the perinatal period but also follow every aspect of the child's subsequent maturation.

Beard: I think everyone would agree with that.

BLOOD SUGAR LEVELS IN PREGNANCY

Beard: One of the most worrying developments is the control of blood glucose with insulin in pregnant diabetics at levels that are well below the physiological mean. I think a therapeutic policy of this kind is often more worrying because it is rarely questioned or subjected to the scrutiny of a research protocol. In Europe it has recently been advocated that the mean blood sugar during pregnancy should be kept just above constant symptomatic hypoglycaemia in the mother, as low as 3.5 mmol/l. In Germany recently I saw this policy being pursued by the administration of soluble insulin four or five times a day, accompanied by multiple blood sugar estimations. This worries me a lot because of the possibility of nutritional deprivation for the fetus.

Milner: Why does it worry you?

Beard: Because we may be creating an abnormal environment for the fetus.

Milner: Essentially what Roversi has claimed is that by triple insulin injections per day to keep the mean blood sugar between 3.5 and 5.5 mmol/l he has completely abolished fetopathy due to maternal diabetes (Roversi *et al.* 1977). He is producing babies with a normal birth weight for gestational age. If that experience was expanded and was thereby shown convincingly to have reduced the incidence of congenital anomalies to within the normal range, you would have to argue very hard to convince me that it wasn't a good thing.

Beard: Has Roversi done a control series?

Milner: I don't think he has to do a control series.   His control, if you like, is normality as we understand it.   The results in the multiparous women were compared with their earlier pregnancies and were uniformly better when the women were given a maximum tolerated insulin dosage.

Beard: Looking at Roversi's paper the matter that concerns me is the effects of the therapy on the birth weight of the babies in his series.   Of a total of 476 babies, 229 (48%) weighed less than 3000 g.   If the influence of gestational age is taken into account, using the weight-gestation chart of Thomson *et al.* (1968), then only 9.7% of the babies in the Roversi series would be expected to have a birth weight of less than 3000 g.   Thus I have concluded that there is an excess of growth-retarded babies in the series.

Pedersen: If anyone wants to use Roversi's treatment they have to start again with a controlled series.   In his series are the babies of average normal weight?

Milner: Yes.

Beard: The questions that Roversi's work raises are particularly pertinent because this form of management is being used in many centres in Europe.

Bennett: In this trial is there any evidence for a reduction in congenital anomalies?

Milner: Yes.   In 473 previous pregnancies in 251 women 26 malformed infants had been born: 14 alive and 12 dead.   When these 251 women were subjected to maximum tolerated insulin therapy during pregnancy four malformed infants were born: three alive and one dead.   Even more noteworthy was the observation that in the 251 pregnancies with maximum tolerated insulin therapy there were five stillbirths not malformed, whereas in the previous 473 pregnancies there had been 123.   I am particularly interested in seeing this approach extended in a controlled manner in different centres.   Then one could discover the general validity of the claims.

Bennett: I don't know whether it is good to have lower birth weights or not.   We must have controlled clinical trials and the only person who has ever done controlled clinical trials in this area is Dr O'Sullivan.

O'Sullivan: I am impressed by the size of the problem.   We have spent many years on a controlled trial and in the end we have produced results that should be subjected to validation (O'Sullivan 1975a).   That seems to be the lot of epidemiological studies: you get rid of old saws, you obtain some new information and then you find you have to design another set of investigations